The Genealogy of a Gene

Transformations: Studies in the History of Science and Technology
Jed Z. Buchwald, general editor

The Genealogy of a Gene

Patents, HIV/AIDS, and Race

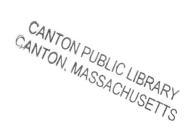

Myles W. Jackson

The MIT Press
Cambridge, Massachusetts
London, England

MIT Press books may be purchased at special quantity discounts for business or sales promotional use. For information, please email special_sales@mitpress.mit.edu.

This book was set in Stone Sans Std and Stone Serif Std by Toppan Best-set Premedia Limited, Hong Kong. Printed and bound in the United States of America.

Library of Congress Cataloging-in-Publication Data

Jackson, Myles W., author.
The genealogy of a gene : patents, HIV/AIDS, and race / Myles W. Jackson.
    p.   cm. — (Transformations: studies in the history of science and technology)
Includes bibliographical references and index.
ISBN 978-0-262-02866-0 (hardcover : alk. paper)
I. Title. II. Series: Transformations (MIT Press).
[DNLM: 1. Genes—genetics. 2. Acquired Immunodeficiency Syndrome.
3. Continental Population Groups—genetics. 4. HIV Infections. 5. Patents as Topic. 6. Receptors, CCR5—genetics. QU 470]
RA643.8
362.19697'920072—dc23
2014029650

10 9 8 7 6 5 4 3 2 1

To all of my students throughout the years, and to a new friend, L. S.

Contents

A Note to the Reader

Portions of this book, which discuss particular aspects of molecular biology, are technical. For those who do not have a background in that field, please refer to the glossary at the back. Illustrations throughout the book accompany and clarify the technical discussions. The more technical sections are necessary to appreciate the ethical, legal, and social implications of gene patenting and race and genomics, as the epilogue makes abundantly clear. Without these discussions, the book would be a history of science without the science, a trend that has become all too common of late.

Only by linking technical bits of molecular biology to intellectual property law or questions of human diversity is it possible to recognize how intriguing and controversial the debates discussed in this work are. I hope that the labor the reader will invest to appreciate the interplay of the technical details of various fields, including molecular biology, intellectual property, government, history, sociology, and anthropology, will be rewarded with a more thorough and sophisticated understanding of the relationship between science and society over the past twenty years.

Acknowledgments

While writing this book, I received numerous forms of funding, including the Inaugural Dibner Professorship of the History and Philosophy of Science and Technology at New York University Polytechnic School of Engineering, funds from New York University- Gallatin School of Individualized Study, and the Alexander von Humboldt Foundation. In 2010, I received the Francis Bacon Award in the History and Philosophy of Science and Technology from the California Institute of Technology. As part of the award, Caltech sponsored a conference on gene patenting in May 2011, and I was the Francis Bacon Visiting Professor of History there during the winter and spring terms of 2012. That conference enabled me to share my work with intellectual property attorneys, including Luigi Palombi, Sandra Parks, and Tania Simoncelli, science and technology studies (STS) scholars, and historians of science. I would like to thank Fran Tise for her assistance during my stay at Caltech. Discussions with Robert L. Gallo on intellectual property and molecular biology were very helpful, particularly with respect to the tropism tests that are discussed in chapter 6. And Jack Spiegel provided me with invaluable information on gene patenting relevant to chapter 4.

The manuscript has benefitted tremendously from various colleagues in numerous disciplines who kindly read earlier versions and provided me with useful comments and criticisms. They include Ken Alder, Rochelle Dreyfuss, Troy Duster, Robert Kohler, Andrew Warwick, Nasser Zakariya, and the three referees. A number of the scientists working on various aspects of the *CCR5* gene allowed me to interview them, including Robert Doms, Ned Landau, Dan Littman, John Novembre, and Victor Torres. Robert Doms read an earlier version of several of the relevant chapters. I thank them all for their time and assistance. I would also like to thank Vincent Lannoy of Euroscreen, who granted me an interview in Brussels on the CCR5 patent portfolio. He also read early portions of the manuscript.

Numerous colleagues in the history of science and STS have helped me think about my project over the years. They include Peder Anker, Karl Appuhn, Mario Biagioli, Jed Buchwald, Gene Cittadino, Moti Feingold, John Heilbron, Sheila Jasanoff, Dan Kevles, Diana Kormos-Buchwald, Michael Lynch, Guy Ortolano, Robert Silverman, Matt Stanley, Noel Swerdlow, and Nicolás Wey Gómez. While at Caltech, I had the opportunity to discuss various aspects of my works in the history of science with a number of scientists. They include Frances Arnold, David Baltimore, Eric Davidson, Alice Huang, Elliot Meyerowitz, Dianne Newman, David Politzer, and Ellen Rothenberg. I would also like to thank Sam Galison for creating figures 1.2 and 1.3.

I am indebted to the comments and questions from numerous audiences when presenting various earlier portions of the manuscript, including those at Ben Gurion University, the California Institute of Technology, Cambridge University, Cornell University, the Fraunhofer Institute for Industrial Mathematics, the German National Academy of Sciences Leopoldina, Harvard University, Hebrew University, New York University, Northwestern University (particularly Bonnie Honig, who suggested the title), Tel Aviv University, the University of California at Los Angeles, the University of Washington, and Yale University.

1 The Story of the *CCR5* Gene

Enough! 'tis granted thee! Divert
This mortal spirit from his primal source;
Him, canst thou seize, thy power exert
And lead him on thy downward course.
—Johann Wolfgang Goethe, "Prologue in Heaven," *Faust*, part 1

Prologue, But Certainly Not in Heaven

On a steamy July day in Washington, D.C., in 1992, the scientist-entrepreneur J. Craig Venter left the National Institutes of Health (NIH) to accept an offer from Wallace Steinberg, chair of the Healthcare Investment Corporation of New Jersey, the largest venture capitalist healthcare fund at the time, to run a nonprofit research center, The Institute for Genomic Research (TIGR). TIGR was to have a budget of $70 million over a ten-year period (the actual total amount eventually increased to $85 million) to search the human genome for gene sequences without meddling from the government.[1] Steinberg placed a substantial bet on the future of pharmacogenomics, the nascent technology that focuses on the influence of an individual's genetic makeup on drug response. He summed up the biotech industry's vision: "By the year 2000, [all] drug companies in the world will use genomic data as their Rosetta stone for the development of new drugs and diagnostic procedures. No science will be more important to the future of medicine than genomic research."[2] The era of personalized medicine had begun.

In 1992, Steinberg set up a sister company of TIGR, Human Genome Sciences, Inc. (HGS). HGS was a for-profit biomedical corporation that was headed by its founder, William A. Haseltine, a Harvard Medical School professor who was known for his research on HIV and his entrepreneurial spirit. HGS would be privy to the sequences that TIGR discovered for the first six months. After that period, Venter was free to publish the information so that academics and nonprofit organizations could study those sequences.[3] If HGS thought that a particular sequence was interesting, perhaps it was a gene that might have diagnostic or therapeutic value, HGS had the right to keep that sequence from the scientific community for an additional twelve months. Initially, Venter had thought that only a handful of sequences would fall under that category, but Haseltine invoked the extension clause on every sequence that could be medically important.[4] It was clear from the start that Venter and Haseltine were at cross purposes. Venter thought that he would identify and publish as many genes as possible while Haseltine would oversee financial matters. Haseltine held a different view of their relationship: "The primary goal was to build a new global pharmaceutical company that discovers, manufactures, and sells its own pharmaceutical products, with a market cap of three billion or greater. That was immediately my goal. I don't care what Craig's goal was. He was just a booster rocket."[5] Rockefeller University's Norton Zinder, who discovered genetic transduction, explained that "When he went off with Bill Haseltine, Craig was seen as evil.... The world looked on TIGR as an absolute den of corruption."[6]

While he was working at the NIH, Venter decided to accelerate the sequencing of the human genome by creating expressed sequencing tags (ESTs) of around 500 nucleotides in length from automated partial sequences of complementary DNA (cDNA) clones. cDNA is made from messenger RNA (mRNA), which is translated into proteins: nucleotides that are not coding for the protein are spliced out at the pre-mRNA stage. ESTs can be used to fish for new human genes and uncover new coding regions in the genome. Because less than 2% of the human genome codes for proteins, this EST technique, published in *Science* in 1991, greatly increased both Venter's gene-hunting efficiency and the value of TIGR's database.[7] It is therefore not surprising that Venter became the leader in the hunt to find and sequence humans genes.[8] Referring to TIGR's databank, Haseltine commented, "An academic can use the data for anything he wants. The only thing they can complain about is that they can't derive income from it. Well, that's life."[9] Venter subsequently left TIGR to head up Celera Genomics in 1998, but he had left his mark on history. He and Haseltine represent a new hybrid of the late twentieth and early twenty-first centuries—the scientific entrepreneur.

As historian of science Steven Shapin has noted, a new breed of investigator, the scientific entrepreneur, emerged by the 1970s.[10] They "were individuals who sought, *by their own efforts*, or those of a small number of coworkers, to turn knowledge into profitable goods or services."[11] Earlier scientists also engaged in the commercialization of their research. Late nineteenth-century physicists assisted the development of the electrical industry, and twentieth-century solid-state physicists, chemists, nutritionists, and agricultural scientists actively worked in the private sector. But by the 1970s, the business end was seen as part and parcel of the new scientific enterprise of molecular biology.[12] Profit-seeking threatened the perceived openness of the scientific enterprise:

For biology, fear and secrecy were largely new. Until the middle of the 1970s, the scientists in molecular biology seemed little different than monks toiling in scholarly poverty and obscurity. Openness was one of the chief virtues practiced. They discussed results openly. They sent one another not only ideas, but also samples of their work in tissue cultures and extracted genes. Graduate students who wanted to work in the field were expected to live on salaries at the poverty line.... As a compensation [compared to lawyers, doctors, and businessmen], the biologists had their intellectual purity. There was a special honor in the poverty of the dedicated researcher, and a suggestion that money could not tempt a talented biologist from the rigors of work. Industrial laboratories were full of secrets and unimagination [sic].[13]

By the end of the 1970s, however, molecular biologists had known sin, to borrow J. Robert Oppenheimer's confessional mea culpa on behalf of nuclear physicists some thirty years earlier. Although secrecy is critical to the viability of commercial enterprises, companies also realized that if they wished to attract top scientists, they needed to permit them to publish. And academic secrecy is certainly not unheard of; now that universities have entered into alliances with industry, it is a far greater problem than it was a generation ago.[14] But industrial secrecy was and still is a real concern for many scientists who claim that it thwarts scientific progress.

During the 1990s, a new type of company began to emerge, and these DNA sequencing firms—such as HGS, Incyte Pharmaceuticals, Inc. (now called Incyte Genomics, Inc.), and Millennium Pharmaceuticals—were headed by these scientific entrepreneurs.[15] They all began operating and trading on what Michael Fortun calls "the promises of forward-looking genetic information."[16] At the time, these so-called platform companies were seen as a new model that encouraged growth in genomics and biotechnology.[17] By the summer of 2000, HGS had obtained over 100 gene patents with another 7,500 applications still pending. Five years later, Incyte, HGS, and Millennium were all in the top ten of the most active biotech patent assignees in the United States, with Incyte first (442 DNA-based patent families by the U.S. Patent and Trademark Office), HGS second (219 patents), and Millennium sixth (167 patents).[18]

Although all were united in the pursuit of biotech research and capital gain, these three companies employed different strategies for profit. HGS, partnered with TIGR, was producing high-throughput technologies for identifying and sequencing genes, creating expressed sequence tags, and mapping gene positions. In 1993, they sold first-rights access to their extensive data bank to SmithKline Beecham (now GlaxoSmithKline) for $125 million.[19] They also sold nonexclusive subscriptions to Pfizer in that same year.[20] Incyte announced that it would shift its focus away from drug development toward its own genomic databanks, such as LifeSeq and ZooSeq. For a fee, researchers could now compare similar genes in different species, avail themselves of recent literature published on those genes, access a genetic map with markers locating the genes' precise locations, and link to protein databases. Rather than sell exclusive rights to a particular pharmaceutical giant, they offered nonexclusive access to Hoffmann-La Roche, Hoechst, Glaxo, Upjohn, and Johnson & Johnson for several years for $15 million to $20 million per company.[21]

In a sense, HGS and Incyte were mirror images of each other. Although HGS slowly began to take on more of a pharmaceutical role, Incyte remained with information technology and emphasized computer algorithms rather than chemical reagents. Incyte was "more like a software company than a biotechnology firm."[22] Despite their antithetical approaches, Incyte and HGS were seen as the common enemy by the leaders of the Human Genome Project (HGP) (discussed in the next chapter), who criticized Incyte and HGS for applying for patents where the role and utility of the gene were unknown or "downloading the public consortium's genome data every night and filing patent applications for any genes they found."[23]

From the start, Millennium Pharmaceuticals covered the gambit of biotechnological research, from gene sequencing information to gene expression, to drug development. By 1996, Millennium had agreements with Hoffmann-La Roche, Eli Lilly, and Astra.[24] In short, HGS, Incyte, and Millennium were new companies for a new age.

These nascent sequencing companies drew on the most advanced instrumentation available. Former Caltech scientist Leroy Hood's laboratory wedded scientific instruments with molecular biology and organic chemistry.[25] Such a marriage was a daring and unstable one during the late 1970s. Drawing on funds obtained by Monsanto and his home institution, Caltech, Henry Huang had attempted for several years to automate the standard techniques of DNA sequencing of Frederick Sanger, Allan Maxam, and Walter Gilbert. The problem lay in the difficulty of detecting DNA's minute signal among a strong background of noise. Huang's efforts did spark the interest of Lloyd Smith, who joined Hood's laboratory from Stanford in April 1982. Smith had implemented lasers and florescent methods to study biological processes, and his expertise in organic chemistry was precisely what Hood's laboratory had lacked.[26]

During this period, an intense collaboration ensued between scientists and engineers at Caltech and the biotech instrument company Applied Biosystems of Perkin Elmer Corporation, whose employee Tim Hunkapiller suggested that four separate dyes be used for each DNA nucleotide. Smith realized that chemical dyes would not be sensitive enough to label the tiny amounts of DNA but quickly surmised that fluorescent dyes would work. In 1986, Applied Biosystems, in collaboration with Hood and Smith, created the first automatic DNA sequencer, the ABI 370A.[27] The new machine could sequence 12,000 letters per day, far more than the most skilled lab technicians could at the time. A year later, other automatic sequencers entered the market, including DuPont's Genesis 2000 and EG&G Biomolecular's machine, the latter of which was suited for small-scale projects. And the Japanese and Europeans were creating sequencing machines of their own.[28] The world of molecular biology was becoming silicon based. These were the automatic sequencers, which formed Venter's sequencing arsenal.

Automatic sequencers were not the only form of the new "dry biology." Programmers developed computer algorithms to identify rapidly similarities between sequences. At the time, there were two types of DNA and protein sequence alignment software programs, FASTA and BLAST. In 1982, FASTA or FAST-ALL (since it can be used to compare quickly a protein or DNA sequence) was developed by David J. Lipman of Pennsylvania State University and William R. Pearson of the University of Virginia. It uses local sequence alignment to find matches of a desired DNA (or protein) sequence with similar databases and libraries. BLAST (Basic Local Alignment Sequence Tool) is also a computer algorithm used to compare DNA and amino acid sequences with preexisting libraries and databases. Created by Eugene Myers of the University of Arizona, Stephen Altschul and Warren Gish of the U.S. National Center for Biotechnology Information (NCBI), and Lipman and Webb Miller of Penn State in 1990, BLAST is often used to seek similar genes in different species.[29] It locates homologous sequences by identifying short matches between two sequences, a process known as seeding. BLAST can produce numerous sequence alignments in a shorter span of time, while FASTA finds only the best alignment and is more sensitive— that is, it misses fewer homologs than BLAST. Computer science had now formed a critical part of biotechnology.

The Origins of *CCR5*[30]

In 1993, The Institute for Genomic Research sent a DNA sequence to Human Genome Sciences: it was one of thousands of sequences that TIGR was obliged to send to HGS. It later turned out to be a particularly interesting and important one. On June 6, 1995, two HGS scientists, Yi Li and Steven M. Ruben, filed a patent application on that DNA sequence (as they had for many others), which they called polynucleotide encoding human G-protein chemokine receptor HDGNR 10. Based on a discovery in a cDNA library derived from human monocytes, a type of white blood cell, the company's computers identified the sequence as a seven-transmembrane receptor protein that was comprised of 352 amino acids.[31] The patent claims included the sequence as found in nature and its cDNA copy (a copy of the mRNA after the removal of introns by RNA splicing), and the latter was deposited in a public depository, which had become standard practice in biotech intellectual property law. As Haseltine recalled in 2000, "Very quickly, we discovered that it was a chemokine receptor … and we used that information to write that description of the gene in a patent."[32] In an age when computers compare DNA sequences with those that code for proteins with known functions, they could predict with reasonable certainty the gene product's function by drawing on the concept of sequence homology using FASTA and BLAST. According to Haseltine, the company ran the standard biochemical assays, or "wet biology," to confirm the computer's prediction of identity and function.[33] As is shown in the next chapter, many scientists were skeptical of such a claim.

Two proteins are said to be homologous (they likely possess similar or the same functions and share an evolutionary history) if a certain percentage of amino acids in their sequences is identical. In proteins that possess 250 amino acids or more, two proteins are considered homologous if 20% of the amino acid sequences are the same when aligned.[34] It turned out that the HDGNR 10 sequence possessed a 70.1% identity and an 82.9% similarity over a 347 amino-acid stretch to another sequence, a chemokine receptor that bound to chemokine MCP-1 (or monocyte chemotatic protein-1).[35] Li and Ruben could thus conclude with a high degree of confidence that their sequence coded for a G-protein chemokine receptor.

Chemokines are small proteins that are about 70 to 130 amino acids in length and that act as messengers among cells of the immune system, whose function is to protect the body from invading pathogens, such as viruses and bacteria. They activate and traffic leukocytes (white blood cells) to areas of inflammation.[36] To date, forty-eight chemokines and nineteen receptors have been isolated.[37] Chemokine receptors (the molecules to which the chemokines bind) are seven-transmembrane proteins and a type of G protein-coupled receptor (GPCR). Most recognize more than one chemokine, and conversely, several chemokines bind to more than one receptor.[38]

Chemokines are divided into four subfamilies: CC chemokines act on lymphocytes, basophils, eosinophils, and monocytes; CXC chemokines influence neutrophils; CXC3 chemokines interact with lymphocytes, macrophages, and dendritic cells; and C chemokines attract T cells to the thymus. All of these cells are types of leukocytes. Ever since the late 1980s, chemokines and their receptors have been the subject of intense scrutiny by immunologists, molecular biologists, and biomedical researchers. The first chemokine isolated was platelet factor 4 (PF4), back in 1961, although its function was not elucidated until 1977.[39] A second chemokine, interleukin-8 (IL-8), was identified in December 1987.[40] The word *chemokine* was coined at the Third International Symposium of Chemotatic Cytokines in 1992 to describe and standardize the nomenclature of the large family of structurally related chemotatic cytokines.[41] In 1995, when HGS filed its application, chemokines were known to result in the activation and migration of monocytes, neutrophils, T-lymphocytes, and fibroblasts. It also was well known at the time that certain chemokines influence a number of physiological responses, including inflammatory responses, hematopoietic stem cell proliferation, and endothelial cell growth. Finally, biochemists and immunologists had implicated chemokines in wound healing, lymphocyte trafficking, allergies, asthma, and arthritis. The HGS patent application summarized what was known about the role of chemokines; however, it did not disclose a specific function of the particular protein coded for by that gene. It was an extremely broad utility patent, "a tool for screening for receptor agonists and antagonists."[42] That is to say: the patent would cover the screening of chemicals and biomolecules to see which ones would bind to the receptor and trigger a physiological response and which ones would bind but not elicit a physiological response. Such a vague statement seems meaningless because it lacks specificity.

HGS waited until its patent was approved. Nearly five years later, on February 16, 2000, HGS president William Haseltine announced to a world still recovering from its millennium celebration that his company's patent application for HDGNR 10 had been approved: it was now U.S. Patent 6,025,154. The announcement made the headlines in major U.S. newspapers. Why would anyone care? Much had transpired in the five years that it had taken to grant the patent.

Identification of the Gene and Its Product

The mid-1990s witnessed the confluence of two critical fields within biomedicine, chemokines and HIV/AIDS, both of which form the gene's scientific lineage in my genealogical study.[43] Researchers attempting to understand HIV infection were struck by two curious observations—the specificity of HIV-1 entry into different types of cells and the suppressive effect on HIV-1 replication by certain chemicals secreted by the body.[44] This work led to the elaboration of the viral cycle of HIV and the chemokine network that regulates immune responses to viral pathogens.[45] As discussed below, scientists determined that the CD4 receptor enables cells to fuse with HIV-1, but only when it is expressed on a human-cell type. They reckoned that a cofactor (or a coreceptor) was required for viral fusion. Other biomedical researchers began to realize that HIV-1 possesses distinct tropisms: various HIV-1 strains were able to infect cells by binding with different chemokine receptors on CD4 cells, a type of leukocyte. In short, *tropism* refers to the type of chemokine coreceptor that is selected by the virus during infection. M-tropic (R5) HIV-1 recognizes CCR5 as a coreceptor, and T-tropic (X4) HIV-1 uses CXCR4 (or fusin) as a coreceptor. CCR5 is predominantly expressed on T cells (namely, memory and activated CD4 cells), gut associated lymphoid tissue (GALT), macrophages, dendritic cells, and microglia. CXCR4 is found on T cells (naïve and resting CD4 cells and CD8 cells), B cells, neutrophils, and eosinophils.[46] Viral isolates during the early stages of HIV-1 infection (that is, before the onset of AIDS) are predominantly R5-tropic, and after symptoms appear, X4-tropic strains are isolated from most patients.[47] Scientists believe that the vast majority (over 90%) of sexually transmitted HIV-1 infects the host cells via CCR5 as the virus can infect CCR5-expressing macrophages and dendritic cells found on the mucous membranes of the genital and gastrointestinal tracts (figures 1.1 and 1.2).[48]

In 1986, the University of California at San Francisco virologist Jay Levy noted a man who routinely came to his laboratory to be tested for HIV.[49] After initially detecting the virus and testing him for five months, Levy could no longer identify it in his blood. Levy conjectured that perhaps the virus had entered into host cells and therefore could not be identified floating in the blood. The obvious candidates were CD8 cells, a type of T cell. When the CD8 cells were removed, the virus reappeared. After the cells were added back in, the virus once again vanished. When individuals are infected with HIV-1, the CD8 cells can control the virus. After they lose that control, HIV-1 begins to kill the CD4 cells. Levy searched in vain for a substance that he assumed was secreted by the CD8 cells, calling it CAF or

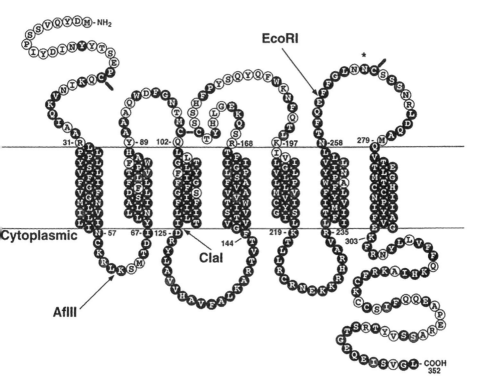

Figure 1.1
The wild type, or normal, CCR5 protein, a 7-transmembrane protein found on CD4 cells. *Source:* Joseph Rucker, Michel Samson, Benjamin J. Doranz, et al., "Regions in β-Chemokine Receptors CCR5 and CCR2b That Determine HIV-1 Susceptibility," *Cell* 87, no. 3 (1996): 437–446, here 443.

CD8 antiviral factor.[50] He was never able to locate it. Nearly a decade later, however, Robert Gallo and Paolo Lusso did.

In December 1995, six months after HGS filed its patent application, Gallo and Lusso's laboratory at the National Cancer Institute of the National Institutes of Health found that three chemokines (the β-chemokines RAN-TES, MIP-1α, and MIP-1β) that were secreted by activated CD8 lymphocytes suppressed HIV-1 replication in vitro.[51] Those three chemokines were most likely Levy's CAF. As critical as this research was, neither Gallo nor Lusso realized that these chemicals blocked the entry of HIV-1: they assumed that they were inhibiting viral transcription. In February 1996, Edward Berger of the National Institute of Allergy and Infectious Diseases of the NIH presented a paper demonstrating that with his utility assay he had

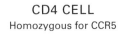

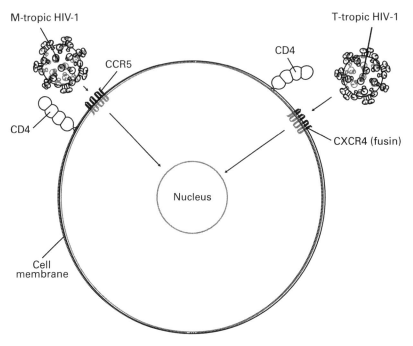

Figure 1.2
The CD4 cell of someone possessing two copies of the wild type (that is, normal) *CCR5* gene. Both CCR5 and CXCR4 (fusin) are present on the cell's membrane. M-tropic HIV-1 binds with CCR5, and T-tropic HIV-1 binds with CXCR4. In both cases, the virus's genetic material enters into the CD4 cell's nucleus.

isolated fusin (now called CXCR4), a chemokine receptor that facilitated the replication of HIV-1 in the human body. That paper was published in *Science* three months later.[52] It was later revealed that the fusin receptor functioned for X4-tropic, but not R5-tropic, HIV-1 strains.[53] As a result of these two papers, the fields of chemokine research and HIV/AIDS research subsequently became intricately and inextricably linked.

Things were beginning to fit together rather quickly. Within two weeks in late June 1996, a number of laboratories in the United States working independently at the National Institutes of Health, the Aaron Diamond AIDS Research Center of Rockefeller University, New York University's School of Medicine, Dana-Farber Cancer Institute, and the University of Pennsylvania School of Medicine, which was collaborating with a laboratory at the

Free University of Brussels, were in a race to announce the discovery of a coreceptor on CD4 cells.[54] Each lab brought various skill sets, experimental techniques, and training to the hunt. For example, John P. Moore of Rockefeller (now at Weill-Cornell School of Medicine) was a classically trained biochemist. NYU School of Medicine's Dan Littman and Nathaniel (Ned) Landau were molecular biologists with an expertise in gene transfer and expression cloning. Richard A. Koup, at the Aaron Diamond AIDS Research Center, was a clinical immunologist. Robert W. Doms's lab at Penn's School of Medicine drew on various techniques in biochemistry, cell biology, genetics and immunology to elucidate membrane proteins that were relevant to the HIV cycle of infection. They generally were cell biologists who were (and are) interested in how cells interact with HIV. Doms had been a postdoc at the NIH from 1988 to 1996, where he had been working on the same floor as Berger.[55]

Researchers from one of the labs of the Aaron Diamond AIDS Research Center and the NYU School of Medicine took human embryonic kidney (HEK) 293 T cells, which were cotransfected with CD4 and various chemokine receptor expression vectors. They demonstrated that CCR5 in concert with CD4 permitted the entry of R5-tropic HIV-1 into the cells. The other Aaron Diamond lab collaborating with biomedical researchers from Progenics Pharmaceuticals, Inc. used various cell biology techniques to assess HIV-1 entry into CD4 T cells from two exposed but exceptionally resistant individuals named EU2 and EU3. They corroborated Gallo and Russo's results that β-chemokines inhibited HIV-1 infection.[56] In a similar fashion, the Penn-Brussels labs showed that the expression of human CD4 in quail QT6 cells, which can be efficiently transfected, failed to support HIV-1 replication; however, CCR5 expression with CD4 in QT6 cells enabled R5-tropic (but not X4-tropic) replication.[57]

At roughly the same time, Berger's lab found that CCR5 enabled nonhuman cells to undergo fusion with the envelope protein of R5-tropic HIV-1 isolates. In addition, the lab tested the effects of chemokines on HIV-1 fusion and replication conferred by vaccina-encoded CCR5 plus CD4 expressed on NIH 3T3 cells. RANTES, MIP-1α, and MIP-1β competitively inhibited R5-tropic strains of HIV-1 infection.[58] Finally, biomedical researchers at the Dana-Farber Cancer Institute in collaboration with scientists from Harvard's School of Public Health and Beth Israel Hospital took HeLa cells, in which HIV-1 isolates do not enter very efficiently, and coinfected them with plasmids expressing cDNA of various chemokines and CD4-expressing vectors. Expression of the CCR5 protein was significantly enhanced as a result.[59]

Unbeknownst to the biomedical researchers, the patent that HGS filed for the gene of the human G-protein chemokine receptor HDGNR 10 was the same gene for the coreceptor, now called CCR5, that the HIV-1 virus (of the R5-tropic variety) recognizes to infect CD4 cells. That so many labs came to the conclusion independently and simultaneously and published the results so quickly was unprecedented. Koup recalls:

You know that you have to work all night, and all weekend, because if you're not one of the first people in print, you're nowhere.... I don't think there's ever been a scientific discovery where the data were generated as quickly, and were out in print as quickly, as this. And by so many people. It was just amazing.[60]

Landau, Koup's colleague at Aaron Diamond during this period, concurs:

Dan [Littman] and I were writing our paper as fast as possible, sending it back and forth by E-mail. I was sleeping in my office. I have a sleeping bag under my desk. We had arranged a courier to transport the paper overnight to the journal *Nature* in London. He was supposed to come here at three in the afternoon, and we were still working on the paper at two. Then at 2:30 our E-mail system broke down. And the courier showed up. I went crazy, screaming at the computer guy to fix the system. Finally it fixed itself. The manuscript wasn't in good shape, but we sent it anyway.... It was pretty funny when we got the reviews back. One of the reviewers said, "Out of 15 authors, couldn't any of them have proofread this manuscript?"[61]

The competition among these laboratories to be the first to announce the discovery of the coreceptor of HIV-1 was apparently intense and at times acrimonious.

The plot soon thickened. Koup had collected the blood cells of twenty-seven individuals who were had been resistant to HIV-1 infection for over a decade. As discussed in further detail below, two of these twenty-seven men had a specific mutation of the *CCR5* gene known as $\Delta32$.[62] Within a month of determining that CCR5 was the coreceptor for HIV, biomedical researchers discovered that this critical mutation, in which thirty-two nucleotides are deleted, results in a frame shift and the generation of a premature stop codon, truncating the CCR5 protein.[63] In short, the receptor is not present on the cell membrane but remains in the cytoplasm of the CD4 cell; therefore, HIV-1 cannot gain entry into the cells (figure 1.3). In terms of a lock-and-key analogy, if HIV-1 is the key and CCR5 is the lock, then the lock is on the wrong side of the door for HIV-1 to enter into and infect the cell. Marc Parmentier and his postdoctoral assistant Michel Samson of the Free University of Brussels and their colleagues at the University of Pennsylvania School of Medicine were all credited with the codiscovery and later the patenting of the $\Delta32$ mutation. It turns out that Parmentier had a technician in his laboratory who was homozygous for the $\Delta32$ mutation.[64]

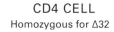

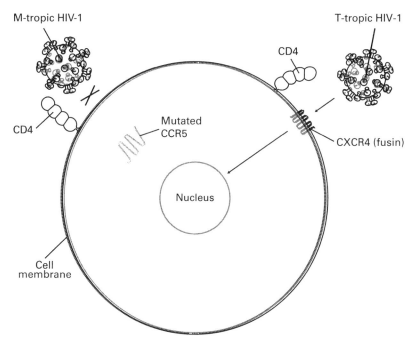

Figure 1.3

The CD4 cell of someone who possesses two copies of the *Δ32* allele. The protein product of *Δ32* is not present on the cell membrane but remains in the cell's cytoplasm. Therefore, M-tropic HIV-1 cannot recognize it and infect the cell with its genetic material (as denoted by the X in the figure). T-tropic HIV-1, however, is unaffected by the *Δ32* mutation. It still can bind with CXCR4 (fusin) and insert its genetic material in the nucleus.

In 1994, Parmentier, who was a molecular biologist and whose lab cloned the *CCR5* gene in late 1995 by screening a human genomic DNA library with the mouse MOP020 clone, had launched Euroscreen, a preclinical stage biopharmaceutical firm, which is a spin-off company of the Free University of Brussels. One of Doms's graduate students at Penn, Benjamin J. Doranz, had read Parmentier's article on the cloning of *CCR5* and asked for and obtained the clone. Those two groups then began what became a very fruitful collaboration. After Parmentier isolated and cloned the gene, the two groups identified the receptor and determined its function. Like everyone else, however, they were unaware at the time of the HGS patent application. Both Parmentier's and Doms's groups also collected blood samples from individuals around the globe whose lifestyles put them at risk for the disease but who never succumbed to AIDS, suggesting that they possessed a natural immunity. For example, Doms's group collected blood from sex workers in Bangkok.[65]

Two years later and independent of Gallo and Lusso's work, Doms and Samson reported on the natural ligands that bound to ChemR13 (chemokine receptor 13, now called CCR5) (namely, RANTES, MIP-1α, and MIP-1β) and the concentration levels needed to elicit a biological response.[66] Later research critically showed the ligands inhibiting HIV-1 infection of CD4 cells at those same levels of concentration: HIV-1 clearly recognized CCR5. On April 9, 1997, Euroscreen filed a patent application with the U.S. Patent and Trademark Office for an "active and inactive CC-chemokine receptor"—the wild-type CCR5 protein and the mutated Δ32 receptor.[67] The wild-type (that is, the normal or nonmutated) protein, it turned out, was, in principle, the same as the one that was encoded by the gene sequence in the Human Genome Sciences application, which had not yet been granted. Indeed, HGS's application had not been made public until eighteen months after the application deadline, December 6, 1996.[68] The Belgians, however, stated that the wild type is recognized by HIV-1.

In addition to the Euroscreen researchers, three scientists—Patrick W. Gray, Vicki L. Schweickart, and Carol J. Raport (from ICOS, a for-profit biotech company in Seattle)—also filed a patent on the CCR5 gene and receptor (which they initially called chemokine receptor 88-C) on December 20, 1995, U.S. patent application 575,967. Their subsequent article was published less than seven months later and described the isolation of the gene by identifying two yeast artificial chromosomes (YACs) clones that encoded the CCR1 gene. YACs are vectors that are used to clone large DNA sequences. Because CCR2 and the gene coding for another closely related GPCR, V28 (now called CX3CR1) are found in close proximity to the CCR1 gene on human chromosome 3p21, the ICOS scientists used YAC DNA as a template for polymerase chain reaction (PCR), which is a technique used to amplify copies of a DNA millions of times over. The sequence of the primer was based on DNA sequences from the second cytoplasmic domain and the sixth transmembrane domain of these chemokine receptors because they are highly conserved among CCR1, CCR2, and CX3CR1. It turns out that the CCR5 gene was within 150 kilobases of (or rather close to) the CCR1, 2, and 3 genes.[69]

Their patent was for the receptor 88-C sequence, methods of production of the recombinant vector and cell lines, and the screening of ligands for the detection of diseases that were associated with chemokine receptors.

They mentioned numerous maladies, including atherosclerosis, rheumatoid arthritis, asthma, tumor growth suppression, and other maladies; AIDS
was not included. The three ICOS scientists filed a second patent application, 661,393, on June 7, 1996.[70] This one, however, listed AIDS, and it
included broad screening claims. On December 20, 1996, they filed a third
patent application (771,276), which covered monoclonal and humanized
antibodies, which bound to CCR5 in order to halt HIV-1 infection. ICOS,
cofounded in 1989 by George B. Rathmann, cofounder of Amgen, was
Washington's largest biotech company. It specialized in drug development
to treat inflammatory diseases (hence its interest in GPCRs and the manufacture of antibodies for other biotech companies) until it was bought out
by Eli Lilly in January 2007. Finally, Steven M. Ruben and Yi Li filed another
patent for the HDGNR 10 (CCR5) peptide and its corresponding nucleic
acid on behalf of Human Genome Sciences on November 18, 1998. The
application corrected the DNA sequence that was listed in the initial application, and it included the claim that the gene product was the HIV-1 coreceptor. The responses of biomedical researchers and Wall Street executives
to these patents are the subject of chapter 2. Although the history of the
CCR5 patent is itself fascinating, it can be used as a heuristic tool to probe
the boundaries between science, technology, and society. The chapters of
this book investigate the themes that form the complete genealogy of the
CCR5 gene—intellectual property, natural selection, big and small pharma,
human diversity studies, personalized medicine and ancestry studies, and
race and genomics.

The *CCR5* Gene and Intellectual Property

Can a gene be considered a product of human hands if it is merely isolated
from the genome? Chapter 3 addresses the patentability of genes as natural
products. Patenting natural processes (rather than products) started in the
1860s and 1870s with BASF's process patent for synthesizing the natural
dye alizarin and with Louis Pasteur's process patent for producing yeast
cultures. During the first decade of the twentieth century, the isolated and
mostly purified compound adrenaline, called Adrenalin, was patented by
Parke-Davis, and that patent was upheld by United States District Court
Judge Learned Hand in 1911. His decision was an attempt to assist the
fledgling U.S. pharmaceutical industry in competing with its German counterpart. Thanks to the Plant Patent Act, new varieties of plants, excluding
sexual and tuber-propagating ones, were deemed patentable in 1930. By the
1950s, "sex hormones had become biotechnological 'goods.'"[71] Steroids,

vitamins, and antibiotics followed suit. In 1980, Chakrabarty's artificially created *Pseudomonas* bacterium was deemed to be patentable subject matter by the U.S. Supreme Court.

One therefore might argue that gene patenting is the inevitable next step in the commodification of natural processes and products. Historian of science Edward Yoxen dates the origins of the technological capitalization of life back to the 1920s.[72] Intellectual property scholars Peter Drahos and John Braithwaite maintain that "The patenting of genes, which through the 1990s increasingly drew more public attention, was the culmination of a business approach that had been evolving in the chemical, agricultural, seed and pharmaceutical sectors for all of the 20th century."[73] However, the patenting of genes raises critical concerns that distinguish it from the patenting of other biological entities. These include the inability to patent around the gene and the corresponding ability potentially to block downstream research on diagnostics and therapeutics, as chapter 3 addresses.

Chapter 4 details the numerous critical legal and epistemic issues that are raised by the CCR5 patent in the United States. These include the constitution of a patent claim, the effect of broad utility patents on downstream research on HIV/AIDS diagnostics and therapeutics, the relationship between the written specification and the deposited object, and the sufficiency of computer-determined sequence homology in defining both utility and function of a patented gene product. In a sense, the debate forms another chapter in the saga of the artificial versus the natural. The distinction, which can be traced back to Aristotle, has always been hotly contested and never very clear.[74] In this case, the decision rests with the United States Patent and Trademark Office and various courtrooms.

Although much has been written on the possible effects of gene patenting on future research, I offer a concrete example by investigating the history of the *CCR5* gene, including the history of molecular biology, the sociology of science and technology, and the history of intellectual property law. The goal is to historicize how these moral economies change over time as a result of both political and economic circumstances. I do not accept prima facie that the critiques of commercialization always were as they are today.

Chapter 5 tells the European side of the story. As briefly mentioned, the Belgian company Euroscreen applied for and obtained patents for the gene, its product, the *Δ32* mutation of the gene, and the corresponding mutated protein product. One of its patents was challenged in Europe, and in late 2011, Euroscreen withdrew it. This chapter focuses on the history of torpedoing a patent and sheds light on the important differences between the U.S. Patent and Trademark Office (USPTO) and the European Patent Office (EPO) with regard to gene patents. These differences reflect critical cultural contrasts between Americans and Europeans on the role of corporate interests in healthcare. Such a comparison also demonstrates that there are alternatives. The U.S. system is neither natural nor inevitable.

Chapter 6 discusses how the *CCR5* gene entered into the arena of pharmaceuticals shortly after the discovery that it codes for the coreceptor of HIV-1. In this chapter, I temporarily move away from the esotericism and rarified air of intellectual property law and toward the terra firma of HIV/AIDS research and treatment. CCR5 quickly became the target of a new form of medical treatment using state-of-the-art diagnostic testing, such as structure-activity relationships (SARs) and high-throughput screening (HTS). Just as the understanding of the gene had been the result of cutting-edge research, its protein product subsequently became the object of pioneering developments for drug treatment in the late 1990s. Not surprisingly, intellectual property issues reappear as big pharma enviously guards its patents on HIV/AIDS drugs, much to the dismay and outcry of many. The gene started a new chapter in its life deeply embedded in the world of big pharma.

CCR5's genealogy, however, does not end with intellectual property. The *Δ32* allele also made scientific headlines as biomedical researchers searched for the worldwide distribution of this important allele.

Δ32 and Natural Selection

In 2002, a PBS television program on the Black Death[75] noted that Stephen J. O'Brien[76] (head of the genetics section of the Laboratory of Genomic Diversity at the National Cancer Institute from 1986 to 2011) was struck by the similarity between the Black Death (bubonic plague), which ravished Europe in waves for three centuries starting in 1346, and AIDS. In addition to the severity of the two diseases, both the bacterium responsible for the Black Death, *Yersinia pestis*, and the virus responsible for AIDS, HIV, destroy the immune system's macrophages, which are sent to attack the pathogens. O'Brien learned that Justin Champion, a historian at the Royal Holloway, University of London, who has worked on the history of epidemics, had scoured the London archives to study the effects of the Great Plague of 1665 and 1666 on the city. What Champion found was intriguing: throughout England's capital, there were pockets of survivors surrounded by fatalities of the plague. But how or why did they survive?

To answer Champion's question, the geneticist O'Brien's search took him to Eyam, 20 kilometers southwest of Sheffield, England. This village in the Derbyshire dales is renowned for its brush with the Great Plague. Being far from London, members of the tiny community initially were spared the horrors of which they certainly had heard. That changed in September 1665, when a package of cloth sent from a London warehouse was received by the village tailor, George Vickers, who hung out the cloth to dry. The cloth contained fleas that carried the lethal *Y. pestis*. Vickers was bitten and died within a week of receiving the lethal parcel, and the epidemic spread throughout Eyam. Although some villagers wanted to flee from the outbreak, the village pastor, Reverend William Mompesson, decided to quarantine his parishioners, cutting them off from the rest of the world. Members of nearby villages deposited food at Eyam's periphery in exchange for coins, which had been soaked in vinegar (then seen as a disinfectant of the plague) and left behind by the survivors. Nearly a year after the initial deaths, the first visitors to the village were stunned to see that some residents had survived. Tales of miraculous recoveries and of people who never suffered from any plague symptoms were passed on as part of Eyam lore. Based on his study of the village archives, the historian John Clifford calculated 433 Eyam survivors.

For O'Brien, Eyam was the perfect site for a natural history experiment that studied the intersection between the plague and genetic resistance. Because he had been working on the *CCR5* gene since 1996, O'Brien postulated that people who currently lived in Eyam and whose ancestors lived in the village in the 1660s had the same *Δ32* mutation that greatly diminished HIV-1 infection. O'Brien, the University of Oxford geneticist (now at Duke University)— David B. Goldstein, and their colleagues tested those descendants to see if they had the *Δ32* allele and found that 14% of the DNA samples from the villagers' epithelial cells contained the allele. To see if the *Δ32* frequency was a legacy of the plague survivors, they needed to compare the frequency of the allele in Eyam with those in other populations. After creating an international team of scientists, O'Brien and his colleagues checked the allele's global distribution and quickly concluded that its frequency was far from equal among the world's various populations. Indeed, given their limited sampling size, they did not find the allele among Native Americans, East Asians, Africans, or Indians. Other biomedical researchers, including those of the aforementioned labs at the Free University of Brussels and Penn's School of Medicine, conducted similar studies. It soon became clear that there was a wide range in frequencies of the *CCR5-Δ32* allele. On the Estonian Island of Dagö, or Hiiumaa, for example, the frequency is as high as 18%. In China, the frequency is 0.1%, and the allele has yet to be found among Han Chinese. It also cannot be found among indigenous populations of western and central Africa, and it is rare among South African blacks. Biomedical researchers argue that the presence of the allele at all in sub-Saharan Africa and western China is a result of admixture with Caucasians. American Caucasians possess about a 10% allele frequency, with 1% being homozygous for the trait (or possessing two copies of the allele), whereas African Americans have an allele frequency of 2% with only 0.04% of them being homozygous. Such a discrepancy is striking. In addition, among European populations, the *Δ32* allele frequency mapped nicely onto the areas hit hardest by the plague.

Goldstein, O'Brien and their colleagues then decided to date the *Δ32* allele, which can be done by scrutinizing many DNA samples and locating nearby microsattelites, a type of genetic marker. They employed mathematical models, which revealed that the allele arose around seven hundred years ago at the time of the Black Death in Europe. They were overjoyed, concluding that the descendants of those resistant to the plague throughout the Middle Ages and into the seventeenth century were resistant to the modern AIDS epidemic, thanks to the *Δ32* mutation. Most of those homozygous for the *Δ32* allele will not develop AIDS, whereas those heterozygous for *Δ32* allele show a slower progression of two to four years to AIDS.[77] This seemed to parallel the circumstances in Eyam in which some exhibited no symptoms (presumably homozygous for *Δ32*) and some suffered from the symptoms but recovered (presumably heterozygous for *Δ32*).

This might sound too good to be true, and it turns out not to be true. O'Brien's hypothesis linking *Δ32* to the Black Plague was somewhat premature, as is discussed in chapter 7. Although the hypothesis was subsequently shown to be fallacious, the story is important because it marks the confluence of molecular biology, population genetics, demography, epidemiology, and the history of biology and medicine. O'Brien's project signaled a new type of interdisciplinary collaboration that arose in the 1990s. The *CCR5* gene's *Δ32* allele became a focal point in scientific debates about genes, natural selection, and human diversity. This represents yet another lineage in this gene's remarkable genealogy.

Δ32 and Race

As soon as the allele was discovered by scientists using wet biochemical and molecular biological techniques in 1996, *Δ32* became immediately and inextricably linked to race and ethnicity.[78] Since then, a small number of molecular and evolutionary biologists, population geneticists, and biomedical researchers have begun to query whether race can be established definitively by the use of a group of genetic markers. Such a move has resulted in a spirited controversy among scientists and scholars in the social sciences and humanities. As a result of the skewed frequencies of *CCR5* gene's various alleles, including but not limited to *Δ32*, questions arose as to whether race could or should be reintroduced at the molecular level. Numerous studies in the sociology and anthropology of medicine warned of genetic essentialism and the privileging of race as a category of human difference.

How do scientists deal with human diversity? Genetic diversity and how it is defined and characterized fuel pharmacogenomics as scientists claim that single nucleotide polymorphisms (SNPs) that are found throughout the genome may explain specific responses to medications. Do the differences in SNPs between various human populations map onto race? Is race the only lens through which we should study human variation? What factors drive the importance of race in understanding differences between humans at the DNA level? The same SNPs and other genetic markers that are used by scientists who are working at federal organizations such as the National Institutes of Health to study human diversity and the effects of natural selection on various populations are also employed by big and small pharma and personal genomics companies[79] to offer their clients a glimpse into their genealogical past and their medical future. *Δ32* is one of the most popular tests that these personal genomics companies provide, and they advertise the allele in terms of both HIV infection and race.

The last chapter of this book scrutinizes the confluence of public and private institutions that has given rise to the debate about the so-called molecularization of race.[80] Federal institutions, such as the NIH, are trying to include people of color in the creation of medical diagnostics and therapeutics in light of the Revitalization Act of 1993. Since 1988, the Food and Drug Administration has been calling for more reports of drug differences based on race, sex, and age.[81] The private sector exploits this knowledge of the genome for commercial gain. In addition, rather than passively waiting for assistance, patient advocacy groups have successfully brought their own interests to the attention of the government. In the spirit of inclusion and civil rights, various groups with genetic ailments have mobilized and played an active and critical role in the diagnosis and treatment of diseases.[82]

Race has now become a commodity as big and small pharma, patient advocacy organizations, and the federal government support, for very different reasons, the inclusion of those who have been medically marginalized in the past. Because of that historical exclusion, some of the strongest advocates of race-based medicine, including politicians and biomedical researchers, are people of color. Although the intentions of current biomedical research are not malicious and discriminatory as was the case with early twentieth-century eugenics, the ramifications of genetic essentialism could be grave.

This book gestures toward the role of history in public policy in the spirit of works in the history and sociology of science.[83] Over a quarter of a century ago, sociologists of scientific knowledge focused on scientific controversies to illustrate how nature can never be used as a final arbiter when a controversy is still ongoing. Nature is called on by both sides, and after the debate is resolved, nature can be ascribed retroactively to the victor.[84] As informative and fruitful as those studies have been, my book is about having the historian at the table while the controversy is ongoing.[85] This is a story about the instability of scientific, legal, racial, and ethnic claims. In one sense, it is similar to the work of sociologist of science Sheila Jasanoff on the political coproduction of both science and the social order.[86] Waiting until after the controversy has been settled disenables the historian from intervening. We historians are good at illustrating that controversies have histories. The argument that today's technological innovations and entrepreneurship are so different from the past that history is irrelevant is as fallacious as it is dangerous. But assuming that history repeats itself is equally treacherous and misguided. Today's world has unique elements, and yet how we arrived at this moment is informative. There always are alternatives. Biological entities were not always patentable or seen as commodities. Similarly, human variations do not necessarily need to be equated with so-called racial differences. Historians need to point out that neither the patenting of genes nor the categorization of human difference as racial is inevitable. We are obliged to inform others of times when alternatives were presented only to be erased from the collective memory.

Donald MacKenzie's pioneering work, *Inventing Accuracy: A Historical Sociology of Nuclear Missile Guidance*, examines the scientific legitimacy of a public policy (nuclear missile guidance systems, in his case) that was presented to the U.S. public as being grounded in good science, technology, and economics.[87] In reality, it was not. As he shows, nothing was either natural or inevitable about the rise of certain technologies over others. There were alternatives, and he argues that social interests fueled the support of some technologies over others.[88] In addition, his work provides a blueprint for intervening in the world today.

Historians also need to explain why certain choices were made over others. Biocapitalism has guided much but not all biomedical research into genes over the past thirty years. A number of scholars in science and technology studies (STS) and cultural studies have argued that we are in a new age of capitalism.[89] Like race, genes and healthcare are also commodities. Genes are accorded value, and therefore they encourage investment in their owners. Biocapitalism is the product of biotechnology, which sees biological entities, such as genes, as part of scientific projects of profit-making and profit-seeking.[90] On the one hand, it harkens back to Karl Marx's *Das Kapital* and his analysis of the dynamics of labor and commodities, which form the basis of producing and marketing entities, such as today's biomolecules.[91] Biocapitalism also gestures back to Michel Foucault's concept of biopower in the first volume of *The History of Sexuality*. The word *biopower* refers to the ability of nation-states to govern and manage their subjects' bodies.[92] In this book, however, the discussion of biocapitalism goes beyond references to Marx and Foucault.

Corporate capitalism and biotechnology are shaping twenty-first-century America.[93] As Hannah Landecker has argued, "Cultured cells ... function within a well-established system of labor and exchange; they are normalized in and by these systems; yet they also represent profound and recent change to a new state of being, as routine tools, alienable commodities, and sites of production."[94] Rebecca Skloot's account of HeLa cells describes how Henrietta Lacks's cells have been purchased worldwide over the past half century for pioneering research in molecular biology without any financial benefit to the possessor of those cells or her descendants.[95] The means of production in biocapitalism are raw materials, natural entities, and legal and technical tools (in this case, intellectual property law, which results in the commodification of the so-called subjects of labor). These legal and technical tools structure the social relationships of those in the biotech world. Private enterprise is assisted by a laissez-faire government, and the benefits are reaped by the members of that group. Those whose DNA sequences have been patented are alienated from the means of production. They do not share in the governance of biomedical research or reap the profits.

The word *biocapital* also is used by big pharma to proclaim the arrival of a new age in pharmaceuticals and medical treatment. The biomedical sector (including big pharma) and the governments of developed countries have created and sustained biocapitalism. As the British sociologist and social theorist Nikolas Rose has argued:

Energized by the search for biovalue, novel links have formed between truth and capitalization, the demands for shareholder value and the human value invested in the hope for cure and optimality. A new economic space has been delineated—the bioeconomy—and a new form of capital—biocapital. Old actors such as pharmaceutical corporations have been transformed in their relation with science on the one hand and stock markets on the other.[96]

The political and economic backdrop to this study is the rise of biocapitalism from the 1970s to the 1990s. Critical decisions by the U.S. federal government, specifically by the U.S. Patent and Trademark Office and the various lower courts, have catered to the interests of private industry, such as pharmaceutical giants and nascent personal genomics companies. This period witnessed the fall of communism and the reappraisal of the role of public institutions in scientific research and development. The story is in part about the increased role that is played by the privatization of biomedical research. The public-private worlds have now become a hybrid.

As a historian, I need to see how much of the history of the *CCR5* gene and its protein product is one of biocapitalism. Uncritically and myopically analyzing the gene's history solely through that lens would conflate the numerous intricacies of the gene's history and paint too simplistic a picture. I therefore seek to determine which parts of the CCR5 story are owed to biocapitalism and which are not.

My story details how the *CCR5* gene is defined and redefined by various communities. It was not invented at the moment of its definition, and as a historian, I do not care about it as a *Ding an sich*. The definition and emergence of the *CCR5* gene were predicated on capital, laboratory practices, computer algorithms, statistical analyses, population genetics and biomedical studies, and historical and sociological studies.[97] The gene was embedded and often entangled in numerous scientific, cultural, economic, and social networks. As historian of science Ted Porter correctly points out, "Scientific objects are not made only by scientists.… [T]hey are shaped by the interests and expectations of diverse actors."[98] Histories of scientific objects are therefore by their nature interdisciplinary.[99] Although the French sociologist Bruno Latour has complained that most historians of science do not provide stories of "nonhuman nature," I do not claim that scientific objects, such as the *CCR5* gene, have their own agency.[100]

My study represents the brief history of a particular object and its cultural, sociopolitical, and ethical aspects by providing glimpses into facets of the gene's history. I wish to eschew any ontological or metaphysical commitment.[101] Scientific objects can be used as heuristic tools to probe the boundaries between science and society, and their stories track the histories of those ever-changing contours. The story of the *CCR5* gene links a myriad of diverse topics in ways that a biography of a person (or indeed a prosopography of a particular group) cannot.

Although this book resembles earlier studies on the biographies of objects, including scientific objects,[102] this is not a biography of the *CCR5* gene. The gene's story is still unfolding. Rather, this book focuses on a period of about twenty years of the gene's life from the early 1990s to the present. I am interested in understanding where we are today and why, and the *CCR5* gene provides a vehicle for that analysis. This account is not about the progress of science. Likewise, this historical narrative does not offer a progressive view of history that inexorably, inevitably, and naturally leads to the present day. In these respects, my book is similar to Friedrich Nietzsche's and Michel Foucault's notions of genealogy.[103] It is a "history of the present," to borrow Foucault's phrase[104]—an effective history (*wirkliche Historie*, as Nietzsche called it), as opposed to a traditional history:[105]

An entire historical tradition (theological or rationalistic) aims at dissolving the singular event into an ideal continuity—as a teleological movement or a natural process. "Effective" history, however, deals with events in terms of their most unique characteristics, their most acute manifestations.[106]

Genealogy also works at other levels as well. I map a genealogy of the *CCR5* gene, including its major allele, *Δ32*, tracing its lineage of descent throughout history among large population groups, categorized by some biomedical scientists as race, and addressing its importance to those who wish to see if they have a greatly reduced risk of succumbing to AIDS. Nietzsche spoke of both *Herkunft*, or descent based on bloodline as well as cultural traditions, and *Rassen*, or races.[107] Genealogy therefore links the body and history.[108] In short, the gene's genealogy is a complex and intertwined one, including lineages of biocapitalism, the sciences of chemokines and HIV/AIDS, the Human Genome Project and the HapMap, intellectual property law, big and small pharma, personal genomics companies, and race. Perhaps it is time for historians of science once again to realize the political relevance of their work, not simply to suggest a link to the present but to substantiate such a link and intervene in the present. It is also time for historians of science to re-engage with scientists.

2   The CCR5 Patent(s)

The Human Genome Project Sets the Tone

Although gene patents had been awarded for nearly a decade before its existence, the Human Genome Project (HGP) (1990 to 2003) brought human genes and intellectual property issues to the fore. An international collaboration that was started and led by the United States, the HGP had an ambitious goal—to sequence the entire human genome, which is made up of 3 billion base pairs of DNA.[1] Planning started in 1984 with the work of Charles DeLisi, a physicist and director of the Office Health and Environment at the Department of Energy, and Robert Sinsheimer, a Caltech molecular biologist and chancellor of the University of California at Santa Cruz. Sinsheimer wanted to create a genome project at UC Santa Cruz to determine the details of the human genome, and DeLisi was interested in drawing on the Department of Energy's "Genbank" at Los Alamos National Laboratory to probe the feasibility of sequencing all 3 billion base pairs.[2] The HGP produced many of the techniques that have been developed or refined for DNA sequencing.

In 1987, a committee of the National Research Council of the National Academy of Sciences, chaired by Bruce Alberts, voiced its support for the massive sequencing initiative and urged Congress to appropriate $3 billion to the Department of Energy and the National Institutes of Health over a fifteen-year period for the mammoth undertaking.[3] In 1990, Congress approved the recommendation and set a target completion date of 2005.[4] In 1996, after the initial phase of mapping the human genome was near completion, the actual sequencing commenced. Soon sequencing laboratories sprang up at the Massachusetts Institute of Technology, Stanford University, Baylor University, the University of Washington, the University of Texas Southwest Medical Center, the University of Oklahoma, the Institute for Systems Biology (Seattle), Cold Spring Harbor Laboratory, and Washington University. These centers were joined by laboratories in Cambridge, United Kingdom; Jena, Berlin, and Brunswick (Braunschweig), Germany; Yokahama, Japan; Beijing, China; and Evry, France. A total of twenty centers worldwide took part.[5] In addition, the private sector, such the Institute for Genomic Research and later Celera Genomics, both headed by J. Craig Venter, joined the sequencing, resulting in controversy and animosity.[6]

The specter of intellectual property protection for newly discovered human DNA sequences loomed over the planning stages of the HGP. In 1987, Harvard's Walter Gilbert claimed he would raise capital for the Genome Corporation by copyrighting and selling gene sequences. This move provoked strong responses against commercialization. As two European scientists, Lennart Philipson and John Tooze, complained: "the prospect of private capital financing this work and then keeping secret the sequence information and restricting access to the libraries of clones from which it was obtained, in order to generate corporate profits, is too obscene to find many supporters."[7] Or so they hoped.

In the late 1980s, questions of intellectual property were continually raised at genome conferences. As journalists focused on the more egregious and pernicious ethical issues generated by the HGP (such as fears of eugenics practices and the sharing of individuals' genetic information with interested parties, such as employers and insurance companies), a lively debate concerning intellectual property was raging away from the media's spotlight. The debate centered around how to navigate between a strict intellectual property protection (which would stymie downstream research) and an absence of any patents (which would keep secret some information that was relevant to biomedical research and also discourage researchers from pursuing critical investigations). Money was the issue. Two quotes reflect this apparent dichotomy of knowledge sharing and profit. George Cahill of the Howard Hughes Medical Institute queried, "What is the bucks-to-ethics ratio here?"[8] And an intellectual property scholar from the University of Michigan School of Law, Rebecca Eisenberg, summed up the conflict: "The patent system rests on the premise that scientific progress will best be promoted by conferring exclusive rights in new discoveries, while the research scientific community has traditionally proceeded on the opposite assumption that science will advance most rapidly if the community enjoys free access to prior discoveries."[9]

The gene-patenting issue became public in July 1991 at a Senate hearing on the Human Genome Project's progress. At that meeting, hosted by Senator Peter Domenici (Republican, New Mexico), Venter announced that his National Institutes of Health lab had been filing for patents on small fragments of DNA that were isolated from brain tissue using the expressed sequencing tag (EST) technique that was described in chapter 1.[10] Reid G. Adler, who at the time was the head of the NIH's Office of Technology Transfer, had received an anxious call from a fellow lawyer at Genentech. His colleague expressed concern that if Venter and the NIH made the gene sequences available to the public, then companies such as Genentech might not be able to patent their own gene-sequence discoveries.[11] Adler therefore felt that perhaps the NIH should patent these sequences, permit university scientists to use them royalty free, and offer them to for-profit companies at a fair cost.[12] This would prohibit biotech companies from patenting them and charging exorbitant royalties or licensing fees. Both the Pharmaceutical Manufacturers Association and the Industrial Biotechnology Association predictably and forcefully argued that the NIH should not patent gene sequences because the federal organization might make them public at no cost.[13] Although Venter originally opposed the idea, Adler pointed out that the Bayh-Dole Act (which, among other things, required scientists who received federal funds to patent their work) strongly suggested that they should at least try to patent the ESTs.[14] Venter agreed, although the U.S. Patent and Trademark Office initially rejected the applications on the grounds that they lacked utility.

Many of Venter's colleagues were dismayed by the move to file patent applications on ESTs. Nobel laureate James Watson then was director of the Human Genome Project at the NIH and therefore technically Venter's boss, and he argued in front of Senator Domenici and the press that it was insane to patent gene fragments because the information contained in their sequences was incomplete. In addition, automatic gene sequencers "could be run by monkeys"; the process was obvious and therefore not patentable. Finally, anyone who patented a gene fragment could potentially block downstream research on that gene.[15] In April 1992, or eighteen months after the HGP's inauguration, Senator Mark O. Hatfield (Republican, Oregon) expressed his concerns regarding the ethics of gene patenting and called for a moratorium on such patents until thorough studies could be conducted.[16] His fears were somewhat assuaged when Senators Dennis DeConcini (Democrat, Arizona) and Ted Kennedy (Democrat, Massachusetts) agreed to chair a committee on gene patenting for the Senate Judiciary Committee.[17]

The debate about patenting genomic research was unresolved when the Human Genome Project began,[18] and some contradictory and confused views surrounded intellectual property issues germane to the HGP.

In 1988, the Office of Technology Assessment concluded that "genome projects raise no new questions of patent or copyright law"[19] but failed to consider how technology-transfer issues would apply to the sequence data that the HGP generated.[20] Although the National Research Council queried whether a central agency of the federal government should own patents for commercially available clones, it argued that genome sequences should not be copyrighted.[21] Many factors—the extraordinary output of nucleic-acid sequencing data without much information about their products' functions, a lack of understanding of the applicability of patent law to genes, and the lag time for the effective implementation of the federal technology-transfer laws—resulted in a mess of nucleic-acid patents in the 1990s. The issue of human gene patenting took center stage after Venter left the National Institutes of Health in 1992 to head the Institute for Genomic Research and collaborate with Human Genome Sciences, Inc.

HGS's CCR5 Patent and the Responses

By 2000, the year in which their patent for CCR5 was approved, Human Genome Sciences, Inc. (HGS) owned thirteen patents on chemokine receptors.[22] Patenting the genes of these receptors signaled a critical shift in intellectual property. Inventions no longer possessed intrinsic value; they now had potential value as therapeutic targets.[23] Despite the five years it took to approve this particular patent, examiners spent an average of seventeen hours to review a patent as they struggled to work through a backlog of applications.[24] Overpatenting is a problem at the U.S. Patent and Trademark Office. Examiners are encouraged to award patents because they provide sources of constant revenue. From 1990 to 1991, patent processing fees rose from $175 million to $290 million. Two years later, the number had risen to $423 million, and by 1997, it had skyrocketed to $674 million.[25] In addition, patent attorneys do their best to have their clients' patent applications approved. At the time, an examiner's rejection of an application might have resulted in a hearing of the Board of Patent Appeals and Interferences with the examiner's supervisor.[26] And compared to the European Patent Office, the U.S. Patent and Trademark Office had a very high turnover rate of examiners. Between 1992 and 2004, one out of every two examiners left, so many examiners lacked experience, and only 45 percent had more than five years' experience on the job.[27] Finally, examiners follow the courts on the patenting rules, and if the courts are silent about a particular issue, then the applicant receives a patent unless the examiner can show that the claims are false. The burden of proof lies with the examiner, not the applicant. This might begin to explain why the grant rate of the USPTO on patents (excluding design patent applications) from 1981 to 1998 rose from 60% to 76% and then dropped to 74% in 1999 and to 71% in 2000.[28] After conducting extensive interviews with patent examiners from numerous patent offices worldwide, the Australian intellectual property scholar Peter Drahos remarked on "how little patent offices care about the social costs of the uncertainty that they are generating by granting so many patents."[29] He suggests that the financial incentives for patent offices to behave like businesses threaten to undermine their social contract with the citizenry.[30]

The particular patent for HDGNR10, later to be called CCR5, was granted by Garnette D. Draper of the USPTO. The overwhelming majority of the patents that Draper reviewed were chemical, biochemical, molecular biological, and pharmaceutical in nature.[31] In essence, this agency accepted a certain type of patent to assist the biotech industry's financial growth. The patent abstract reads:

Human G-protein chemokine receptor polypeptides and DNA (RNA) encoding such polypeptides and a procedure for producing such polypeptides by recombinant techniques is [sic] disclosed. Also disclosed are methods for utilizing such polypeptides for identifying antagonists and agonists to such polypeptides and methods of using the agonists and antagonists therapeutically to treat conditions related to the underexpression and overexpression of the G-protein chemokine receptor polypeptides, respectively. Also disclosed are diagnostic methods for detecting a mutation in the G-protein chemokine receptor nucleic acid sequences and detecting a level of the soluble form of the receptors in a sample derived from a host.[32]

On February 16, 2000, a day after the USPTO approved the HGS patent on CCR5, company president Haseltine remarked, "the discovery of the *CCR5* receptor gene is another example of the power of genomics' approach to drug discovery. It was one of many genes that we found early in our discovery program. Experiments confirmed that the CCR5 receptor played a key role in the biology of the immune system and as an AIDS virus receptor."[33] HGS's initial patent application, however, did not mention HIV or AIDS.

The stock market responded positively to Haseltine's announcement. The company's shares saw a 21% increase in value on that first day and 50% in the two trading sessions following the announcement. The gene went from being a potential commodity to an actual one because it now was defined in part by market forces. HGS's stock reached an all-time high.[34] In early 2000, Haseltine sold $525 million in bonds convertible into stock at prices as high as $109 per share and was able to raise over $900 million in another offering in November of that year at $75 per share.[35] He made it clear that even though HIV was not mentioned in HGS's patent application, any company that used this receptor for drug treatment programs after February 15, 2000, without paying royalties to HGS would be subject "not just to damages, but to double and triple damages."[36] HGS licensed its patent to pharmaceutical companies, such as Praecis Pharmaceuticals, Inc. (now a part of GlaxoSmithKline) of Cambridge, Massachusetts, for AIDS drug development based on "peptide mimetic drugs," and HGS itself worked on monoclonal antibodies to block viral entry into CD4 cells.[37] Haseltine did add that "We would not block anyone in the academic world from using this for research purposes."[38] He later repeated that sentiment: "we do not use our patents to prevent anyone in academics or the non-profit world from using these materials for whatever they want, so long as it is not commercial."[39] HGS entered into licensing agreements with drug companies in the United States, Japan, France, and Germany.[40] In addition to Praecis Pharmaceuticals, Inc., these companies included Pfizer, AstraZeneca, Boehringer-Ingelheim, and Monogram Biosciences.[41]

Although Wall Street welcomed the news of Human Genome Sciences' patent, many scientists did not. In 1997, Edward Berger had confirmed that the gene sequence revealed by HGS's international patent filing WO 96/39437 was indeed the gene coding for CCR5.[42] The controversy was announced in a short piece in *Science* but did not become public until after the patent was awarded. Despite Haseltine's comments, academics were unsympathetic, and some were incensed. Robert Gallo, who at the time was director of the Institute of Human Virology at the University of Maryland, Baltimore, protested: "If the patent office awards a patent to someone who clones a gene, even though they have no notion of its function and no real idea of its use, that would be like saying, 'I found a fungus, therefore I should get credit for penicillin.'"[43] The patent "takes my breath away. As a society, we have to ask if it's fair" to reward a company that simply sequenced the gene but did not perform the labor necessary to determine its precise function.[44] Eric Lander, founding director of MIT and Harvard's Broad Institute, admonished the USPTO for "creating a thicket of patents," giving them out "willy-nilly for very, very slight investments." He feared that "in the long run that's a big mistake," concluding that "you can discover all sorts of things pretty easily by computer, and our patent policy hasn't yet caught up with that."[45] Dan Littman of New York University School of Medicine, who was one of the scientists who determined that HIV-1 recognizes CCR5 as a coreceptor, was also dismayed: "Now you have companies coming from a completely different direction and not even trying to understand function before seeking patents.... They can just sit there and wait for others to do the research for them."[46] Littman was interested in patenting the *CCR5* gene as well; however, he was dissuaded by NYU's Technology Transfer Office.[47] Biomedical researchers feared that the CCR5 patent would be a classic "submarine patent"—one that was submerged out of site at the USPTO and that appeared only when other scientists' work gave the patent significance.[48]

Haseltine defended his company's research and financial interests: "you are rewarded for speculation. If you teach what to do and you are right, you don't have to show it yourself. You are rewarded for intelligent and correct guesses.... The patent office does not reward perspiration. They reward priority. They don't care if someone spent 20 years to find an invention or 20 minutes." He wished to differentiate his company from those that simply mined the genome for profitable genes: "We did real biology. We didn't just find a gene and patent it."[49] He continued by arguing that "we did a lot of work."[50] Although many scientists noted that such research "require[s] little scientific insight or creativity,"[51] HGS's chief scientific officer insisted that computational gene searchers required much effort.[52] In addition, HGS's chief patent counsel, Robert Benson, remarked, "Scientific credit is one thing; patent law is another."[53] Scientists were not the only ones who were outraged. Gregg Gonsalves, policy director for Treatment Action Group (TAG), which is a New York lobby group for AIDS research, was displeased: "These guys are the robber barons of the genetic age. They are going to patent everything they can get their hands on and squeeze as much money out of it they can. This is not about making progress on AIDS; it is about making money."[54]

A month later the controversy intensified. Not only did HGS fail to list HIV-1 recognition in the patent application, but in a rush to file, the company's sequence was incorrect. It made errors in the noncoding and coding regions of the DNA. After the patent was approved and made public, researchers at the National Institutes of Health and Rockefeller University compared the patented sequence with the one that they isolated. Christopher C. Broder, who had been a member of the NIH team led by Berger and Philip Murphy that codiscovered CCR5's role in HIV infection, noticed that a number sequence errors resulted in different amino acids in the protein.[55] He, too, was shocked by the announcement of HGS's patent ("I am flabbergasted") and stated that he could not believe that the USPTO awarded a patent for "armchair" biology research.[56] He continued: "it is rather upsetting to all of us to learn that this company is obtaining patents, despite the fact that we made the discovery first."[57]

Broder noted four errors in the amino acid sequence—one at amino acid position 21, which had a proline where a glutamine should have been; one at position 59, which had a glutamine where a lysine should have been; one at position 62, where a glutamic acid was recorded where a lysine should have been; and an isoleucine at position 130, where a valine should have been. The first switch is near the NH_2 terminus in the extracellular space and is a switch from a hydrophilic amino acid (one in which the side chain is polar) to a hydrophobic one (in which the side chain is nonpolar). The second was in the first inner membrane loop and was a switch from a positively charged amino acid to a hydrophilic amino acid. The third was just three amino acids away inside the CD4 cell with a switch from a positively charged amino acid to a negatively charged one. And the fourth was in the second intracellular loop of the protein and was a switch from one hydrophobic amino acid to another.

Broder alerted John P. Moore about the errors. Moore postulated that HIV-1 would not recognize the protein coded for by the HGS sequence, surmising that one of these switches would affect the protein's folding. As is shown in figure 2.1, the first amino acid switch is next to a cysteine that forms a weak disulfide bridge with the cysteine at amino acid position 269. Glutamine and cysteine are both polar (hydrophilic) amino acids; hence, glutamine will repel cysteine, enabling it to form a weak disulfide bond with the other cysteine at 269. In the HGS patent, proline, which is a nonpolar (hydrophobic) amino acid, replaces glutamine. That repulsion no longer exists; therefore, the weak disulfide bridge will most likely not form. The protein encoded for in the HGS patent would in principle fold differently than the correct protein. Because receptors and their ligands are similar to locks and their corresponding keys, it became clear that the HGS's lock was different from the actual CCR5. Consequently, HIV-1 might not be the appropriate key. So Moore decided to test his hypothesis. Tatjana Dragic, who was a postdoctoral student in his lab and the lead author of one of the five key papers announcing CCR5 as the HIV-coreceptor, synthesized the protein coded for by the HGS patented sequence. She then attempted to hybridize HIV-1 to the protein. Some seven years later, she recalled, "I don't believe it worked."[58] Moore protested that the patent should not be granted: "It's like patenting an airplane that doesn't have a tail. They know it won't fly, but they'll stop everyone who has an airplane with a tail."[59] Dragic concurred: "They [Human Genome Sciences] use sophisticated equipment and computers that analyze the utility of a gene sequence. It isn't the hard work. It isn't the innovative work. It's not fair for others to have to pay licensing fees just because they got lucky."[60]

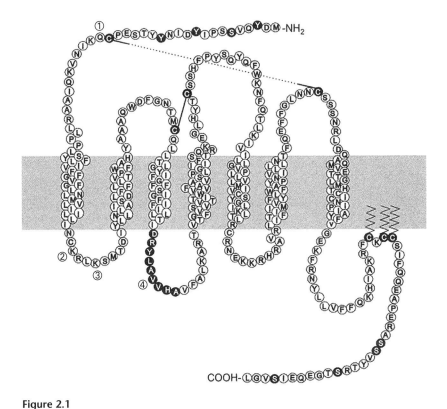

Figure 2.1
The initial Human Genome Sciences patent application for CCR5 contained numerous errors, including four that resulted in amino acid switches—proline glutamine at 21, glutamine lysine at 59, glutamic acid lysine at 62, and isoleucine valine at 130. The protein depicted in this figure is the wild type (or normal) protein. *Source:* Martin Oppermann, "Chemokine Receptor CCR5: Insights into Structure, Function, and Replication," *Cellular Signaling* 16, no. 11 (2004): 1201–1210, here 1202. The first switch (a proline rather than a glutamine) is critical because it disrupts the formation of a weak disulfide bridge (dotted line in the upper portion of the figure), thereby affecting the folding of the protein.

Haseltine, however, did not despair over the errors. HGS insisted that despite the errors, which it admitted, it was still entitled to any and all royalties from anyone who used the gene for profit, particularly in the search for new treatments, such as producing molecules to bind the receptor, thereby blocking the virus's entry into the cell. He and other company officials argued that any errors in the company's description (or sequence) and its corresponding protein were irrelevant because the HGS patent referred to a copy of the gene in a living cell that HGS deposited in the American Type Culture Collection (ATCC) in Manasas, Virginia. According to Haseltine, "When we file a patent, we don't claim the sequence as the invention. The invention we claim is the gene we deposit with the ATCC. We know that our sequence and most sequences are not perfect. Anyone who wishes can go to the ATCC. It's the same as the olden days, when inventors used to deposit a little model of their inventions."[61] As is shown in chapter 4, Haseltine might be correct that depositing a gene in a public depository trumps any errors in the written specification.

At the time, however, intellectual property lawyers disagreed about the importance of those errors. Not surprisingly, HGS's lawyers publicly declared that the mistakes were irrelevant. John H. Barton, a professor of intellectual property at Stanford School of Law, disagreed: "A patent must claim the invention in enough detail so that the public knows what is and is not protected. If you don't make the written patent final—subject, obviously, to some arrangement for correction if there really is a clerical error—then the rest of the world doesn't know what is patented, and that isn't right."[62] Craig Jepson, an intellectual property specialist from Franklin Pierce Law School in New Hampshire, thought that HGS would win if the patent were challenged: "It sounds like the patent may have problems, but I couldn't say they are fatal."[63]

To make the story even more interesting, on September 10, 2002 (two years and seven months after the granting of the Human Genome Sciences patent), the USPTO awarded U.S. Patent 6,448,375 to Euroscreen for the nucleic acid and protein sequence of CCR5.[64] This patent was examined by Jeffrey Stucker and Jegatheesan Seharaseyeon.[65] It covered the complete wild-type amino acid sequence of the receptor, amino acid sequences of 80% homology, and the defective receptor of the $\Delta32$ mutation, and unlike the HGS patent, Euroscreen's patent disclosed the receptor's relevance in HIV-1 infection.[66] Although there was a disagreement about whether HGS did any wet biochemistry, no such confusion shrouded the Belgians' work. The Belgians were aware of the HGS patent.[67] In addition, ICOS's patent applications (see chapter 1) also had been approved—U.S. Patent 6,265,184 on July 24, 2001 (examined by Prema Mertz); 6,268,477 on July 31, 2001 (also examined by Prema Mertz); and 6,797,811 on September 28, 2004 (examined by Yvonne Eyler and assisted by Joseph F. Murphy).[68] The patent application that was filed by Yi Li and Steven M. Ruben of HGS (with the sequence correction and the listing of HIV-1 as a coreceptor for the protein) was also approved as U.S. Patent 6,800,729 on October 5, 2004. It cited the early HGS patent as being a "Related U.S. Patent Document."[69] Draper, who was the examiner of the initial HGS patent, also examined and approved a related ICOS patent on August 3, 1999, "providing purified and isolated polynucleotide sequences encoding a novel human macrophage-derived C–C chemokine designated MDC, and polypeptide analogs thereof."[70]

But how can the U.S. Patent and Trademark Office give a patent for the same gene to three different entities? In fact, a single gene may have multiple patents, and a single patent usually contains numerous claims. In the case of HGS and that of Euroscreen and ICOS, the sequence was theoretically for the same gene, but there were two different sequences because the original HGS sequence was incorrect. All the patent applications were filed before the announcement of CCR5 as the HIV coreceptor was published in either the patent or the written literature.[71] Finally and perhaps most important, different patent examiners sometimes unwittingly grant patents that claim the same subject matter. Reviewing the massive amount of claimed prior art is a huge challenge,[72] so the USPTO conducts annual quality-control testing of patents awarded and reports an error rate between 4% and 6%.[73]

So who was the inventor? Human Genome Sciences was the first to submit a patent application (which was not as important as the first to invent under U.S. patent law at the time), yet shortly after the announcement of the granting of the patent, it was known that the sequence was wrong. ICOS could be seen as the inventor, as could Euroscreen. Both unquestionably performed the requisite biochemical experimentation in gene isolation and identification, although Euroscreen was the first to determine the function/utility of the protein as the HIV-1 coreceptor. What counts as an invention for each claim, such as the sequence, the protein product, and the determination that the protein product is the HIV-1 coreceptor? Was the inventor the one who merely performed computer sequence searches? Was it the company that first patented the correct sequence? The first to claim a broad utility? The first to claim a specific utility? What is the difference between a discovery and an invention? Although historians and philosophers of science have struggled over this distinction, the U.S. Patent and Trademark Office, unlike the European Patent Office, offers patents to both discoveries and inventions. The USPTO awarded patents to all three companies. It would be up to the companies themselves—with, if necessary, the assistance of the Board of Patent Appeals and Interferences (BPAI) of the USPTO—to sort things out. The Commissioner of Patents also could declare an interference, even if the parties involved wished to settle, should he or she feel that the claims were not allowable. At the time, the Commissioner had the power to order a reexamination if he or she was made aware of new substantial grounds for unpatentability.

Because at the time patents were granted to the first to invent in the United States, one company could have in theory initiated interference proceedings to determine priority issues. That would have provided the legal answer to the question "Who is the inventor"? The BPAI is the quasi-judicial branch of the USPTO and is comprised of administrative patent judges. They find interferences fairly rarely and declared only sixty-four new interferences in 2011.[74] In the case of the CCR5 patent, no interference was filed either by the parties involved or by the Commissioner, and the Commissioner never declared a reexamination.

Euroscreen, ICOS, and Human Genome Sciences decided that rather than seek infringement and litigation, they would join forces. At first, there were several patent estates worldwide. In the United States, HGS owned the *CCR5* sequences (wild-type and mutations), antibodies produced to CCR5, and screening with CCR5. ICOS also owned the *CCR5* sequences and antibody production, and Euroscreen owned the *CCR5* sequences and screening methods. With its patent in hand, Euroscreen was in a position to negotiate. In December 2002, Euroscreen and ICOS combined their CCR5 patent estates, and in January 2007, HGS joined the two, with Euroscreen acting as the exclusive licensor in the nonantibody field of the CCR5 patent portfolio. In January 2008, a year after Eli Lilly bought ICOS, Euroscreen was assigned ICOS's CCR5 patent rights. The portfolio is now shared between Euroscreen and HGS, which was acquired by GlaxoSmithKline in August 2012. As a result of this combined patent portfolio, GlaxoSmith-Kline and Euroscreen now own the patent rights covering the wild-type *CCR5* nucleic acid and the human CCR5 protein sequence, the cDNA of *CCR5*, the *Δ32* allele and the corresponding mutated receptor, the antibodies to the protein products of those wild-type and mutant sequences, the CCR5 cell lines, and the use of the wild-type CCR5 protein for screening agonists and antagonists for use in HIV diagnostics and treatment.[75] Because the details of the licensing agreements are secret, the amount of money that Euroscreen and HGS have earned from the CCR5 patent portfolios has never been publicly disclosed.[76] If they can be forged, licensing agreements are always the way forward because patent litigation can be time consuming and costly for all parties involved. Indeed, the average litigation rate in the United States is less than 2%.[77]

According to Vincent Lannoy of Euroscreen, this is the "patent portfolio which we are sublicensing to companies who are developing therapeutic drugs that block the ability of HIV to bind to the CCR5 receptor and therefore to infect the target cells. Portions of the portfolio are also being licensed to companies developing and selling CCR5-based diagnostic tests for the direction of such CCR5-directed therapeutic drugs."[78] Pierre Nokin, Euroscreen's president and chief executive officer at the time, commented immediately after the announcement of their patent:

> This patent award is a significant milestone in the development of Euroscreen, as it represents and justifies many years of outstanding work performed by our scientists. Several companies already use the CCR5 receptor as a target for the development of novel anti-HIV drugs, and the award of this patent will enable Euroscreen to generate future revenues from licensing this target to such commercial partners.
>
> Euroscreen owns all intellectual property rights to the CCR5 receptor and its role in HIV infection, however, research into preventing HIV infection is an important focus of the scientific and medical community, and such fundamental studies will be allowed to continue unrestrained by this award.[79]

Because of the importance of chemokine receptors to physiological processes and a myriad of diseases, sequencing companies that are interested in licensing their patented sequences to major pharmaceutical companies have played a prominent role in the discovery of genes coding for those receptors. G protein-coupled receptors (GPCRs) are ideal targets for future blockbuster drugs, so companies that hold the gene patents for them possess the potential for great reward. The sequencing company Celera Genomics (under Venter's direction and with the recommendation of Celera's intellectual property lawyer, Robert Millman) filed provisional patent applications on genes with sequences that were similar to ones coding for GPCRs. This gave Celera a lead (albeit a brief one) in filing before they sent the information to biotech firms (such as Amgen, Novartis, and Pharmacia-Upjohn) that paid for early access to Celera's database.[80] GPCRs, which include chemokine receptors, constitute a disproportionately large share of the prescription drug market.[81] Prozac and Claritin are two current therapeutic drugs that target GPCRs.[82] Patent protection is critical for companies and universities, which possess the genes that encode those receptor proteins. In addition to Human Genome Sciences, patent owners of DNA sequences of various chemokine receptor sequences include the U.S. Department of Health, the Regents of the University of California, Merck, Glaxo and

SmithKline Beecham (which now are GlaxoSmithKline), Schering, Brigham and Women's Hospital, Arena Pharmaceuticals, Incyte Pharmaceuticals (now Incyte Genomics), ICOS (now Eli Lilly), Genentech, the Theodor-Kocher Institute of the University of Bern, and the New York Blood Center Institute.[83] Most of these patents were filed between 1997 and 2000. The importance of GPCRs as drug targets is evinced by the statistic that nearly 25% of the top two hundred best-selling drugs worldwide in 2000 regulated GPCR activity.[84] Not surprisingly, they are the subjects of much controversy.

The patenting of the *CCR5* gene illustrates how lenient the U.S. Patent and Trademark Office was in granting patents. Human Genome Sciences had the incorrect sequence in its patent application. It merely listed the gene's function as a chemokine receptor and wished to use it to screen it for antagonists and agonists. There was no mention of HIV/AIDS in HGS's initial patent application, just vague statements about the physiological roles of chemokines, which were well known at the time of their application. It was unclear how much "wet biochemistry" HGS scientists actually performed. Thousands of the early gene patents in the 1990s were filed by sequencing companies, which often did not perform the standard biochemical assays but simply relied on computer-generated sequence homology to deduce function. HGS's gene happened to be associated with an important ligand, which was the virus responsible for the greatest epidemic of our time. An unimaginable backlog of patent applications coupled with a patent office that was encouraged to be patent friendly to assist the biotech sector gave rise to a number of highly questionable gene patents in the 1990s. DNA sequencing companies were able to exploit the situation to their advantage. These companies wanted to lock up as many genes as possible with patents to convince investors of their viability in an extremely competitive market. All of this came with a price, which was shoddy science. Many scientists were angered by the HGS patent and felt that the capitalism of biocapitalism was trumping the bio.

3 Gene Patenting and the Product-of-Nature Doctrine

The CCR5 patent has become emblematic of the ways that intellectual property law has changed the conduct and content of scientific knowledge and the social, political, and ethical implications of such a metamorphosis. The resolution of these issues signaled the willingness of the U.S. Patent and Trademark Office to assist the biotech sector. This chapter and the next two continue to trace the *CCR5* gene's intellectual property lineage. As a historian, I am wary of teleological histories. The astute reader will quickly identify a tension, particularly evident in this and the next chapter, between the teleology of gene patenting as lawyers perceive the situation from historical cases and the historically contingent and contextual accounts of those cases. I am interested in understanding how it can be argued that genes are (or are not) patentable entities. This requires a close reading of the precedents that lawyers point to and read to construct their cases. As I recount this history, readers will see that these cases were meant to solve contemporary problems and frame future legal decisions. Often distinctions that lawyers and judges now draw are established well after the fact.

"How can I patent my genes?" is a query that I often hear when I lecture on the subject. Even university scientists have interrupted me to explain that natural products are not patentable. Other incredulous statements and queries quickly ensue: "Genes are not inventions but discoveries." "How can another person or entity 'own' my genes?" "Can I patent my own genes before someone else does?" Eventually, the conversation turns to issues of impact: "How does this affect scientific and medical research?" "Does gene patenting encourage innovative research?" "Does it challenge the objectivity of science, which is claimed to be free from commercial interest?" "Does it foster collaboration or thwart it by means of secrecy?" These are crucial questions. As for the answers, in many cases, the proverbial jury is still out. As a historian, I argue that before we can begin to understand them, we need to review the history of how we arrived at a point when it became permissible to patent genes. Without a precedent that establishes that genes are not patentable and given the statutes that govern the USPTO, a number of lawyers have argued that the decision to patent genes is not unexpected.

The U.S. patent system is predicated on article I, section 8 of the U.S. Constitution, which stresses the importance of technological advances to a national economy: "To promote the Progress of Science and useful Arts, by securing for limited Times to Authors and Inventors the exclusive Right to their respective Writings and Discoveries."[1] Patents are awarded to defend an inventor's intellectual property and are divided into four categories—processes or methods, machines, articles of manufacture, and compositions of matter, or improvements thereof.[2] Generally, there are three types of patents—utility patents, which protect an invention's useful process, machine, manufacture, or composition of matter; design patents, which cover the physical appearance of objects; and plant patents, which are granted for all plants except sexual and tuber-propagating ones.[3] They must satisfy a number of criteria. First, the invention must be novel. Before the passing of the Patent Reform Act of 2011, others must not have known about it or used it previous to the filing of the patent application.[4] Until the reform, a patent application needed to be filed prior to one year after the time it was publicly disclosed or used. Second, the invention must possess a utility. Third, it must not be obvious to someone skilled in the art. Fourth, the invention needs to be described and explained in a manner that allows one who is skilled in the art to make and use the invention. Fifth, the claims of the patent must be clear and specific. And the entity must be considered patentable material, which is the theme of this chapter. Laws of nature, physical phenomena, and abstract ideas have been deemed not patentable.[5] A patent provides a limited monopoly, normally twenty years after the filing of the application. The inventor agrees to make public the invention so that others may use it for their own work after paying a fee, thereby enhancing innovation and economic growth. In exchange, the government agrees to protect the invention from infringement. In a sense, patents are the antithesis of trade secrets, in which an inventor decides not to disclose the invention to the public.

Perhaps the first question that is raised in gene patenting in general is whether genes are patent eligible. Do they fit the category described by 35 U.S.C. section 101, which defines patentable subject matter as "any new and useful process, machine, manufacture, or composition of matter, or any new and useful improvement thereof"?[6] These words owe much to the quill of Thomas Jefferson, who added "composition of matter" in 1793, a phrase that was absent from the initial Patent Act of 1790, which had defined patentable subject matter as "any useful art, manufacture, engine, machine, or device, or any improvement therein not before known or used."[7] He had chemical inventors in mind with the addition of that phrase.

Gene Patenting, Profit, and Biomedical Research Funding

In March 1982, the U.S. Patent and Trademark Office awarded the first patent for a human gene inserted into a bacterial cloning vector, the adrenocorticotropin-lipotropin precursor gene. The application had been filed in December 1978. Other genes quickly followed, including those coding for insulin and human chorionic somatomammotropin.[8] These early gene patents were human-produced complementary DNA (cDNA) molecules that were cloned in a vector: the patent claimed a recombinant DNA plasmid vector containing the cDNA.[9] This move paved the way for literally thousands of patents on human genes. The isolation and purification (that is, simply making a cDNA copy of the gene's mRNA after the RNA splicing removes the introns) of the gene apparently rendered it a product of human agency. By 1984, the USPTO was granting patents for DNA sequences themselves rather than the cDNA copy. The sequences were the same nucleotide sequences as those found in nature.[10] The first patent using the phrase "isolated DNA" was issued in 1987.[11] Some of the subsequent patents were on the genes without the cloning vector. Less and less human intervention seemed to be required.

In an attempt to clarify and standardize the international stance on gene patenting, in 1988 the U.S. Patent and Trademark Office (USPTO), European Patent Office (EPO), and Japanese Patent Office (JPO) composed a joint communiqué declaring isolated biological materials to be chemical compounds and therefore patentable:

Purified natural products are not regarded under any of the three laws as products of nature or discoveries because they do not in fact exist in nature in an isolated form. Rather, they are regarded for patent purposes as biologically active substances and chemical compounds and eligible for patents on the same basis as other chemical compounds.[12]

This sentiment was echoed some ten years later by John J. Doll, who was the former director of the USPTO's Biotechnology Patent Examination Group and later Commissioner of Patents and acting director of the USPTO: "in order for isolated DNA sequences to be distinguished from their naturally occurring counterparts, which cannot be patented, the patent application must state that the invention has been purified or isolated or is part of a recombinant molecule."[13] Rebecca Eisenberg discussed the patentability of genes, stating that "if the DNA sequence is identical to a sequence that exists in nature, it may still [be patented] if the patent applicant has made the sequence available in an isolated or purified form that does not exist in nature."[14]

From 1987 to 1988, the number of patents awarded in U.S. Patent Class 935, which is the class of genetic engineering patents, rose from around a hundred a year to just under three hundred. In 1988, the USPTO established a new unit to deal with biotechnology patents.[15] From 1990 to 1995, the number of patents stabilized at around 350 patents per annum, with a substantial increase after 1995 due to the implementation of new cloning techniques, which made gene isolation much easier and more efficient (figure 3.1).[16] Throughout the 1970s, only 123 DNA-based patents had been awarded by the USPTO.[17]. By spring of 2009, 50,000 patents on DNA sequences had been awarded by the USPTO, and a year later the Office announced a backlog of 30,000 biotech patents. The numbers had risen dramatically during the late 1990s and early 2000s.[18] A 2005 study showed that nearly 20% of around 23,000 human genes coding for proteins were already patented, with thousands more pending the USPTO's approval and 63% of the patented human genes owned by private companies.[19] A more recent study suggests that 41% of our genes have now been patented.[20]

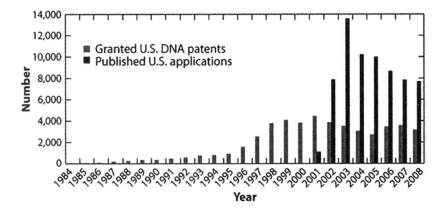

Figure 3.1
Granted U.S. DNA patents (1984 to 2008) and published U.S. DNA patent applications (2001 to 2008). *Source:* Robert Cook-Deegan and Christopher Heaney, "Patents in Genomics and Human Genetics," *Annual Review of Genomics and Human Genetics* 11 (2010): 383–425, here 384.

Not surprisingly, most of these genes are ones whose mutations give rise to serious illnesses that are pervasive in the industrialized world.[21] Although the USPTO has awarded more gene patents than all other patent offices combined, the EPO and the JPO also began granting gene patents by the early 1980s.[22] That decade was a banner one for the worldwide biotechnology industry.

The private sector has been funding an ever-increasing percentage of biomedical research over the past two decades. In 1965, for example, the federal government accounted for nearly two-thirds of the total spending on biomedical research. By 1993, that number had shrunk to 39% of $30 billion in contrast to 50% for industry-based funded research and development.[23] A year later, the amount of federal funding for biomedical research fell by 5%. By 2000, the total sum of money spent on biomedical research (both basic and applied) in the United States was $71 billion, 24% of which ($17.1 billion) was from the National Institutes of Health; 7% ($5.2 billion) from other federal sources; 5% ($3.5 billion) from state and local governments; 5% ($3.4 billion) from foundations, charities, and other private sources; 30% ($21.4 billion) from pharmaceutical firms; 20% ($14.2 billion) biotech firms; and 9% ($6.3 billion) from medical device firms.[24] Although the federal government still spends a great deal of money on biotech research and development (and still funds a majority of basic research in the United States), it has been eclipsed by for-profit firms in the total funding of biomedical research.[25] Sheldon Krimsky has shown that leading research universities in the United States are obtaining more of their research funds from industry and has discussed the ramifications of that increased dependency.[26]

American biotech start-up companies flourished, albeit rather ephemerally for most, increasing in number to 1,457 by 2002. Their revenues climbed from $8 billion in 1993 to $20 billion in 1999 and to $27.6 billion by 2001.[27] By 2002, the U.S. biotechnology industry had purportedly furnished over 437,000 jobs, generated $47 billion in revenue, and added $10 billion in taxes to the coffers of federal, state, and local governments in taxes.[28] Reid G. Adler, who initially was the director of the Office of Technology Transfer of the National Institutes of Health and later became a technical law clerk to the Honorable Giles S. Rich of the U.S. Court of Appeals for the Federal Circuit, summed up the benefits of the biotech industry: "The biotechnology industry presently sponsors academic research, conducts elegant independent studies, relieves academia of repetitive and technical tasks, provides employment opportunities for postdoctoral scientists, and offers the promise of revolutionizing medicine and agriculture."[29] It all seemed perfect.

Private and state interests were not simply blurred: they overlapped considerably and at times appeared to be indistinguishable. Nikolas Rose labels it "a virtuous alliance of state, science, and commerce in the pursuit of health and wealth."[30] He explains:

Projects to govern the bioeconomy in almost every geographical region are characterized by novel alliances between political authorities and promissory capitalism. An apparently virtuous connection between health and wealth mobilizes the large budgets for research and development invested by national governments and private foundations, the dealings of the commercial health care and health management industries, the operation of the pharmaceutical and biotechnology companies, the flows of venture and shareholder capital.[31]

Starting in the early 1990s, federal support for biotechnology was a boon to the private sector. Federally funded biomedical research sought to strengthen American pharmaceutical and health biotechnology industries against foreign competitors. The government financed a large amount of basic pharmaceutical research so that private companies did not need to.[32] Support for the biotech sector spanned the Democrat-Republican divide. President Bill Clinton's support of biotechnology was obvious during his second administration. In January 2000, he proclaimed "Biotech Month" and requested $340 million for research for the fiscal year 2001 to fight bioterrorism.[33] A year later, his administration released new gene-patenting guidelines, which were welcomed by those who were in favor of gene patenting. William Haseltine heralded them as "the Magna Carta of biotechnology."[34] He claimed that the guidelines "establish clearly and in the most dramatic fashion the patentability of human genes."[35] Krimsky, a leading critic of gene patenting, reluctantly concurred: "If anything, the document reinforces the move toward economic colonization of the human genome and other biochemical substances found in nature."[36]

Early History of the So-called Product-of-Nature Doctrine

As Lewis Hyde has eloquently argued, the Founding Fathers of the United States were deeply committed to the notions of the commons and commonwealth.[37] They abhorred unlimited monopolies, equating them with the tyranny from which they sought to extricate themselves. They were dedicated to a cultural commons and were tacitly committed to a natural commons that allowed community access to nature. Benjamin Franklin and many other eighteenth-century Americans felt that knowledge of nature and technological innovation were generated by communal efforts.[38] But were their sentiments on the nonpatentability of natural products shared by the U.S. legal system throughout the nineteenth century?

The product-of-nature doctrine was not well defined in nineteenth-century litigation. Subsequent cases selected historical precedents that in hindsight might appear to address the patentability of natural products but that at the time of the original cases actually did not.[39] Two U.S. Supreme Court cases of the late nineteenth century serve as examples. The first decision was *American Wood-Paper Company v. Fiber Disintegrating Company* (1874) (henceforth *American Wood-Paper Patent*),[40] which revolved around the question of whether paper pulp (cellulose) that was extracted from wood through chemical processes and through vegetable substance by means of chemical and mechanical processes could be patented. The mechanical process involved a machine that shred the wood or vegetable substance into shavings, and the chemical processes included reactions such as chlorination, boiling in a strong alkali solution under high temperature and pressure, and washing to remove the hydrochloric acid.

Two key considerations of the Court in *American Wood-Paper Patent* were the nature and patentability of the extract (pulp). Justice William Strong argued that

in cases of chemical inventions, that when, as in the present case, the manufacture claimed as novel is not a new composition of matter, but an extract obtained by the decomposition or disintegration of material substances, it cannot be of importance from what it has been extracted.

There are many things well known and valuable in medicine or in the arts which may be extracted from divers substances. But the extract is the same no matter from what it has been taken. A process to obtain it from a subject from which it has never been taken may be the creation of invention, but the thing itself when obtained cannot be called a new manufacture.[41]

Pulp from wood and paper was known and commonly used before the invention of the extraction process. As Judge Strong continued, "Thus, if one should discover a mode or contrive a process by which prussic acid could be obtained from a subject in which it not now known to exist, he might have a patent for a process, but not for prussic acid."[42] The Court ruled that pulp was not patentable—not because it was a product of nature but because it was already known at the time of the patent. It failed due to prior art, meaning that relevant information that was specified in the patent application was already known and available before the application was filed.[43]

Ten years later, the Supreme Court ruled on another case that was relevant to the patenting of a natural substance, *Cochrane v. Badische Anilin &*

Soda Fabrik (1884).[44] The German firm BASF owned a U.S. patent for synthetic alizarine (alizarin), an important dye that was obtained from coal tar. It had long been known that naturally occurring alizarin could be isolated from the root of a madder plant. The plaintiffs argued that the patent was not new because it was chemically equivalent to the natural substance. The novelty claim overlapped with the product-of-nature argument.[45] The Court concluded that

the article produced by the process described was the alizarine of madder, having the chemical formula $C_{14}H_8O_4$. It was an old article. While a new process for producing it was patentable, the product itself could not be patented, even though it was a product made artificially for the first time, in contradistinction to being eliminated from the madder root. Calling it artificial alizarine did not make it a new composition of matter, and patentable as such, by reason of its having been prepared artificially, for the first time, from anthracine [anthracene], if it was set forth as alizarine, a well known substance.[46]

Similar to the Court ruling in *American Wood-Paper Patent*, the new method of production was patentable; however, a composition-of-matter claim could not be upheld for artificial alizarine, not because it was a natural product but because it was chemically identical to the natural dye that was used in prior art. It was an "old product" that was obtained by a new method. The Supreme Court by and large ignored the product-of-nature arguments.[47]

The USPTO's Commissioner of Patents did deal with a case that directly related to the patentability of natural products. In 1888, William Latimer applied for a process patent to extract the fibrous core from the center of the pine needles of longleaf pines (*Pinus australis*). He also included a composition-of-matter claim on the pine needles themselves because their centers could be used in the burgeoning textile industry. Echoing the logic of the aforementioned Supreme Court cases, the examiner argued that although the process was patentable, the product was not. The examiner, however, ruled that it was not patentable because it was a product of nature and therefore not an invention. The U.S. Patent Commissioner affirmed the examiner's rejection in his *Ex parte Latimer* ruling of 1889, citing *American Wood-Paper Patent* and *Cochrane*.[48] As the legal historian Beauchamp has shown, however, a number of patents on natural products were granted after *Ex parte Latimer*, such as a patent for extracted clam juice that was subsequently filtered and boiled, the isolation of a chemical compound from the orris root used to make a perfume, and sheep thyroid glands.[49] Beauchamp argues that "any product-of-nature prohibition was in practice extremely narrow, and that any substance subjected to the slightest human alteration or processing was treated as a regular invention and assessed by standard criteria of novelty and inventiveness."[50]

The Twentieth Century

By the turn of the twentieth century, courts began to establish what Beauchamp calls the "useful difference" doctrine: an isolated natural substance was patent eligible if the isolation process rendered that substance more useful than its natural homolog.[51] This doctrine became evident in 1910 in *Kuehmsted v. Farbenfabriken of Elberfeld Co.* (known as the aspirin case). Kuehmsted infringed on Bayer's patent on aspirin (acetylsalicylic acid), which was based on a naturally occurring compound, salicylic acid. Bayer's chemist Felix Hoffmann, however, had created "a medicine indisputably beneficial to mankind—something new in a useful art, such as our patent policy was intended to promote."[52]

Parke-Davis & Co. v. H. K. Mulford Co. (1911)[53] is a patent-infringement case that raises the issue of patentability of biological entities. This decision, written by Judge (Billings) Learned Hand, has been referred to in the legal literature as the primary precedent for the early cases of gene patenting until Federal Circuit Judge Alan D. Lourie argued the contrary in 2011.[54] The case begins by affirming that a "substance extracted from animal tissue for medicinal use, which is new, practically and therapeutically may be patentable, although it differs from the previous preparations only in its degree of purity from other portions of the tissue."[55] The key question was whether the Parke-Davis biochemist Jokichi Takamine's purification of adrenaline was sufficient to render it new therapeutically and commercially and therefore patentable.[56]

Patent examiner James B. Littlewood was responsible for adjudicating the original patent application for Adrenalin, which was the commercial name for the mostly purified, patented adrenaline in 1900. As Jon M. Harkness has shown, Littlewood denied the patent multiple times after various revisions by the applicant on the grounds that it was "a product of nature, merely isolated by applicant, and hence is not drawn to such patentable invention as required by statute."[57] Littlewood finally granted the patent on the seventh review on June 2, 1903. The critical point, as Harkness points out, was that

Takamine's lawyers did not succeed in convincing Littlewood that an isolated or purified product of nature was worthy of a patent (in fact, they never really attempted to argue this position). Instead Takamine's legal team finally convinced—or wore down—Littlewood to accept the idea that "Adrenalin," the medical product, was something different than a purified or isolated version of "adrenaline," the hormone.[58]

Adrenalin proved to be an important medical product. Parke-Davis & Co. actively enforced its patent and in 1905 engaged in a priority dispute with H. F. Mulford. The case now became one of patent infringement, and little was said about Adrenalin being a product of nature. The experts brought in by both sides did not address this issue of patenting natural products: they were interested only in matters of priority. As Harkness argues, "Questions about whether an invention was not eligible for a patent because it was nothing more than a pre-existing natural substance were rare. Indeed, the examiner who had originally refused Latimer's product claim acknowledged the exotic nature of the issue: 'This exact question, so far as [I am] aware, has never been considered by the courts or by [Patent] Commissioners.'"[59]

Priority was critical because during the early years of the twentieth century, a number of adrenaline-based products were being sold in the United States and Europe. Hoechst of Germany was marketing Suparenin. But Parke-Davis & Co.'s Adrenalin was relatively pure, safe, and efficacious in contrast to Suparenin.[60] At that time, chemical and pharmaceutical substances were not patentable in Germany. The first pan-German patent law was created after unification and passed in May 1877. It stated that the following inventions were excluded from patent protection—those "consisting of food, stimulants or therapeutic agents, as well as the invention of substances produced by means of chemistry if the invention does not include a specific production process."[61] Unlike patent laws in the United Kingdom, France, or the United States, the German Patent Law of 1877 prohibited the patenting of chemicals, including drugs.[62] Such a decision was seen to be in the interest of the public good because, in part, a monopoly on drugs was deemed to be dangerous to the public welfare:

On the one hand, therapeutic agents have such an important value for the well being of the people in general, and for public health in particular, that it seems impossible to grant a drug's inventor a right that would include the possibility of limiting access or increasing the price. On the other hand, the attribution of such a patent would increase the risk that this form of legal protection on the substance to be marketed would mislead the public to use dangerous substances. The decision to exclude drugs and their use from patent protection has therefore two grounds. Patents can however protect production processes. The law thus seeks to keep the public from being misled into believing in the therapeutic value of an invention, and to make preparation processes public. By so doing, it does not damage access and use but facilitates them.[63]

The patenting of pharmaceuticals also seemed superfluous to bright synthetic organic chemists. German chemists could invent a myriad of processes, which could be patented, to produce a pharmaceutical, so companies could create a wall of patent protection around a particular drug.[64] German chemists from August Wilhelm von Hofmann to Paul Ehrlich and Carl Duisberg were renowned for their abilities in synthetic organic chemistry.[65] In short, German organic chemists could easily use process patents to circumvent the official ban on pharmaceutical product patents.[66] This also encouraged innovation because more methods were devised to create chemicals. German governmental officials worked closely with chemical company officials to draft and tailor the nation's patent law to the interests of the pharmaceutical industry.[67]

During the early twentieth century, the American Pharmaceutical Association lobbied the federal government for weaker patent protection. They argued that they were facing unfair competition from German companies, which obtained product patents of their pharmaceuticals in the United States.[68] American pharmaceutical companies advocated for changing the law so that only patents for processes and not the pharmaceutical products themselves could be patented. The problem was serious enough that three bills were introduced in Congress: the Mann Bill of 1904 and the Paige and Edmonds Bills of 1915 sought to eliminate product patents on drugs and require any drug-related patent to be worked in the United States within two years of granting the patent.[69] None of the bills passed.

Lacking a strong tradition in chemical synthesis, the burgeoning U.S. and British pharmaceutical industries were centered around the extraction and purification of natural substances rather than the organic synthesis of artificial substances: "on the isolation, purification, and chemical and physiological characterization of naturally occurring compounds such as hormones and vitamins, much more important work was done outside of Germany between 1900 and 1935."[70] Something needed to be done legally to recognize such efforts and to save the American chemical and pharmaceutical companies. Not surprisingly, these industries turned to patent decisions, which starting with Judge Learned Hand's ruling, permitted the patenting of natural substances that were isolated and purified.[71] Purification was crucial. The U.S. introduced drug regulation in 1902 with the Biologics Control Act that required the Hygienic Laboratory, later to become the National Institutes of Health, to test and monitor new vaccines and antitoxins for their safety and efficacy.[72] As British business historian Joseph Liebenau argues:

In 1902 the first American Act regulating the manufacture of new medicines and licensing their producers was passed.... The 1902 Act for the first time called on the government to monitor the production of new medicines by a permanent laboratory of trained medical scientists who would have inspection and licensing powers over all producers who sold biological products across state lines. This Act was possibly the single most influential stimulus for the establishment of pharmaceutical laboratories in American drug companies.[73]

American scientists were able to combine synthetic organic chemistry techniques gleaned from their research with their German colleagues with natural-product chemistry, fermentation, and endrocrinology.[74] Natural-product-based companies, such as Parke-Davis, began to compete with the well-established German pharmaceutical companies.[75] Starting with World War II, the patenting of products of nature—in the form of antibiotics, hormones, and vitamins—was dominated by the United States and, to a lesser extent, the United Kingdom.[76] Two different patent regimes helped foster two different research traditions. In the Anglo-American world, which includes the United States, the United Kingdom, and Canada, pharmaceutical research centered around physiological chemistry and the isolation and purification of natural products from plants, animals, and humans, whereas in Germany and Switzerland, synthetic organic chemistry was carried out not only in universities but also in research laboratories of the dyestuff industries.[77] German and Swiss chemists created synthetically the active principles found naturally in plants and animals and improved on their natural analogues for use as medications.[78]

On April 28, 1911, Judge Hand of the District Court for the Southern District of New York ruled in favor of Takamine's patents:

> But, even if it [Adrenalin] were merely an extracted product without change, there is no rule that such products are not patentable. Takamine was the first to make it available for any use by removing it from the other gland-tissue in which it was found, and, while it is of course possible logically to call this a purification of the principle, it became for every practical purpose a new thing commercially and therapeutically. That was a good ground for a patent.... The line between different substances and degrees of the same substance is to be drawn rather from the common usages of men than from nice considerations of dialectic.[79]

Hand's ruling undoubtedly benefited the U.S. pharmaceutical companies in gaining the lead over their German counterparts. As Dutfield points out, "the Patent Office was often flexible in its application of the doctrine to the extent of allowing purified or isolated natural products to be protected. In addition, the courts sometimes interpreted the law in ways that favored owners in cases where the patentability boundaries relating to new kinds of product were unclear and needed to be demarcated."[80] This case paved the way for the subsequent patenting of sex hormones, steroids, vitamins, antibiotics, and genes in the United States.[81]

In 1930, Congress passed the Plant Patent Act, which awards a patent to an inventor "who has invented or discovered and asexually reproduced a distinct and new variety of plant, other than a tuber-propagated plant."[82] Congress initially asked whether this act would contradict the product-of-nature doctrine, whether a new variety of plant would be considered an invention or discovery, and whether the breeder would be considered an inventor or discoverer.[83] The House Committee on Patents argued that although a new plant variety found in the field was a product of nature and therefore not patentable under article I, section 8, a new variety of plant that was cultivated was created through human intervention and therefore patent eligible.[84] The link between biological and chemical entities was established early on because the House Committee insisted on the analogy between "the part played by the plant originator in the development of new plants and the part played by the chemist in the development of new compositions of matter."[85]

The House Committee on Patents was at the time mindful of the product-of-nature doctrine. During the 1920s, 1930s and 1940s, the U.S. courts began to crack down on patents in general, including those on natural products, as the Antitrust Division of the Department of Justice pursued a number of corporate giants. The government's attitude was one of deep skepticism and suspicion with regard to patents.[86] In this period, the circuit courts for the first time used strong language opposing product-of-nature patents. In 1928 the Circuit Court of Appeals for the Third Circuit underscored that a patent could not be awarded for a product of nature.[87] General Electric's William D. Coolidge, the inventor, applied for a patent on an improved vacuum tube possessing pure tungsten, which he referred to as a new metal. His process of creating the element consisted of converting the oxides of tungsten into pure tungsten. The tungsten oxides were initially heated in a gas furnace to liberate oxygen, carbon, and chemical impurities. The resulting product was then heated electrically, which changed the substance from the yellow oxide to the blue oxide, to the bronze oxide, and then finally to pure tungsten. These various oxides of tungsten were different and possessed distinct properties from pure tungsten. However, the court denied his claims on pure tungsten:

What he produced by his process was natural tungsten in substantially pure form. What he discovered were natural qualities of pure tungsten. Manifestly he did not create pure tungsten, nor did he create its characteristics. These were created by nature and on that fact finding the reasoning as to the validity of the product claims will be based.[88]

Despite the rulings by the lower courts against the patents on products of nature, members of the U.S. Patent and Trademark Office still seemed to equivocate. In 1939, Pasquale Joseph Federico, mathematician, longtime director of the USPTO, editor of the *Journal of the Patent Office Society*, and one of the primary architects of the Patent Act of 1952, concluded an article entitled "Patents for New Chemical Compounds" by asking whether isolated and purified products of nature should be patent eligible:[89]

If a substance, hitherto not known to exist, is discovered in some plant or animal material, extracted in concentrated or pure form, and demonstrated to be highly useful, can the product be patented? Or can a patent for the product be obtained by the first one to isolate in pure form a substance which has been known and used but only in a crude state accompanied by its natural impurities? The remarkable progress made in biological chemistry in discovering, concentrating and isolating vitamins, hormones and the like has increased the importance of questions such as these. A categorical answer of "No, because the substance is not really new," cannot be made. The problem is not as simple as all that. Patents for products of this kind have been granted by the Patent Office in some situations, and in other situations patents for the products have been refused. A full study and analysis of this and other fields of patent law relating to chemistry would be beneficial.[90]

He cites *Parke-Davis v. Mulford* for the example of patents on pure adrenaline and adrenaline salts and *Kuehmsted v. Farbenfabriken of Elberfeld Co.* for the aspirin patent.[91]

In 1948, the Supreme Court decided *Funk Brothers Seed Co. v. Kalo Inoculant Co.* Kalo Inoculant sued Funk Brothers for patent infringement, citing their patent for the product and process of creating a mixture of root-nodule bacteria for inoculating legumes. Funk Brothers argued that the patent was invalid. Kalo's patent included six strains of naturally occurring bacteria, each of which could be used to fertilize legumes. The patent holder combined these strains so that a farmer could purchase one fertilizer for various plants rather than one for each.[92] The bacterial strains did not inhibit one another. The Seventh Circuit ruled that the inventor had produced a new and different composition of noninhibitive strains, which possessed utility.[93]

The Supreme Court disagreed, arguing that the implementation of a natural principle or phenomenon was not patentable. The properties of the patented bacteria were exactly those exhibited in nature:

We have here only product claims. [Varley Sherman] Bond does not create a state of inhibition or of non-inhibition in the bacteria. Their qualities are the work of nature.

Those qualities of course are not patentable. For patents cannot issue for the discovery of the phenomena of nature.... The qualities of these bacteria, like the heat of the sun, electricity, or the qualities of metals, are part of the storehouse of knowledge of all men. They are manifestations of laws of nature, free to all men and reserved exclusively to none. He who discovers a hitherto unknown phenomenon of nature has no claim to a monopoly of it which the law recognizes. If there is to be invention from such a discovery, it must come from the application of the law of nature to a new and useful end.... The Circuit Court of Appeals thought that Bond did much more than discover a law of nature, since he made a new and different composition of non-inhibitive strains which contributed utility and economy to the manufacture and distribution of commercial inoculants. But we think that the aggregation of species fell short of invention within the meaning of the patent statutes.[94]

Along with the eighteenth-century American Founders, the Supreme Court seemed to privilege the natural commons.

In addition, the patent failed to disclose an invention. Theirs was an obvious and trivial use of a natural product. As the Court argued:

The combination of species produces no new bacteria, no change in the six species of bacteria, and no enlargement of the range of their utility. Each species has the same effect it always had. The bacteria perform in their natural way. Their use in combination does not improve in any way their natural functioning. They serve the ends nature originally provided and act quite independently of any effort of the patentee.[95]

The Court continued:

Even though it may have been the product of skill, it certainly was not the product of invention. There is no way in which we could call it such unless we borrowed invention from the discovery of the natural principle itself. That is to say, there is no invention here unless the discovery that certain strains of the several species of these bacteria are non-inhibitive and may thus be safely mixed is invention. But we cannot so hold without allowing a patent to issue on one of the ancient secrets of nature now disclosed. All that remains, therefore, are advantages of the mixed inoculants themselves. They are not enough.[96]

It should be said, however, that this decision dealt with the ineligibility of patents for natural phenomena rather than natural objects.

The lower courts seemed more sympathetic to product-of-nature patents after the Patent Act of 1952 was passed, and the Antitrust Division abated its attack against large corporations. *Merck & Co. v. Olin Mathieson Chemical Corporation* (1958) was the first relevant case for patentability that was tried after the passing of the act.[97] In 1926, scientists discovered that patients suffering from pernicious anemia could benefit from adding a large quantity of cattle liver to their diets. Some twenty years later, new liver extracts could be administered to patients; however, they were expensive, and not

all patients could tolerate them.[98] Biochemists of the period could not isolate or identify the specific agent that was responsible for the improvement
in the patients' health. Mary S. Shorb, a bacteriologist at the Department
of Agriculture and later at the University of Maryland, developed an assay
with a microorganism, *Lactobacillus lactis Dorner* (or LLD), to discover this
unknown agent. In 1947, she entered into a collaboration with scientists
at Merck, one of whom was Thomas R. Wood, who had been working on
this therapeutic compound since 1938. Wood hired a chemist, Edward L.
Rickes, and in October 1947, they isolated a pinkish compound, which
after further purification and concentration turned out to be a red crystalline material, which they subsequently named vitamin B_{12}.

In 1957, the district court, echoing the decisions during the 1920s
through 1940s, ruled that the patent of vitamin B_{12} was invalid on the
grounds that it was a product of nature and that there was a lack of invention. In reversing the decision a year later, the U.S. Court of Appeals for the
Fourth Circuit addressed the product-of-nature defense. The court interpreted the Patent Act of 1952 as authorizing patents for

"any new and useful composition of matter," provided only that the conditions of
patentability … are met. There is nothing in the language of the Act which precludes
the issuance of a patent upon a "product of nature" when it is a "new and useful
composition of matter" and there is compliance with the specified conditions for
patentability. All of the tangible things with which man deals and for which patent
protection is granted are products of nature in the sense that nature provides the
basic source materials. The "matter" of which patentable new and useful compositions are composed necessarily includes naturally existing elements and materials.[99]

The court ruled that unlike the situation in *American Wood-Paper Patent*,
the vitamin B_{12} produced was new, and it possessed unique properties that
were not in the naturally occurring substance: "As found in "natural" fer-
mentates, it has no utility, therapeutically or commercially, until converted
into compositions comparable to the patented products."[100] Later, the court
ruled that "Until the patentees produced them, there was no such B_{12} active
compositions. No one had produced even a comparable product…. The
new product, not just the method, has such advantageous characteristics
as to replace the liver products. What produced was, in no sense, an
old product."[101] One precedent on which the court drew was *Kuehmsted v.
Farbenfabriken of Elberfeld Co.*, discussed above.[102]

The court also drew on the Adrenalin patent as a precedent:

Illustratively, in Parke-Davis & Co. v. H. K. Mulford Co., … the product claims of
a patent upon adrenalin were sustained. Adrenalin is a concentrate of the blood

pressure raising principle in the suprarenal glands of living animals. It certainly is a product of nature in the sense the B_{12} active compositions here may be said to be products of nature.[103]

The court cites Judge Hand's ruling. The court incorrectly identified Adrenalin as a natural product. Littlewood finally relented on granting the patent after Takamine's lawyers spent two years convincing the examiner that Adrenalin was not a product of nature. As William Kingston has shown, the U.S. pharmaceutical industry lobbied to ensure that the Patent Act of 1952 would permit the patenting not just of vitamins but of discovered antibiotics as well as the techniques of their mass production and screening.[104] The vitamin B_{12} patents were the subjects of yet another legal case in 1967. The court upheld the composition-of-matter claim for a purified natural substance as long as that substance could pass the requirements for nonobviousness and utility.[105]

Throughout the 1960s and 1970s, more rigorous agricultural intellectual property statutes were being sought in the United States due to the Green Revolution shepherded by Norman E. Borlaug as well as the rising domestic seed industry.[106] On December 2, 1961, an International Conference for the Protection of New Plant Products in Paris created the Union Internationale pour la Protection des Obtentions Végétales (UPOV). Initially, it sought intellectual property protection of plant varieties by means other than patents.[107] Because the United States declined to join unless patents were included in such protection, the UPOV acquiesced, and in 1978, referring back to the U.S. Plant Patent Act of 1930, patents were allowed on plants internationally by "any member state to give patent and varietal protection to the same genus or species of plant if both types of protection were in place before 31 October 1979."[108]

Meanwhile, plants seemed not to be the only living objects that the lower courts wished to patent. *In re Bergy* is a case from the mid-1970s that was advanced by Malcolm E. Bergy and colleagues, who applied for a patent on a purified strain of *Streptomyces vellosus* that produced the antibiotic lincomycin.[109] The examiner rejected the patent claim, stating that the bacterium was a product of nature. The Board of Appeals upheld the decision, albeit for a different reason. It argued that the patent sought to cover a living organism that was not covered by the Plant Patent Act, thereby setting a dangerous precedent. In 1977, the U.S. Court of Customs and Patent Appeals ruled three to two in favor of Bergy. Judge Giles S. Rich, who wrote the majority opinion, reckoned that pure cultures of living organisms were "much more akin to inanimate chemical compositions such as reactants, reagents, and catalysts than they are to horses and honeybees or raspberries and roses."[110] The U.S. Patent and Trademark Office was not impressed and appealed to the U.S. Supreme Court. At that point, Bergy pulled out of the process.[111] This case has been used to support gene patenting.

A second ruling used to support gene patenting was *In re Bergstrom* (1970). This case dealt with the patenting of purified prostaglandins PGE and PGF from human prostate glands. The Court of Customs and Patent Appeals ruled that the purified hormones were not natural substances. The key issue was whether they were novel. Ultimately, the court felt that purified materials were indeed new.[112] In short, only cases decided in the lower courts—*Parke-Davis & Co. v. H. K. Mulford Co.*, *Merck & Co. v. Olin Mathieson Chemical Corporation*, *In re Bergy*, and *In re Bergstrom*—have been used as legal precedents for gene patenting. *In re Bergy* was rendered moot by *Diamond v. Chakrabarty* (discussed below), which does not mention *In re Bergstrom*.[113] None of these cases argued that natural products are patentable simply when they are merely extracted or isolated from their impure, natural environments. They are rendered patentable only if human hands bring about the isolation and purification and the new substance is *"different in kind* from the natural product," echoing Hand's sentiment.[114]

A number of Supreme Court decisions from the 1970s and 1980s on algorithms and computer programs have become relevant to issues of patentable subject matter and gene patenting. As Eisenberg argues, "DNA sequences are not simply molecules, they are also information. Patent claims to information—even useful information—represent a fundamental departure from the traditional patent bargain."[115] Genes are similar to mathematical algorithms because they carry information. They offer a blueprint for their replication and the synthesis of proteins; they code for information that carries out a sequence of processes. Such information, however, is the handiwork of nature, not scientists. In *Gottschalk v. Benson* (1972),[116] the Supreme Court found that the implementation of an algorithm was trivial, denying a process claim for a numerical algorithm and arguing that it would be equivalent to patenting an abstract idea. *Parker v. Flook* (1978) dealt with a patent for a "Method for Updating Alarm Limits."[117] The method contained a mathematical algorithm that provided instructions for performing a series of operations. The Court ruled that the process patent claim did not have an inventive step: "Even though a phenomenon of nature or mathematical formula may be well known, an inventive application of the principle may be patented. Conversely, the discovery of such a phenomenon cannot support a patent unless there is some other inventive concept in its application."[118] Although the lower courts and the U.S. Patent and Trademark Office initially resisted the granting of patents to information technology, the trend has been reversed.[119] In *Diamond v. Diehr* (1981),[120] the Court decided that a physical process that controlled a computer program was indeed patentable: a machine or process that utilizes a mathematical algorithm is distinct from an invention that claims the algorithm in the abstract. The time period bookended by *Gottschalk v. Benson* and *Diamond v. Diehr* witnessed the rapid growth of an industry that was seen to be patent driven. The Supreme Court decided to uphold software patents because it was thought that software was the type of invention, which the drafters of the initial Patent Act and framers of the Constitution would have protected. This was precisely Judge Hand's view on patenting isolated and purified natural products with respect to the U.S. pharmaceutical industry.

The 1980s and 1990s: The Post–*Diamond v. Chakrabarty* World

Diamond v. Chakrabarty[121] (1980) is the only U.S. Supreme Court case that is cited as precedent for the patenting of genes. While working at General Electric, the microbiologist Ananda M. Chakrabarty created a new bacterium of the *Pseudomonas* genus. The original utility claimed by Chakrabarty for this artificial bacterium was the production of proteins from the degradation of hydrocarbons.[122] Later work revealed that this bacterium also possessed the coveted attribute of being able to break down crude oil into biodegradable materials, which was a quality that could be applied to oil spills. At the time of his patent application, there were four known species of bacteria that could metabolize oil. These species competed with each other, however, thereby limiting the amount of oil that they could convert. Chakrabarty took four genes coding for the proteins that degrade different components of oil and cloned them in bacterial vectors. While irradiating the bacteria with ultraviolet light after introducing the genes into the recombinant DNA vectors, he discovered a method for cross-linking that allowed all four genes to be present in one bacterium. This newly created bacterium could degrade multiple parts of crude oil with a far greater efficiency than the four original species. This bacterium is clearly the product of human hands because it did not exist before Chakrabarty's invention.

The case was initially read both as dealing with the product-of-nature doctrine and overturning *Funk Brothers Seed Co. v. Kalo Inoculant Co.* (1948). The facts of both cases are strikingly similar: both inventors isolated materials and then packaged them. Scientists at Kalo Inoculant isolated different, noncompeting strains of bacteria and packaged them as a fertilizer. Chakrabarty isolated genes and packaged them in bacteria. Over time, however, this view has changed, and most people have focused on Justice Felix Frankfurter's opinion in *Funk*. The Court contrasted Chakrabarty's artificial bacterium with the mixture of bacteria in the failed patent of Kalo Inoculant: "Here, by contrast, the patentee [Chakrabarty] has produced a new bacterium with markedly different characteristics from any found in nature and one having the potential for significant utility."[123] As Frankfurter argued, Kalo Inoculant was attempting to patent the idea of putting mutually noninhibiting bacteria into a single package. Chakrabarty, on the other hand, was patenting the bacterium that he created.[124] The genes encoding the proteins that metabolized oil were not part of the patent. Finally, critical to the attempt to use Chakrabarty as a precedent for gene patenting, "nowhere did the Court refer to the 'isolation' or 'purification' of the artificial bacterium nor to its production in a carefully controlled laboratory as being indicia of 'invention.'"[125] As a result, *Diamond v. Chakrabarty* is no longer seen as a product-of-nature case. The Supreme Court stressed that Chakrabarty's "discovery is not nature's handiwork, but his own; accordingly it is patentable subject matter under §101."[126] A significant amount of human intervention was required, and such intervention needed to render the artful product sufficiently different from other types of naturally existing *Pseudomonas* bacteria.[127] Although it cannot be accurately claimed that the case serves as a legal precedent for gene patenting, it can be argued that *Diamond v. Chakrabarty* set the milieu for the patenting of genes because it signaled an extension of the range of patent eligibility. As Dutfield points out, "The decision in *Diamond v. Chakrabarty* was the first success in a campaign by industry to clarify (and later to change) patent rules in the biotechnology field in ways that suited their interests."[128]

The next round of biotechnology's successes occurred two years later. Intellectual property lawyers persuaded the U.S. Patent and Trademark Office and the courts that genes were chemical compounds; hence, chemical intellectual property could be applied to biotech patents.[129] The analogy between genes and chemicals seemed a perfect one for the USPTO because patent law in the United States had by this time reached a stage where the patenting of isolated and purified natural products was well established.[130] This decision went unchallenged until the late 1990s, when scientists from leading research institutions began to question the sagacity of reducing genes to chemical compounds.[131]

Diamond v. Chakrabarty paved the way for the patenting of life forms. In 1988, the USPTO granted a patent on a living animal for the first time in the office's history: Harvard's oncomouse was a genetically engineered rodent that was predisposed to cancer.[132] DuPont Corporation, which had given Harvard $6 million to fund research on the oncomouse, enjoyed an exclusive license for its use.[133] Much like Chakrabarty's *Pseudmonas* bacterium, the transgenic mouse did not exist in nature. Although it was clearly a living mammal, it was the creation of human hands in the laboratory. As Fiona Murray points out, the oncomouse changed the so-called cycles of credit in the academy.[134] DuPont's commercial economy based on its exclusive license seemed to many to be antithetical to the scientific, moral economy of knowledge sharing. Or perhaps the moral economy of knowledge sharing was now an antiquated model. By 1988, many academic scientists owned patents in this new age of academic economy of credit. Patents establish a new type of credit distinct from and in addition to published works.

During the last decade of the twentieth century, two cases decided by the U.S. Court of Appeals for the Federal Circuit were indirectly relevant to gene patenting. In *Amgen Inc. v. Chugai Pharmaceutical Co.* (1991), the Court of Appeals for the Federal Circuit, echoing earlier arguments, concluded that "a gene is a chemical compound, albeit a complex one"[135] and that a claim on a "purified and isolated DNA sequence" was novel and therefore valid.[136] The court was referring to the 1988 joint communiqué of the U.S. Patent and Trademark Office, European Patent Office, and Japanese Patent Office: it was the only court case that addressed the issue of the patentability of isolated DNA, albeit indirectly. Patent infringement, rather than subject-matter patent eligibility, was the primary issue.[137]

In *Schering Corp. v. Amgen Inc.* (2000), the Court of Appeals for the Federal Circuit accepted a district court's interpretation of "substantially pure DNA sequences" in a patent claim as including "both naturally-occurring and non-naturally occurring sequences."[138] Schering Corporation and Biogen, Inc. sued Amgen Inc. for patent infringement of its U.S. Patent 4,530,901 on interferon and its production. Again, infringement, not patent validity, was at issue, and the influence of the aforementioned joint communiqué was again clear. As is discussed in greater detail in chapter 4, using chemistry as the precedent for biotech intellectual property law has caused a number of serious problems.

In conclusion, the history of patenting natural products is convoluted, and those who wish to unearth a clear trajectory or stance will be disappointed. Nineteenth-century cases, which retrospectively served as precedents in the twentieth century, rarely addressed the patent eligibility of natural substances directly. As Beauchamp concludes, "before the twentieth century, there was no jurisprudential category of natural products, only a set of rules about novelty and distinctiveness from the prior art that applied across technologies, without regard to natural origin."[139] Judge Learned Hand's landmark decision that Parke-Davis's patent for Adrenalin was legitimate proved critical to the development of the U.S. pharmaceutical industry. Although the U.S. Patent and Trademark Office generously granted patents on natural products that had been isolated or minimally modified, the courts were becoming more skeptical. From the 1920s through the 1940s, corporate giants were the bugbears of the Department of Justice, which sought antitrust litigation. During that period, stricter product-of-nature statements were uttered by the federal circuit courts. After the Patent Reform Act of 1952, however, the lower courts warmed up once again to patents, particularly on modified natural products, as the green revolution and the biotech sector successfully asked the USPTO to increase intellectual property coverage. The historical contingencies of the views on patenting natural products indicate how various intellectual property regimes are not inevitable but are historically contingent.

4   The CCR5 Patent and Intellectual Property Law

The previous chapter analyzes the patentability of natural products, which is relevant to all gene patents. The lack of legal clarity described in that chapter is also the theme of this one. The CCR5 patent is particularly fascinating because it also raises a number of concerns with other aspects of intellectual property law. Using the CCR5 patent as a guide, this chapter analyzes how various legal precedents based on chemistry have proven to be inappropriate. Gene patents are controversial not simply because of their eligibility for intellectual property protection. This patent is particularly interesting because it occurred at a time when the status of patenting genes was being renegotiated, when the accuracy of computer sequencing for determining the function and utility of a gene product was being challenged, when the role of broad-utility patents to downstream research was being debated, and when the nature of the deposited object and its written specification were being redefined (aspects that are cued by chapter 1). In short, this is a story about the simultaneous instability of a patent claim and the instability of the validity of a scientific technique in establishing a scientific claim.[1]

Patenting the Incorrect Nucleotide Sequence

One intriguing issue in the history of the *CCR5* gene is the frequency of patents on the incorrect sequence. If a patent application contains an incorrect sequence, then it would seem that the application must be rejected because the correct invention is not being disclosed. In 2004, the European Patent Office initially revoked Myriad Genetics' patent on one of its breast-cancer genes, *BRCA1*, because the company had patented the incorrect sequence. It was too late to correct the errors because the proper sequence had already become common knowledge; it was publicly accessible in a gene databank.[2] The patent was annulled because it now failed the nonobviousness criterion of patentability. Four years later, however, the highest board of European appeal reversed the EPO's revocation after Myriad agreed to limit the scope of the claim to frame-shift mutations resulting in either the substitution of incorrect amino acids or early chain termination. The board ruled that an exact sequence is not necessary to detect these sorts of mutations.[3] The patent was never challenged in the United States.

Haseltine might well have been correct in arguing that the nucleic acid deposited at the American Type Culture Collection (ATCC) trumps the information described in the specification as long as the object is referred to by that specification. Claim 1c of Human Genome Sciences' (HGS) patent application states that "a polynucleotide encoding a polypeptide having the amino acid sequence encoded by the cDNA contained in ATCC Deposit No. 97183."[4] Corrections may be made to a patent specification even after the patent has been granted as long as the scope of the claims is not enlarged (unless the application has been submitted within two years after the patent was awarded), no new matter has been introduced, and the initial patent has not expired.[5] As noted in chapter 1, HGS filed a subsequent patent on the *CCR5* gene with the corrected sequence in 1998, which was three years after the submission of the initial patent application and fifteen months before the patent was granted. In addition, as is typical with gene patents, the patent claims the particular sequence as well as

the polynucleotides of the present invention includ[ing] the polypeptide SEQ ID NO:2 (in particular in the mature polypeptide) as well as polypeptides which have at least 70% similarity (preferably at least 70% identity) to the polypeptide of SEQ ID NO:2 and more preferably a 90% similarity (more preferably at least 90% identity) to the polypeptide of SEQ ID NO:2 and still more preferably a 95% similarity (still more preferably at least 90 [sic-95]% identity) to the polypeptide of SEQ ID NO:2 and to portions of such polypeptide with such portion of the polypeptide generally consisting at least 30 amino acids and more preferably at least 50 amino acids.[6]

An error of four nucleotides in the coding region of 1,056 nucleotides and three more in noncoding regions (totaling 1,414 nucleotides) is well within the preferred interval of identity. This configuration owes much to patenting of chemicals. So-called Markush structures are a class of structurally related chemical compounds that are deemed functionally equivalent and are used in patent claims. As the legal scholar Burton Amernick notes:

In claims that recite compositions and the components of compositions, it is sometimes important to claim, as alternatives, a group of constituents that are considered equivalent for the purposes of the invention, or for a particular function thereof, even though this group does not belong to a recognized chemical group.... It has been permissible to claim such an artificial group, referred to as a "Markush Group," ever since the inventor in the first case ... won the right to do so.[7]

Thousands of compounds can be subsumed into a generic category, including compounds that do not exist at the time of the patent application. The language used in DNA sequence claims is based on the Markush notation.[8]

Written Description, Disclosure, and Biological Deposits

In addition to the requirements that a claimed invention must be useful, new, and nonobvious, the patent specification must support the claimed subject matter by an adequate written description that will enable anyone who is skilled in the art to make and use the invention and that discloses the best mode known to the inventor. According to 35 U.S.C. section 112, first paragraph:

The specification shall contain a written description of the invention, and of the manner and process of making and using it, in such full, clear, concise, and exact terms as to enable any person skilled in the art to which it pertains, or with which it is most nearly connected, to make and use the same, and shall set forth the best mode contemplated by the inventor of carrying out his invention.[9]

The specification serves three functions—to disclose the invention's features and components, to instruct one skilled in the art how to make and use that invention, and to inform the users about the best mode for carrying out the invention.[10]

As is the case with many aspects of intellectual property law, the written description requirement originates with chemical and mechanical claims; however, it is a statutory requirement applicable to all categories of invention, including biotechnology.[11] The inadequacy of written description for biotechnology inventions first arose in the context of plants and microorganisms that were isolated from nature in *Guaranty Trust Co. v. Union Solvents Corporation* (1931).[12] Because of the difficulty of providing a detailed written description that is sufficient to enable the production of complex living organisms, the courts approved the submission of a sample of living material with a public depository and held that disclosure in the specification of an accession number corresponding to the deposit was sufficient to satisfy the specification requirement.[13] The sufficiency of deposits as a written description was first tested in *In re Argoudelis* in 1970. The invention involved a process for synthesizing two new antibiotic compounds by cultivating the bacterium *Streptomyces sparsogenes var. sparsogenes*. The court focused on the inability of a written description by itself to enable the practice of the invention when the invention is an organism that has been isolated from nature. The written word was insufficient to disclose how to obtain the requisite starting material.[14] The court ruled that since "there can be no description in words alone of how to obtain the micro-organism from nature,"[15] the deposit of the microorganism was sufficient to satisfy section 112, first paragraph, if (among other requirements) it was placed in a public depository before the filing date of the patent application and the depository and accession number were referenced in the application.[16] The key is the reduction to practice, which requires that the claimed invention work for its intended purpose.[17]

How important is the biochemical composition to the written description? *In re Fisher* (1970) had for decades often served as a precedent case when applying section 112 to biologically active proteins.[18] The relevant claim recited an adrenocorticotrophic hormone (ACTH) preparation containing the active component of a polypeptide of a specified sequence of at least twenty-four specified amino acids from the protein's N-terminus. The claim was initially rejected because it contained an insufficient written disclosure of this later claimed subject matter. The parent application merely disclosed a process for extracting ACTH for the pituitary glands of various animals.[19] The U.S. Court of Customs and Patent Appeals (CCPA),[20] however, agreed with the patent applicant, ruling that "a written description of such a biotechnology invention does not require that the specification recite the nucleic acid sequence of a gene invention, or the amino acid sequence of a polypeptide product."[21] Because the written description requirement was satisfied by a specific biological function, a precise description of its structure did not need to be given or known by the applicant.[22] In theory, a reduction to practice can be enabled simply by depositing a protein or DNA sequence in a plasmid without knowing anything about that sequence. The assumption is that someone may go to the depository and analyze (that is, sequence) it.[23] In short, *Fisher* established that "the deposit alone is sufficient to satisfy the written description requirement, both for the deposited DNA and the protein that it will inherently produce."[24]

In a case that was similar to the CCR5 patent, *Ex parte Maizel* (1992), the Board of Patent Appeals and Interferences rejected a deposit, deeming that it was insufficient to provide a written description of a deposited DNA plasmid encoding for the protein, B-cell growth factor, because the specification failed to disclose the correct DNA coding sequence. The *Maizel* ruling is the antithesis of the one rendered in *Fisher*. The original sequence of the DNA in the patent application contained three errors, two of which were serious.[25] These two errors of the nucleotide sequence corresponding to the positions +185 and +196 resulted in reading frame shifts that dramatically altered the protein's content.[26] Maizel had deposited two cell-line plasmids with the American Type Culture Collection, and he attempted to correct the disclosure by adding the correct sequence to the patent. The Board of Patent Appeals and Interferences decided that the specification did not describe the deposited DNA and could not be corrected "because the amino acid sequence set forth as a descriptive parameter in the original specification was erroneously deduced and the protein was not purified and/or isolated."[27] On reconsideration, the Board did not change its stance, ruling that the description requirements for both the DNA and its protein product were not satisfied and that there was no evidence that if those skilled in the art had the deposited material, they would have been aware of the DNA structure of the growth factor and its corresponding protein.

A 1993 Federal Circuit Court decision continued in this tradition of rendering an opinion that contradicted *Fisher*. *Fiers v. Sugano* involved the date of invention. The court ruled that a written description of DNA necessitated a "precise definition, such as by structure, formula, chemical name, or physical properties."[28] Federal Circuit Judge Lourie agreed with the earlier decision of the Board of Patent Appeals and Interferences that the written specification failed constructive reduction to practice because it lacked the specific DNA sequence, remarking that "one cannot describe what one has not conceived."[29] The critical question here is whether it was possible to reduce an invention to practice simply by isolating a protein from its natural environment or by depositing a genetic sample or whether the precise sequence needed to be possessed and specified.[30] *Fisher* on the one hand and *Fiers* and *Maizel* on the other offer mutually exclusive answers to that query. The judges seemed to take a minor requirement that previously was used to determine the date of invention and place it in a new, prominent role. This resulted in a major change in law and created a great deal of confusion and controversy.[31]

In 1997, the Court of Appeals for the Federal Circuit ruled on a case that dealt with the sufficiency of the written description claims. The case, *Regents of University of California v. Eli Lilly & Co.* (henceforth *Eli Lilly*), involved generic claims of cDNA segments of vertebrate, mammalian, or human insulin. Although the cDNA claim for human insulin was specific, the corresponding claims reciting vertebrate and mammalian cDNAs "were broadly generic."[32] The plaintiff argued that the defendant had infringed on its patent for the recombinant DNA plasmids and microorganisms that produce human insulin.[33] The defendant's specification merely described a single cDNA sequence of rat insulin with no written description (that is, sequence) of either vertebrate or mammalian insulin.[34] Because of the redundancy of the genetic code,[35] vertebrate and mammalian insulin cDNAs covered a vast number of sequences. The court ruled that an adequate written description "requires a precise definition, such as by structure, formula, chemical name, or physical properties." Accordingly, "an adequate written description of a DNA requires more than a mere statement that it is part of the invention and reference to a potential method for isolating it; what is required is a description of the DNA itself."[36] This ruling was based on the *Fiers* case.[37] Lourie, who wrote on behalf of the court in both *Fiers* and *Lilly*, argued that "[a] description of a genus of cDNAs may be achieved by means of a recitation of a representative number of cDNAs, defined by a nucleotide sequence, falling within the scope of the genus or of a recitation of structural features common to the members of the genus, which features constitute a substantial portion of the genus."[38] Kenneth Burchfiel, an attorney who has extensively researched the Court of Appeals for the Federal Circuit's patent decisions, points out that

Following the Federal Circuit's decisions in *Fiers* and *Eli Lilly*, it appeared that the Federal Circuit had created a written description standard which required the disclosure of an exact nucleotide sequence for a claimed DNA. The seemingly inflexible written description requirement applied in *Eli Lilly* raised questions of invalidity for many patents containing broad generic claims to DNAs defined by their coding function. In addition, if a sufficient written description requires the disclosure of a specific nucleotide sequence, this rule could invalidate patents which issued prior to Eli Lilly, even where the applicants had deposited biological materials containing the claimed nucleotide sequence, and thus clearly "possessed" the invention described by accession number in the specification.[39]

In 2001, the U.S. Patent and Trademark Office's "Guidelines for Examination of Patent Applications under the 35 U.S.C. 112, ¶ 1, 'Written Description' Requirement" reaffirmed that the written description requirement ensures that the applicant can convince those who are skilled in the art that the applicant actually was in possession of the claimed invention at the filing date.[40] The key requirement is that the description is sufficient to verify that the deposited biological material is in fact what is described in the application. In response to those arguing that the written description should include the complete sequence of DNA, the Guidelines said that "Describing the complete chemical structure, i.e., the DNA sequence, of a claimed DNA is one method of satisfying the written description requirement, but it is not the only method.... Therefore, there is no basis for a *per se* rule requiring disclosure of complete DNA sequences or limiting DNA claims to only the sequence disclosed."[41] Despite numerous complaints that *Fiers* and *Eli Lilly* were antithetical rulings, the USPTO disagreed and stressed that *Eli Lilly*, a precedent that they were required to follow for the written description requirement, used the phrase "such as" and then gave examples.[42] The USPTO decided that such language left the door open to other ways in which a written description could be deemed as adequate. Its flexibility enhanced the likelihood of patentability but soon proved to be problematic.

Perhaps this aforementioned threat to gene patents with broad generic claims in the written specification (which includes Human Genome Sciences' CCR5 patent) explains in part the decision of the Federal Circuit Court to reverse its opinion some five years later. The importance of having a deposit with the written description was revisited in the Federal Circuit case of *Enzo Biochem, Inc. v. Gen-Probe Inc.* (2002).[43] Enzo Biochem claimed three nucleic acid probes that hybridized to three strains of gonorrhea-causing bacteria and not the homologous three strains that cause meningitis.[44] Rather than identifying the DNA sequences of the probes in the specification, they simply deposited them at the American Type Culture Collection (ATCC) at the time of the filing. Sued by Enzo Biochemical for infringement, the defendants (Gen-Probe Inc.) argued that Enzo's patent did not fulfill the written-description requirement. They claimed that it was invalid because its specification described the three probes only in terms of function (hybridization to *Neisseria gonorrhoeae*) rather than by structural composition (that is, sequence). The U.S. District Court of Southern New York rejected Enzo's assertion that the deposit of their probes at the ATCC "inherently disclosed that the inventors were in possession of the claimed sequences"[45] and ruled in favor of Gen-Probe Inc. The Federal Circuit Court initially upheld the District Court's decision, applying the precedent of *Eli Lilly* (that a description of the probes by function alone is insufficient): "a deposit is not a substitute for a written description of the claimed invention."[46] In addition, the court held that "references in the specification to the ATCC deposits alone did not satisfy the WD [written description] requirement."[47] The dissenting decision reasoned otherwise: public deposit (and therefore disclosure) of the probes "provide a precise and unmistakably clear description of the invention that is accessible to the public."[48] Although a deposit is sufficient to demonstrate possession, it does not necessarily demonstrate enablement or the disclosure of a claimed invention that is sufficiently clear and detailed for someone skilled in the art to carry out the invention.

Three and a half months later, however, the Federal Court readdressed the issue of whether deposits were a sufficient description of their sequences.

In *Enzo II*, the court reversed its initial ruling. The Federal Court concluded that "reference in the specification to a deposit in a public depository, which makes its contents accessible to the public when it is not otherwise available in written form, constitutes an adequate description of the deposited material sufficient to comply with the written description of §112, ¶ one."[49] Such a move narrows the scope of the patent. In the early days with models, the patents were claimed centrally, so judges needed to determine how far their scope extended. Now the written description determines the scope, and a deposit gives rights only to what was actually deposited—nothing else.[50] The court cited *Amgen Inc. v. Chugai Pharmaceutical Co.*: the depositing of samples was necessary in the patenting of antibiotics because (as had been the case since the 1930s with biological materials) inventors could not always successfully employ words to explain how to obtain the starting material from nature.[51] This ruling contradicted those rendered in *Fiers* and *Eli Lilly*. From 2002 to 2010, the Federal Circuit Court retreated from its previous insistence that inventors divulge detailed characterizations of biological materials in the written descriptions before claiming them.[52] In short, whereas the rulings in *Enzo I* and *Eli Lilly* underscore that the written-description requirement is distinct from the enablement requirement, *Enzo II* conflates possession and enablement.[53]

Enablement versus Possession, Post-CCR5 Patent

The *Enzo II* ruling was highly controversial. One outraged legal scholar exclaimed, "*Enzo* was perhaps the worst example of judicial legislation from the Federal Circuit in recent years."[54] The Court of Appeals for the Federal Circuit's decision on the "written description" raised a deeper and more important question: what are the nature and purpose of this requirement with regard to biotechnological inventions? The Federal Circuit expanded the role of biological deposits beyond the traditional one of satisfying the companion enablement requirement under U.S. patent law.[55] This ruling allowed an inventor to dispense with a description of the structure of a chemical compound (the nucleic acid sequence) on the premise that someone skilled in the art would be able to ascertain the structure by going to the public depository.[56] In essence, this rendered patenting of biotech materials easier because the written description did not need to be as rigorous. Judge Randall R. Rader of the Federal Circuit disagreed with *Enzo II*, arguing "the written description requirement as created and applied for thirty years does not apply to this case."[57] He concurred with the decision of *Enzo I*, asserting that the written description is really a test of enablement. He feared that a dangerous trend could be set using *Enzo II* as a precedent—that the written description requirement would be applied as a general disclosure doctrine in place of enablement against the specification for priority. In that case, the public would not truly know what had been invented because the patent relied solely on the written description for that information.[58]

Judge Lourie, who wrote the majority report, was basically substituting the written description for determining patentable subject matter. By privileging the deposit, he was narrowing the scope and thereby aiming to avoid dampening downstream research. This leaves applicants with a scope limited to the nucleic acid (or protein) sequence. In addition, there was the fear that the DNA sequence could be easily deduced from the protein sequence or that a therapy could be guessed from prior art and that the patent applicant therefore would contribute nothing new to the art. Lourie felt that the written description mitigated that problem. Federal Judge Radar disagreed. The purpose of the specification, in his view, was to inform the public about the metes and bounds of the invention and the ways that it is to be used. Using it to inform other policy issues is problematic.[59]

In a more recent case, however, the U.S. Court of Appeals for the Federal Circuit ruled that section 112 required a distinction between the written specification requirement and the enablement requirement. In *Ariad Pharmaceuticals v. Eli Lilly Co.* (2009), the plaintiff claimed patent infringement of U.S. Patent 6,410,516 for the transcription factor NF-kB in the U.S. District Court for the District of Massachusetts.[60] The Federal Circuit decided that a written description requirement is separate from an enablement requirement even after the introduction of claims, following the U.S. Supreme Court's summary of the three requirements for section 112, first paragraph: "the patent application must describe, enable, and set forth the best mode of carrying out the invention."[61] A researcher must now perform the labor and identify the compound by composition and by its effects.[62]

So was Haseltine's declaration that his company's incorrect specification is irrelevant correct? It might be. At the time of the granting of the patent, *Eli Lilly* would have been the obvious, new precedent case against the CCR5 patent. However, the *Enzo II* decision would have supported the patent, and *Ariad* suggests that it would have had problems if someone had challenged the patent after it was granted. What constituents a patent claim, particularly the relationship between the written description and a deposit, seems to have been (and still is) a highly unstable area with much legal maneuvering and negotiating. And gene patenting has added to the confusion. Perhaps former Federal Circuit judge Arthur J. Gajarsa best summarized the frustration and confusion when he complained that the district courts and practitioners "are currently left to trudge through a thicket of written description jurisprudence that provides no conclusive answers and encourages a shotgun approach to litigation. Yet, this thicket is the result of our best efforts to construe an ambiguous statute; only Congress wields the machete to clear it."[63]

Patenting Based Solely on Sequence Homology

The next issue that is raised by CCR5 patent deals with utility claims solely based on sequence homology. In 2001, the U.S. Patent and Trademark Office's revised examination guidelines for the utility requirement solidified its stance on the patentability of genes, declaring that if a patent specification discloses a use for a gene or its product, then "an inventor's discovery of a gene can be the basis for a patent on the genetic composition isolated from its natural state and processed through purifying steps that separate the gene from other molecules naturally associated with it."[64] DNA isolated in this fashion is not a product of nature "because that DNA molecule does not occur in that isolated form in nature."[65] This section of the chapter is concerned with broad utility claims that are inferred by sequence homology rather than demonstrated by "wet" biochemistry. The use of sequence homology to identify these receptors has radically changed the process of identifying a protein's function. Classical experimentation to determine a receptor's function is seen by many to take too much time in the mercurial world of patenting. Given the number of sequence databases, scientists can determine sequence homology by searching the Internet.[66] Human Genome Sciences' CCR5 patent is not the only one whose utility was based solely on sequence homology. As Linda L. McCabe and Edward R. B. McCabe have argued, of the six thousand human gene patents that were granted to Celera and similar sequencing companies, "many were based on sequence information alone, with no demonstrated functional data."[67]

So what is necessary to prove utility? Someone of ordinary skill in the art needs to show that the invention has utility based on what he or she has been shown. Is sequence homology sufficient here? How accurate and reliable are the arguments of a protein's function based on sequence homology? What are scientists' responses to such accuracy and reliability? What were the USPTO's guidelines for permitting patents based on sequence homology when the CCR5 patent was being reviewed? And given that the function of a gene can be inferred based on sequence homology to a known protein, is that not obvious, thereby failing section 103 of the patent requirement?

Example 10 of the U.S. Patent and Trademark Office's "Revised Interim Utility Guidelines Training Materials of 1999" dealt with DNA fragments encoding a full open reading frame (ORF), which is a sequence of DNA that does not contain any stop codons; transcription proceeds, and a complete protein is produced.[68] The specification disclosed a cDNA library that was created from human kidney epithelial cells. Five thousand members of this library were sequenced, and ORFs were identified. One member of that cDNA library (SEQ ID NO: 2) had a high level of homology to a DNA ligase, which was an enzyme that anneals single-stranded breaks in complementary DNA strands. The complete ORF of SEQ ID NO: 2 encoded a protein— SEQ ID NO: 3. Aligning SEQ ID NO: 3 with known amino acid sequences of DNA ligases revealed a high level of sequence conservation among the various ligases. The level of sequence similarity between SEQ ID NO: 3 and the consensus sequence was relatively high with a similarity score of 95%. A search of the prior art indicates that SEQ ID NO: 2 had a high homology to DNA ligases encoding nucleic acids. As a result of the sequence homologies, the specification claimed that SEQ ID NO: 2 encoded a ligase. The training manual posed the following question to the examiner: "Based on the record, is there a 'well established utility' for the claimed invention?"[69] The manual provided an answer:

there is no reason to doubt the assertion that SEQ ID NO: 2 encodes a DNA ligase. Further, DNA ligases have a well-established use in the molecular biology art based on this class of protein's ability to ligate DNA. Consequently the answer to the question is yes. Note that if there is a well-established utility already associated with the claimed invention, the utility need not be asserted in the specification as filed. In order to determine whether the claimed invention has a well-established utility the examiner must determine that the invention has a specific, substantial and credible utility that would have been readily apparent to one of skill in the art. In this case SEQ ID NO: 2 was shown to encode a DNA ligase that the artisan would have recognized as having a specific, substantial and credible utility based on its enzymatic activity.[70]

It concluded the section by informing the trainee that the utility rejection based on 35 U.S.C. sections 101 and 112 does not apply; the utility has been satisfactorily demonstrated.

On March 22, 2000, Jack Spiegel, who at the time was director of the Division of Technology Transfer and Development of the Office of Technology Transfer at the National Institutes of Health, wrote to Q. Todd Dickinson, director of the U.S. Patent and Trademark Office, criticizing the new training materials that were accompanying the *Revised Interim Utility Guidelines* because they did not sufficiently communicate a number of critical issues.[71]

Of particular concern to Spiegel and the NIH were theoretical utilities that were based on sequence homology, or the aforementioned example 10 of the *Revised Interim Guidelines*. No evidence gleaned from biochemical analysis concerning a specific biological property, activity, or function was provided because the USPTO decided that the "sequence homology is sufficient to provide reasonable confidence that the protein encoded by the ORF would have a well-established function."[72] The NIH, however, admonished the USPTO, asserting that this was not the proper standard for determining utility.

In making his argument, Spiegel drew on *Brenner v. Manson*, a 1966 U.S. Supreme Court Case.[73] Manson was a chemist who invented a procedure for manufacturing a type of steroid. He applied for a patent on this procedure but was denied by the patent examiner, who argued that the chemicals that Manson's method generated possessed no specified utility. Manson appealed, claiming that the steroids were being screened for their efficacy in cancer therapies. He argued that an adjacent homolog of his steroid had been shown to possess tumor-inhibiting properties in mice. The Board of Patent Appeals and Interferences upheld the decision, arguing, "It is our view that the Statutory requirement of usefulness of a product cannot be presumed merely because it happens to be closely related to another compound which is known to be useful."[74] He therefore decided to appeal to the Court of Customs and Patent Appeals, which reversed the decision, asserting that it was not necessary to show a utility for the product. One merely needed to demonstrate that the product was not harmful to the public interest. The USPTO's Commissioner of Patents at the time, Edward J. Brenner, appealed to the U.S. Supreme Court, which overturned the CCPA's reversal. The Supreme Court considered the skill level and predictability in the art of manufacturing steroids in its decision.[75] It was convinced by expert witnesses—in this case, steroid chemists who demonstrated that minor changes in the structure of a steroid would result in the chemical possessing significantly different biological activity. The Court consequently ruled that "inference of similar function from homologous compounds was by itself insufficient for purposes of demonstrating a specific and substantial utility."[76] Manson needed to demonstrate that utility of tumor inhibition via experimentation, not homology. The Court reasoned that because a patent is predicated on the concept of quid pro quo, a strict standard of specific and substantial requirements for utility was required:

The basic *quid pro quo* contemplated by the Constitution and the Congress for granting a patent monopoly is the benefit derived by the public from an invention with substantial utility. Unless and until a process is refined and developed to this point—where specific benefit exists in currently available form—there is insufficient justification for permitting an applicant to engross what may prove to be a broad field.[77]

The Supreme Court therefore felt that giving him a patent for a process that produced no useful chemical would discourage others from finding uses for that chemical. Since the 1990s, however, the USPTO has not used the stringent requirement of utility as established in *Manson*.[78]

Although *Brenner v. Manson* serves as the controlling case for patents that assert specific and substantial utility based solely on homology, as Spiegel points out, two subsequent cases are relevant—*In re Folkers* (1965)[79] and *In re Brana* (1995).[80] *In re Folkers* demonstrates that some uses can be gleaned immediately from reciting structural properties, and *In re Brana* asserts that experimental evidence of success in structurally similar compounds is important in determining whether someone skilled in the art will be persuaded by the particular claimed utility.[81] Both cases in a sense confirm the primacy of *Brenner v. Manson*.

In *In re Folkers*, the Court of Customs and Patent Appeals decided that Folkers had invented certain quinone and hydroquinone compounds. It had been well accepted in the art that those compounds possess electron transfer activity: Folkers' patent was therefore successful. But why was Folkers' successful, and Manson's was not? The difference lay in the predictability in the art. According to steroid chemists, a slight change in structure of the steroid can result in a substantial difference in biological activity or function. The same is not true of electron transport compounds. After it was established that Folkers' compounds possessed the property of electron transport, the legal question became whether these were well-established utilities known to someone skilled in the art.[82] Although the outcomes of the two cases were antithetical, "the methodologies pursued and the application of law in both cases are both consistent."[83]

In re Brana dealt was a case in which the chemist and his colleagues disclosed in the specification the use of 5-nitrobenzo[de]isoquinoline-1,3-dione compounds as antitumor drugs. Brana and his colleagues used both in vitro and in vivo mouse-model systems to test the efficacy of these drugs for tumor treatment and compared the results of their chemicals to those that had already been established in the art for possessing this property. Their chemicals were superior. They were required to show that their tests were specific enough to establish utility and that their asserted utility was credible based on this test, because the level of predictability in the art did not permit them to infer this property based solely on structural homology.[84]

Their tests were indeed deemed to be specific enough to establish utility. As for the credibility of the asserted utility, the CAFC needed to determine if one skilled in the specific art of dione production would recognize such a utility.

The key point in all three legal cases is that one skilled in the art decides whether specific properties require empirical substantiation (unpredictable arts) or whether they can be inferred merely via sequence or structural homology (predictable arts). What is the level of unpredictability in the art of genomics? Spiegel, on behalf of the National Institutes of Health, argued that "[t]he DNA and protein arts are recognized as unpredictable, such that minor changes in the nucleotide or amino acid sequences of these molecules may produce profound changes in biological activity."[85] Spiegel reminded the USPTO that

In almost all cases one is not able to predict the functional significance of particular sequence polymorphisms. The direction of the CAFC over the past nine years has been to recognize this unpredictability in the DNA art, and to require gene-related molecules be defined by their sequences and/or other distinguishing physical properties.[86]

He feared that granting DNA patents based on sequence homology alone was threatening this trend. The USPTO seemed to be ignoring the CAFC here:

Despite this direction from the courts, this art has not yet been able to decipher predictable and workable relationships between DNA/protein sequence polymorphism and functional activity. The biotechnology community has not been able to establish a workable counterpart to structural homology (structural obviousness), whereby a measure of sequence similarity is recognized in the art to imply a reasonable expectation of functional equivalence.[87]

Even an extremely high sequence homology cannot guarantee the same function. Mismatches between proteins may be irrelevant or crucial. Do they occur randomly throughout the protein? Are they at the points of biological activity (at the so-called active sites)? How drastic of a structural change results from switching one amino acid to another? That depends. For example, if a cysteine amino acid that is involved in a disulfide bridge with a second cysteine amino acid is switched to another amino acid, the bridge will be lost, thereby dramatically changing the protein's structure. This was the case with Human Genome Sciences' initial CCR5 patent. On the other hand, a switch from one hydrophobic amino acid to another in the transmembrane portion of the protein, for example, might have no effect. The art is highly unpredictable. Even a high degree of structural similarity may correspond to a high degree of functional difference. According to the National Institutes of Health, gene expression and an empirical characterization of the resulting protein are required to determine function. The adoption of chemistry as the paradigm for intellectual property issues germane to DNA is the problem here. In certain branches of chemistry (but certainly not all, as has been shown with steroid chemistry), as a result of literally thousands of cases, one may define with confidence that "homologs (compounds differing regularly by the successive addition of the same chemical group, e.g., by -CH_2- groups) are generally of sufficiently close structural similarity that there is a presumed expectation that such compounds possess similar properties."[88] Adjacent homologs are generally considered to be structurally similar enough to infer a common or similar function.[89] However, genes are more complicated than this. A precise percentage of similarity correlating to similar or exact function cannot be given because one nucleotide difference in a thousand, if occurring in a section that codes for the active site of its corresponding protein, may result in a totally different structure or function of that protein.[90]

The art is becoming increasingly aware that numerous genes have significant stretches of the same sequence, yet their protein products have very different functions. Examples of such genes include ones that code for numerous membrane-associated proteins (such as G protein-coupled receptors [GPCRs], including chemokine receptors), kinases, DNA helicases, zinc finger proteins, and traffic ATPases.[91] George Corey, an intellectual property attorney, also has criticized the use of sequence homology to determine function. He listed three examples of proteins that possess sequence homology but have very different functions—the epidermal growth factor receptor (EGF-R) and the neu oncogene, GPCRs for dopamine and serotonin, and nuclear hormone receptors.[92] Corey continued by citing Human Genome Sciences' CCR5 patent, arguing that "this is like patenting a hydroplane with a propeller and then claiming that the patent covers airplanes because both have propellers, wings for lift and cut through the air."[93] As Spiegel claimed, "To afford specific utility based on shared homology to the transmembrane domain is to encourage patents that provide the public no more utility than it already possessed from knowledge of the broad subject class. This does not satisfy the *quid pro quo* of the patent grant and, therefore, fails the specific utility standard required by *Brenner v. Manson*."[94]

Spiegel then took issue with example 10 of the Training Materials, arguing that the U.S. Patent and Trademark Office's logic is flawed. The applicant provided no evidence that the DNA ligase art was more predictable than the general DNA/protein art. There was no empirical evidence to support the protein's activity and no hint that the state of the art was even considered, so it cannot be concluded that someone skilled in the art would accept the assumption that the protein of SEQ ID NO: 3 possessed DNA ligase activity. Spiegel concluded with a warning: "Granting patents based upon the highest known homology at the time of filing undermines confidence in the patent system by giving an already unpredictable art the appearance of a patent guessing game."[95]

The National Institutes of Health was not alone in encouraging the USPTO to toughen its utility criteria:

> The PTO has heard from Nobel Laureates, the Director of the Human Genome Project, the National Academy of Sciences, the Association of American Medical Colleges [AAMC], academic scholars and representatives of industry. Each cautioned against granting broad patents on gene sequences (particularly sequence fragments) based upon asserted general and theoretical utilities that are not considered specific and substantial utilities.[96]

The rift between the USPTO on the one hand and the NIH, the Association of American Medical Colleges (AAMC), and the National Advisory Council for Human Genome Research (NACHGR) on the other became public in May 2000, when David Dickson published a brief article in *Nature* on the issue of the patenting of genes based on sequence homology.[97] The AAMC, for example, correctly stated that researchers simply use automated programs to guess the identity and function of a gene's product based on homology to known genes and their products. Similarly, R. Rodney Howell, then president of the American College of Medical Genetics (ACMG) wrote to Administrative Patent Judge, Mark Nagumo on March 20, 2000 that "The PTO must decide the criteria to be used to determine whether or not a DNA sequence meets the standard for specific, substantial and credible utility."[98] The ACMG agreed with the NIH that claims of a predicted utility for a gene or its encoded protein based only on sequence homology with other proteins and genes should not be permitted. Jordan J. Cohen, president of the AAMC at the time, queried the creativity of such a process:

> Automated programs and databases frequently enable researchers to infer, or "guess," the identity and function of a protein encoded by a gene based on the similarity of a fragment to other known genes. Such suppositions of utility are technology driven, and require little scientific insight or creativity, and do not characterize a specific, substantial and credible utility.[99]

In 2000, the biotech companies were divided on the issue.[100] Generally, gene-sequencing companies (such as Human Genome Sciences) stood to reap the benefits of the U.S. Patent and Trademark Office guidelines, whereas pharmaceutical companies wishing to undertake therapeutic or diagnostic research feared that such patents could stymie innovation. Charles E. Ludlam, vice president for governmental relations of the Biotechnology Industry Organization (BIO), admitted that

There is a difference of opinion among BIO members as to whether different types of inventions will or will not satisfy the utility requirement. For example, some BIO members believe that utility of most proteins cannot be exclusively demonstrated until the protein has been expressed and biologically characterized. Other BIO members believe that utility can be based on a prediction of biological activity and on the basis of homology to existing classes of polypeptides and proteins.[101]

Not surprisingly, these diverse opinions map onto business interests. Those companies interested only in gene hunting stressed the accuracy of sequence homologies, and pharmaceutical companies that need to pay licensing fees to those sequencing companies argued that experimental biochemistry should be mandatory for utility claims. Ludlam recommended that the view of scientists who are skilled in this area at the time of the patent filing should determine utility based on homology. Sean A. Johnston, vice president of intellectual property at Genentech, feared that a person who was skilled in the art could not accurately predict utility based on homology alone. Rather, "it will be necessary to express the polypeptide and to confirm that it possesses the relevant biological characteristics. Simply put, computer-based homology analysis should not be regarded as a generally reliable prediction of the biological function- and hence, the utility of genes or polypeptides."[102] Former director of Biotechnological Patent Examinations for and former acting director and former Commissioner of Patents of the U.S. Patent and Trademark Office John J. Doll, however, insisted that "there is no scientific evidence to reject claims solely because they are based on computer homology data.... [F]our times out of five, the computer models are correct."[103]

The National Advisory Council for Human Genome Research, on the other hand, was unified against the U.S. Patent and Trademark Office guidelines, "Finding partial sequence similarity is an obvious and non-inventive step."[104] This point is critical. Because the USPTO maintained at the time that sequence homology was sufficient for utility claims, the patent should fail the criterion of nonobviousness. If someone can simply ascertain the sequence homology from accessing DNA databanks on the Internet, the patent applicant would no longer be permitted to claim nonobviousness.[105] The USPTO seems to want to have it both ways. In 1993, a number of patent attorneys conceded in an interview that "after the discovery of the DNA molecule and some of the early technology relating to recombinant DNA[,] most of what had been done in biotechnology was pretty well obvious, meaning noninventive. Setting the bar of inventiveness at too high a level would have meant, however, that many corporate players would have failed to obtain patents in these fields."[106] The USPTO did not want to impede corporate control of biocapitalism; however, it most likely did not realize how that stance on utility would affect other relevant parties.

Broad Utility Claims

The final issue arising as the result of the CCR5 patent was the scope of the patent—the granting of broad utility patents. Since the early 1990s, concerns were raised about the patenting of genes that were found by sequencing companies. Stanford University's professor of intellectual property law John Barton warned that genes could be discovered before their functions were known. In this case, sequences are discovered and not invented.[107] Gene patents are perched on a precarious precipice, the legally ill-defined distinction between discovery and invention.[108] Historically, courts permit patents with broader scopes and wider ranges when a field is new: they reason that such practice encourages innovation and development.[109] This granting of biotech patents with broad scopes was certainly true in the 1990s. One patent attorney in 1999 quipped, "You get utility if you can spell it."[110] Despite the Supreme Court's ruling in *Brenner v. Manson* that patents are not meant to be hunting licenses, many gene patents had become precisely that.

Whereas previous sections of this chapter have discussed issues of gene patenting that have been contested, there is no contestation on this issue here in the United States. In December 2004, however, Germany and France implemented provisions in their patent law for purpose-bound protection for human DNA sequences.[111] Purpose-bound protection limits patent coverage to the specific functions that are described in the patent. This move by the two European nations is highly controversial and goes against the Directive on the Legal Protection of Biotechnological Inventions (European Biotech Directive) as well as the Agreement on Trade-Related Aspects of Intellectual Property Rights (TRIPS).

It turns out that that patenting a gene sequence before knowing all the functions is not a problem as long as one specific function can be demonstrated. The key question then becomes, What counts as specific? Merely stating that a gene encodes a chemokine receptor apparently was specific enough for the U.S. Patent and Trademark Office. As we have seen, DNA sequences are treated like chemicals,[112] and in the world of chemistry, product (or composition-of-matter) claims are often granted. Composition-of-matter claims cover all properties of the patented substances, regardless of whether they are described in the patent specification. Only one single commercial application needs to be stated to receive exclusive control of the substance and all of its properties. As the Report of the Secretary's Advisory Committee on Genetics, Health, and Society explains: "A significant distinction between composition of matter/manufacture claims to isolated nucleic acid molecules and method claims is that claims to molecules cover all uses of the molecule, including uses outside of diagnostics, while a claim to a method of using a molecule would not prohibit one from using that molecule for another method."[113] As Human Genome Sciences' outside intellectual property attorney, Jorge A. Goldstein, remarked, "Whoever is the first to patent a DNA sequence—for any use—can lock up subsequent uses."[114] He continued: "In chemical patent law for over 100 years, everywhere in the world, if you discover a compound that has any use, even a marginal one, you are entitled to a patent on the compound.... Biotech hasn't changed anything."[115] Barton concurs:

This is a result of applying traditional chemical patent law principles to biotechnology. Under chemical patent principles, a patent on a novel chemical covers all uses of that chemical, whether or not discovered by the original patent holder. The discoverer of a new use may have a right to file a further patent, claiming use of the chemical for the particular new purpose, but will still have to obtain a license from the initial patent holder before using the chemical for the new purpose.[116]

Or as Doll explains:

a patent might be granted for compound X, which is disclosed to have a specific use (such as a headache remedy). If other investigators find that X has a new and unexpected use, perhaps in combination with compound Y, for treatment of heart arrhythmias, they may have to obtain a license from the individual who first patented compound X in order to sell XY.

In summary, once a product is patented, that patent extends to any use, even those that have not been disclosed in the patent. A future nonobvious method of using that product may be patentable, but the first patent would have been dominant.[117]

So what constitutes acceptable utility? The answer to this query is predicated on how much an inventor knew about her or his invention at the time of the application's submission. In 1995, the same year in which Human Genome Sciences applied for its CCR5 patent, intellectual property law professors Rebecca Eisenberg and Robert Merges were asked by the U.S. Patent and Trademark Office to provide their opinions on the patentability of inventions associated with the identification of partial cDNA sequences.[118] The USPTO sought comments to their guidelines in response to growing concerns that the Biotechnology Examining Group was imposing too strict utility requirements. At a public hearing in October 1994, representatives from the biotech industry complained that the utility requirements were more stringent for biotech patents than for those in other sectors. Many complained that the USPTO was requiring the type of clinical efficacy demanded by the Food and Drug Administration (FDA) for approval for new drug applications to establish utility.[119] According to Eisenberg and Merges,

in recent years biotechnology patent practitioners perceived an increasing strictness on the part of the PTO in its application of the utility requirement, particularly in the context of claims to methods of treatment or to pharmaceutical compositions. A series of decisions from the PTO Board of Patent Appeals and Interferences ... reflects this trend, which may fully be coming to an end in light of very recent developments in the PTO and Federal Circuit.[120]

Eisenberg and Merges pointed to the Patent and Trademark Office Utility Examination Guideline of 1995, which encouraged examiners not to reject a patent for lack of utility if the applicant claimed a utility that would be credible to one skilled in the art or if the invention had a well-established utility.[121] In short, at the time of HGS's CCR5 patent application, "the utility standard for biotechnology inventions" was "receding from its recent high-water mark."[122] It appears as if the USPTO wished to serve the interests of biocapitalism with respect to the utility requirements. As has been shown, however, biocapitalism is hardly monolithic: differing industries in the biotech world have very different interests. What does it mean, then, to serve the interest of biocapitalism when the interests of major players contributing to this ideology are at odds with each other?

Although many scientists focused their attention on the nonobviousness and utility issues, the real battle over the CCR5 patent was over the scope of its claim. A number of scientists feared that such patents could cover a myriad of applications that are unproven or even unattainable. A month after Haseltine's announcement of the Human Genome Sciences' patent, twelve leading scientists from the National Advisory Council for Human Genome Research wrote a letter to Nagumo, warning that the U.S.

Patent and Trademark Office's 1999 guidelines for patenting criteria might fall far short of the mark. Of particular concern were broad utility claims on human gene patents:

[W]e believe a broad allowance of claims is unjustified and will strongly discourage the further research efforts that will be necessary to translate gene discovery into medically important therapies. To avoid stifling scientific discovery and commercial application, we believe that allowances in these instances must be restricted to those utilities that are enabled by the patent.[123]

They continued by making a specific reference to CCR5:   ·

An example of speculative broad claims, which were in our opinion inappropriately allowed, is seen in the recently granted patent on CCR5. Based on sequence similarity, a patent was granted on a new gene that was claimed to be a putative chemokine receptor. No evidence was given to define the ligand or for any biological role for the putative receptor, but broad claims about the utility of the receptor were allowed.... Independent of knowledge of the filing of the patent, other investigators established that CCR5 is the key co-receptor for HIV, making CCR5 a very important potential drug target. That patent taught nothing that contributed to these later important discoveries, but now the holders can dominate the field. Moreover, this broad allowance makes no concession to the discoverers of the key piece of intellectual property, namely that CCR5 is a HIV co-receptor. Allowing broad, poorly substantiated claims create, *de facto*, an unacceptable monopoly on all fields in which the new gene might be found to be of use.[124]

Technology that is critical to the subsequent development of new diagnostics and therapies downstream from the patent might very well be stymied. Recent studies suggest that broad patent claims can deter innovation.[125] Although arguing that "the chilling effects of patenting" do not seem to have been realized, a 2002 study concluded that "in specific areas there is evidence of problems associated with the numbers and breadth of gene patents now being issued. Many consider the rise of patents with reach-through claims problematic and feel that this may require government attention."[126] Once again, part of the problem lies in the USPTO's decision to acquiesce to patent attorneys who argue that DNA should be treated as a chemical. Unlike other chemicals, however, a particular gene cannot be invented around.[127] Because a specific protein is coded for by that gene, patent holders can in theory effectively block subsequent research. Moreover, the notion of science as an open republic that is willing to share information has now been challenged: "For some, this trend [in accepting broad utility claims] stands in contrast to a long-standing norm of life sciences—to ensure the full access to and the use of publicly sponsored research results by making them freely available to the public."[128] The purpose of a patent is thereby thwarted.

Many scientists have expressed concerns that permitting the patenting of a gene whose precise function is unknown at the time of patent application's submission could preclude a product patent by some future research organization that discovers a more detailed and substantial functional role for that gene. The initial patent may interfere with subsequent research, which was the case with the BRCA1 and BRCA2 gene patents held by Myriad Genetics.[129] Nobel Laureate Harold Varmus, director of the National Institutes of Health at the time (currently director of the National Cancer Institute), and Francis Collins, former director of the Human Genome Project and current director of the NIH, wrote to Dickinson on December 21, 1999: "While we were pleased with the PTO's new stance on the utility of polynucleotides for which only generic utilities are asserted, we were very concerned with the PTO's apparent willingness to grant claims to polynucleotides for which a theoretical function of the encoded protein serves as the sole basis of the asserted utility."[130] Lee Bendekgey, general counsel for the sequencing company Incyte, disagreed, claiming that showing a utility is credible by using sequence homology is sufficient under U.S. patent law.[131] Absolute certainty is not required. Doll said that the patent examiners assume that the claims in a patent application are true unless shown otherwise. In addition, the patent system is self-correcting. If a patent utility proves to be fallacious, it will be revoked. Such a cavalier assertion, however, ignores the time, money, and expertise that are needed to torpedo a patent. In short, the utility claims in Human Genome Sciences' CCR5 patent were problematic for three reasons: they were based on sequence homology alone, they were very broad, and as a result of broad utility and because it was a product claim, it locked up all subsequent utilities, including those relevant to HIV/AIDS diagnostics and therapeutics.

The Response of the U.S. Patent and Trademark Office

Although the U.S. Patent and Trademark Office was willing to solicit comments and criticisms from biomedical researchers about their criteria, they were reluctant to accept them. In the revised guidelines published on January 5, 2001, the USPTO addressed numerous concerns, seven of which were relevant to the patenting of the *CCR5* gene. The first concern dealt with the granting of broad utility patents.[132] Some claimed that the USPTO did tighten the requirement and stated that the invention must possess "a *specific*, substantial and credible utility" as determined by one skilled in the art, but some biomedical scientists wanted the USPTO to crack down on broad utility patents. The Office responded by keeping the status quo: "the patentee is required to disclose only one utility.... The patentee is not required to disclose all possible uses, but promoting the subsequent discovery of other uses is one of the benefits of the patent system."[133] In other words, as long as one claim is specific, substantial, and credible, all further uses are locked up by that composition-of-matter claim.

The second concern expressed by the biomedical scientists was that gene patents delay medical research, thereby negating the social benefits with which they generally are associated. Such patents can also, in principle, quell the incentives of others to continue exploratory research.[134] The USPTO asserted the opposite, insisting that "incentive to make discoveries and inventions is generally spurred, not inhibited, by patents. The disclosure of genetic inventions provides new opportunities for further development."[135] It did not wish to differentiate between product claims in gene patents and product claims of other types of patents.

The third and fourth concerns focused on the scope of the patent, arguing that it should be limited to those uses that are disclosed in the patent application and limited to methods and applications, not the composition of matter (that is, DNA) itself. The USPTO, however, reminded the scientists that a patent gives exclusive rights to the composition of matter for a limited time, even if the inventor discloses only a single use for the composition.[136] In essence, its response is the same here as it was to the objections raised against broad utility claims.

In the fifth instance, biomedical researchers queried the originality and ingenuity of patenting genes. Sequencing DNA had become so routine (and indeed automated) by the 1990s that many scientists felt that the procedure was now uninventive and could not fulfill the nonobvious criterion.[137] Similarly, computer searches of databases to find functions of gene products had also become mundane and trivial. Aaron Klug, former president of the Royal Society of Science, and Bruce Alberts, former president of the National Academy of Science, argued that

It is a trivial matter today—using a computer search of public databases—to use DNA sequences to identify new genes with particular types of biochemical functions. In our opinion, such a discovery should not be rewarded with a broad patent for future therapeutics or diagnostics using these genes when the actual applications are merely guessed at.

The intention of some university and commercial interests to patent the DNA sequences themselves, thereby staking claim to large numbers of human genes without necessarily having a full understanding of their function, strikes us as contrary to the essence of patent law.

Those who would patent DNA sequences without real knowledge of their utility are staking claims not only to what little they know at present, but also to everything that might later be discovered about the genes and proteins associated with the sequence. They are, in effect, laying claim to a function that is not yet known or a use that does not yet exist. This may be in current shareholders' interests. But it does not serve society well.[138]

Other scientists have also challenged the notion that gene hunting via computational techniques is sufficiently ingenious to warrant a patent.[139] John Sulston, winner of the 2002 Nobel Prize in physiology or medicine, feared the consequences of blurring the distinction between an invention and a discovery:

Placing legal or proprietary restrictions on genes should be confined strictly to current applications or to inventive steps. Someone else may choose to work on another application and may thus need to have access to the same gene. Inventing human genes is impossible. So every discovery relating to genes—their sequence, functions and everything else—should be placed in the pre-competitive area. After all, one goal of the patent process is to stimulate competition. The most valuable gene-related applications are often far removed from the first easy steps. So this is a matter of science, not just a matter of principle.[140]

He continued this point by referring to Human Genome Sciences' CCR5 patent: "But who took the inventive step? Was it the company that made a lucky match with the right gene? Or was it the researchers who determined that HIV-resistant individuals had a defective gene?"[141] The USPTO was unmoved by HGS's arguments, pointing out that "Obviousness does not depend on the amount of work required to characterize the DNA molecule."[142] It cited 35 U.S.C. section 103(a) that "[p]atentability shall not be negatived by the manner in which the invention was made."[143]

The sixth concern dealt with patenting a gene and its protein product. The scientists felt that genes should be patented only when the complete sequence of the gene and the function of its product are correctly disclosed. The Patent and Trademark Office rebuked this suggestion because the utility of a claimed DNA sequence does not necessarily depend on the function of the gene product. For example, a DNA sequence might hybridize near a disease-associated gene or have a gene-regulating function.[144]

Finally, the last concern expressed by the scientists was the use of computer-based analysis of nucleic acids to assign a function to a given nucleic acid based on homology to prior art nucleic acids found in databases.

Several scientists, as has been shown, argued that sequence homology was no guarantee of function. The USPTO once again declined to adopt the suggestion, claiming both that homology-based assertions of utility were not inherently unbelievable and that the commentators provided no scientific evidence to back up their claims.[145] The asserted utility of a patent claim must be accepted prima facie by the examiner unless the examiner has "sufficient evidence or sound scientific reasoning to rebut such an assertion."[146] Moreover, a "'rigorous' correlation need not be shown in order to establish practical utility; a 'reasonable' correlation is sufficient."[147] In early 2001, the USPTO still acknowledged the use of homology to infer the gene product's function.[148] The guidelines from January 2001 had not changed for sequence homology, the scientists' protests notwithstanding:

Under the new guidelines, which the USPTO has acknowledged raise the bar for patentability, even the complete DNA sequence of an open reading frame encoding a protein would be unpatentable if the utility of the encoded protein is completely unknown. The USPTO will, however, recognize predicted utilities based on sequence homology to known useful proteins.[149]

There are insightful differences between the three major patent offices—the U.S. Patent and Trademark Office, European Patent Office, and Japanese Patent Office—on this issue of the patentability of genes based on sequence homology, although all three offices adjudicate each patent on a case-by-case basis. At the time of the patent examination of Human Genome Sciences' CCR5 patent application, the USPTO did "not have any ab initio requirement for experimental evidence to demonstrate the function or utility of any invention. The burden of proof in the [sic] establishing unpatentability is on the examiner."[150] The EPO, on the other hand, admitted that claims on proteins that are encoded by DNA sequences that have not been expressed in some host "are very likely not to satisfy the enablement requirement for the same reasons that they cannot satisfy the requirement of industrial application" and warned applicants that "mere in silico evidence concerning expression and function of the protein, no matter whether the level of identity with known proteins is low or high, will most likely be insufficient."[151] In those cases, the EPO would request experimental evidence to demonstrate function.[152] The JPO requested experimental evidence "when the claimed polynucleotide is not proved encoding a certain functional protein by written argument or from the common general knowledge as of the filing."[153] In addition, the EPO and JPO "share the same view that the claimed invention does not have [an] Inventive Step."[154] Such a view was diametrically opposed to the USPTO's stance that "the claimed invention has Non-obviousness."[155]

The European Patent Office also applied more stringent requirements for nonobviousness. For example, the EPO reversed SmithKline Beecham's patent on the human $5-HT_2$ serotonin receptor on the grounds that its DNA sequence was obvious to someone skilled in the art when compared with the sequences of other known receptors.[156] The differences between the EPO and USPTO on gene patents, particularly with respect to the CCR5 patents, are the subject of the next chapter.

Later in 2001, questions were raised as to whether G protein-coupled receptors, such as chemokine receptors, threatened to undermine the U.S. Patent and Trademark Office's stance on sequence homology. Yvonne (Bonnie) Eyler of the USPTO admitted that "G protein-coupled receptors are a large and diverse family of receptors with diverse functions and properties, having no well established utility based on family membership."[157] The USPTO realized that sequence homology might not suffice for determining function.

In short, as a result of the increased stringency of the Patent and Trademark Office and the recent Supreme Court decision that struck down patents on genes that are merely isolated from nature (discussed in the epilogue), it seems highly unlikely that Human Genome Sciences' CCR5 patent would be granted today, as a number of intellectual property lawyers assure me. Michele Wales, an intellectual property lawyer who worked with HGS, argues that with the Court's recent ruling, it will be difficult for those early gene-sequencing companies to survive.[158] Many biomedical researchers welcomed the changes in the USPTO criteria during the early years of the millennium but felt that stricter criteria needed to be in place. The USPTO has ceded too much ground to the interests of certain portions of the biotech sector, although there is evidence that this is slowly changing. After being persuaded that DNA is simply a chemical and lacking any unambiguous guidance from the courts with respect to the patentability of genes, the USPTO has made some curious patent decisions in the biotech sector since the 1990s. In addition the USPTO has seemed to ignore the Court of Appeals for the Federal Circuit's view on the predictability of the art of nucleic acids and proteins. Many issues relating to the written description requirement, possession, enablement, and utility had not been (and still are not) settled. Similarly, although many (but certainly not all) scientists were challenging utility claims based on sequence homology, some quarters of the biotech sector benefitted from these instabilities, and others did not. That point merits reemphasis because a number of scholars have

seen biocapitalism as a united front. It is not correct that all for-profit institutions are singing in unison against a unified nonprofit stance. Although
clearly the forces of biocapitalism are at play here, that heuristic tool might
need some refining to help us understand recent developments in biotechnology and molecular biology. Finally, many maintain that the leniency
toward patenting has given rise to biotechnology. I, however, agree with
those who conclude that patent leniency is a consequence, not the cause,
of biotechnology.

5 The European Response to the CCR5 Patent

Thus far I have told the American story of the CCR5 patent. It possesses a European lineage, as well. In chapter 2, it was noted that the Belgian company Euroscreen is the licensing agent for the CCR5 patent portfolio. Patent holders generally apply for patents in (at least) the three major markets—the United States, Europe, and Japan. Euroscreen filed its two European patents on February 28, 1997, both with priority dates of March 1, 1996. The first patent (EP 0883687) was granted for the CCR5 receptor, derivatives thereof, and their uses and had a European Patent Bulletin publication date of October 27, 2004.[1] The second (EP 1482042) was awarded for the active and inactive CCR5, the corresponding nucleic acid sequences, and screening claims and had a publication date of December 1, 2004. This chapter focuses on the anatomy of opposing a European patent and offers an informative glimpse into the world of patent litigation. In this case, several big and small pharma companies wanted the patent rescinded. As was shown in chapter 4, Biotechnology Industry Organization (BIO) is not united on the issue that sequence homology determines utility. Similarly, it would be a mistake to simplify the debate on gene patenting as merely one that BIO supports and nonprofits oppose. Such a polarized view levels in one swoop critical differences among members of BIO and nonprofits alike.

The European Patent Office versus the U.S. Patent and Trademark Office

Europeans have been far more aware and skeptical of gene patents than Americans. Perhaps the European Society of Human Genetics' (ESHG) Working Party on Patenting and Licensing summarizes it best: "The proliferation of patents on human genes has raised practical and ethical concerns, particularly in Europe. Typically, public opinion is against the patentability of human genes."[2] The European Patent Office and the Japanese Patent Office tend to be stricter than the U.S. Patent and Trademark Office: "The more stringent approach of European and Japanese patent examiners, as compared to their U.S. colleagues, already demonstrates a trend in the right direction."[3] Gene patents are more easily obtained in the United States than in Europe or Japan.[4] The World Trade Organization created the Agreement on Trade-Related Aspects of Intellectual Property Rights (TRIPS) with a view to "harmonize" (as lawyers often call it) intellectual property laws around the globe;[5] however, attempts to establish a substantive patent law treaty have failed. There are important differences between the patenting laws of the USPTO and EPO.[6]

Although European patents are granted to the first that files, before the Patent Reform Act of 2011, Americans rewarded the first to invent. Previously, a provisional application was filed in the United States, which permitted an earlier filing date for the subsequent patent application, which needed to be submitted within a twelve-month period after the provisional patent. As a result of the new patent reform, the United States is moving closer to a first-to-file system that is similar to the European system, and interference proceedings over priority will be eliminated in the United States.[7] Each application is now given an "effective filing date," and patentability is judged on whether any prior art or disclosed information relevant to the patent existed before that date. A one-year grace period remains in the United States, but now the patent applicant must be the one that makes the invention public.[8] The EPO does not permit provisional patents.[9] The invention must be truly novel for patentability in Europe, meaning that it must not be publicly available before it is patented. The United States requires the disclosure of the best method to practice the invention (the best mode requirement), and Europe does not. Under the new statute, the best-mode requirement is no longer enforceable. Until November 2000, the USPTO published patents after they were granted. Since that date, the United States, as Europe, has made patent applications known eighteen months after submission, unless the patentee withdraws the application beforehand. If the inventor is applying for only a U.S. patent, it may still request nonpublication. The EPO allows third-party oppositions: within nine months of the granting of a patent, anyone from the public or private sector may file an opposition. The third party must demonstrate that "(a) proceedings for infringement of the same patent have been instituted against him, or (b) following a request of the proprietor of the patent to cease alleged infringement, the third party has instituted proceedings for a ruling that he is not infringing the patent."[10] The patent holder and the opposition then enter into a debate, and the EPO makes a final decision after oral proceedings. There was no third-party opposition in the United

States at the time of the CCR5 patent filings. That too changed with the Patent Reform Act of 2011. Before the reform, if someone opposed a patent, the USPTO performed a reexamination whereby anyone could present evidence and argumentation. Only the patent holder could engage in a direct conversation with the USPTO to establish the patent's validity. Unlike Europe, after a patent is granted, its validity is assumed. Burden of proof lies with the opposition. The property right of a U.S. patent is enforced throughout all fifty states. Patents in Europe are issued in a bundle, depending on where the applicant has asked for protection. A European patent, however, must be annulled separately by each country if the nine-month period after the award has expired. The EPO requires that the invention possess an inventive step, which roughly corresponds with the USPTO's requirement of nonobviousness, yet the inventive step is a more rigorous criterion: "A European patent application involves an inventive step if it solves a technical problem in a non-obvious way. Note that this introduces two extra requirements: it must solve a problem (no problem solved means no inventive step), and that problem must be technical (solving economic problems means no inventive step)."[11]

Biotech journals are quick to make these differences known to their readers.[12] A topic of concern that often is expressed is the written description requirement, which is stricter in Europe. The invention must be clearly and unambiguously disclosed in the written description. It requires patentees to describe the various permutations and combinations of the invention:

As a result of these differences, amendments that will be permitted in the U.S. might not be permitted in Europe, and strategies that might not be possible in Europe might be successful in the U.S. Thus, it might be easier to amend the U.S. claims to avoid unexpected prior art, or to encompass an aspect of the invention that was not the original focus of the application, while similar strategies in Europe may run up against basis rejections.[13]

Perhaps the most significant difference between Europe and the Americans on biotech patents is a historical one. As Sheila Jasanoff has shown, issues of morality have played a much larger role in European patent deliberations.[14] Article 53 of the European Patent Commission (EPC) cites two reasons to negate a patent application:

a) inventions the commercial exploitation of which would be contrary to "ordre public" or morality, provided that the exception shall not be deemed to be so merely because it is prohibited by law or regulation in some or all of the Contracting states; b) plant or animal varieties or essentially biological processes for the production of plants and animals; this provision does not apply to microbiological processes or the products thereof.[15]

The European Union's Biotech Directive on the Legal Protection of Biotechnological Inventions (henceforth the EU Biotech Directive) of 1998 binds only the members of the European Union, not all members of the European Patent Community. Article 5(1) of the EU Biotech Directive states: "The human body, at the various stages of its formation and development, and the simple discovery of one of its elements, including the sequence or partial sequence of a gene, cannot constitute patentable inventions."[16] Articles 5(2) and 5(3), however, state that isolated gene sequences may be patented even if their sequences are identical to those occurring in nature but only if they are derived by a technological procedure and possess an identifiable industrial application.[17] In 2000, France's former Minister of Justice, Élisabeth Guigou, made it clear that the EU Biotech Directive violated France's bioethics law of 1994, which prohibited patenting of human genetic information.[18] A year later, former French president, Jacques Chirac, requested that the EU Commission clarify the meaning of article 5 because France maintained that the mere discovery of a DNA sequence was not patent eligible.[19] As a result of this concern (as was mentioned in chapter 4), France has provisions in its law that narrow the scope of the patent to the recited utility.[20] The same is true of Germany. This curtailing in patent scope applies only to biotech patents.

By 2005, 5,669 patent families, or sets of patents given out by numerous countries for the same invention, claiming human DNA sequences were awarded worldwide in one or more of three major patent offices. Of those, 94% received at least one patent from the U.S. Patent and Trademark Office, while only 13% were granted at least one patent by the European Patent Office.[21] Hopkins argues that the increase in the United States' healthcare market on the one hand, and the time it takes the EPO to review patents as well as its higher bar of patentability on the other contribute to those skewed numbers. The three sequencing companies that are discussed in chapter 1—Human Genome Sciences, Incyte, and Millennium Pharmaceuticals—find it particularly difficult to have their patent applications approved by the EPO. By 2005, Incyte had only four gene patent families granted out of 513 applications, Millennium had three gene patent families out of 286 applications, and Human Genome Sciences had nineteen patent families despite 471 applications. In comparison, Incyte had 442 gene patent families granted in the United States, Millennium had 167, and Human Genome Sciences had 219.[22] The EPO's more stringent requirements for specific utility claims and the insufficiency of sequence homology for functional/utility claims combine to explain those paltry figures.

The Torpedoing of One CCR5 Patent in Europe

In 2005, two pharmaceutical companies, Hoffmann-La Roche AG (big pharma) and Progenics Pharmaceuticals, Inc. (small pharma), and one British service company that provides anonymity to any company wishing to oppose a patent, Strawman Ltd. of Winchester, United Kingdom,[23] filed appeals against Euroscreen's European patent for CCR5, EP0883687 for "C-C CKR-5 [CCR5] CC-Chemikine [sic] Receptors, Derivatives." Why did Hoffmann-La Roche, Progenics, and the anonymous companies represented by Strawman Ltd. wish to have this particular CCR5 gene patent repealed? They have created and are still in the process of creating molecules—either chemical compounds or monoclonal antibodies—that can bind to CCR5, thereby prohibiting HIV-1 from entering into CD4 cells, particularly T-helper cells.

On June 13, 2005, Strawman Ltd. filed an opposition to Euroscreen's patent. Its forty-eight-page report argued that the patent was not new: "*all* of the subject matter of EP '687 [that is, the patent] was already known—or was very obvious—before the filing and priority dates of EP '687."[24] Although the patent was filed after the 1996 papers were published identifying CCR5 as the HIV-1 coreceptor, the patent claimed a priority date (PD1) of March 1, 1996, or 365 days prior to the filing date of February 28, 1997.[25] This predates those essays. Strawman Ltd. insisted that some of the patent's subject matter was not entitled to the claimed priority date and that some of claims were not permissible because they were related to subject matter that had already been abandoned.[26] Among numerous other open sources, Strawman Ltd. cited the publications of Michel Samson, Tatjana Dragic, and Hongkui Deng, which all predated the patent application. If the priority date was judged impermissible, then these works undermined some of the novelty claims.[27] Finally, Strawman Ltd. cited an undergraduate textbook, Charles A. Janeway's *Immunobiology*, to demonstrate that some of the patent claims both lacked novelty and were obvious.[28]

According to Strawman Ltd.'s attorneys, the patent also lacked an inventive step and failed to disclose the invention in a sufficiently clear and complete way for someone who is skilled in the art to carry it out. In addition, the subject matter of the patent extended beyond the content of the application.[29] The patent claimed that two anti-CCR5 sera had the ability in vitro to inhibit HIV binding, one of which possessed only a partial blocking ability. And some sera had no effect whatsoever on the virus's ability to bind to the chemokine coreceptor. Because not all anti-CCR5 sera could inhibit HIV infection of lymphocytes, "the scope of the claims is clearly broader than the teachings of EP '687 and thus there is an undue burden on the skilled person to identify which anti-ligands will work and which anti-ligands will not."[30] The claim of an antibody's blocking the binding between HIV-1 or HIV-2 and CCR5 was never substantiated:

Nowhere in the application as filed is the skilled person taught a method consisting of determining whether an agonist or antagonist inhibits the binding of HIV virus to said peptide. In addition, nowhere in the application as filed is the skilled person taught that the agonists or antagonists identified by such a screening method and which specifically bind to the peptide can also be used in the treatment or prevention of HIV virus infection.[31]

Finally, there was no teaching in the patent that such drugs are to be used to treat HIV-1 or HIV-2.[32]

On July 26, 2005, Hoffmann-La Roche AG of Basel, Switzerland, submitted a letter of opposition to Euroscreen's CCR5 patent.[33] Its main arguments against the patent mirrored Strawman Ltd.'s. First, Hoffman-La Roche's lawyers argued that the invention was not new. They cited the works of Christophe Combadiere, Heidi Heath, and Jianglin He for priority.[34] The claims dealing with the inhibition of the binding of HIV to CCR5 were in their eyes illegitimate because the function of CCR5 as coreceptor was unknown at the time of the priority date and the patent failed to establish that fact.[35] Hoffmann-La Roche's attorneys also claimed that the patent lacked an inventive step.[36]

The patent also failed to disclose the invention in the written description in such a way that someone skilled in the art could reproduce it. Hoffmann-La Roche's attorneys asserted that

The production of an antibody, which is specific for CCR5 *and* inhibits HIV infection, is associated with severe technical difficulties and a very low success rate, as supported by D25 [William C. Olson, G. E. E. Rabut, K. A. Nagashimi, et al., "Differential Inhibition of Human Immunodeficiency Virus Type 1 Fusion, gp120 Binding, and CC-Chemokine Activity by Monoclonal Antibodies to CCR5," *Journal of Virology* 73, no. 5 (1999): 4145–4155] and by Dr. Michael Brandt, scientist at Roche Diagnostics GmbH, Penzberg, Germany, who has informed us of their attempts to obtain mABs [monoclonal antibodies] that exhibit the effect. Merely producing an antiserum by a procedure, without even isolating and characterizing potential antibodies, does therefore not provide a sufficient description. The patent itself reports that the antisera were unreliable and unpredictable in showing the desired effect, and even the one that reportedly did is not reproducible from the description, and no relevant deposit of biological material was made.[37]

In short, there was no sufficient description provided to show how someone is to "determine whether the said anti-ligand inhibits the binding of the ligand [the virus] to said peptide" of CCR5.[38]

A number of patent claims contained subject matter that extended beyond the content of the application. Hoffmann-La Roche's intellectual property lawyers continued by pointing out two examples in which the subject matter claimed could not be performed across the scope of the patent. First, the patent did not provide any specific example of an antibody that inhibits or reduces the binding of HIV-1 or HIV-2 to CCR5. The alleged reproduction of such an antibody would be impossible. Second, neither a monoclonal antibody nor pharmaceutical composition for inhibition or reduction of binding was stated in the patent.[39] And a number of claims that involved the step of isolating a membrane fraction from cells expressing CCR5 and then performing tests on those membrane fractions (some of which were presumed to possess CCR5) were never substantiated.[40]

Other claims also were problematic. The ability of compounds to bind to CCR5 did not necessarily imply that these compounds could be useful as HIV/AIDS drugs. The description therefore did not provide a method for determining whether a compound could be used for treatment or prevention of HIV infection. None of the claims offered a description for the reduction of binding. Merely assigning a specific function of the serum to a hypothetical component was deemed to be mere speculation and not substantiated in the patent.[41]

Hoffmann-La Roche's attorneys also criticized the broad utility of the patent:

On page 11 it goes on to say that the "agonist or antagonist" may be used in the treatment of a variety of conditions, which are specified as: "Inflammatory diseases, including rheumatoid arthritis, glomerulonephritis, asthma, idiopathic pulmonary fibrosis and psoriasis, viral infections including … HIV-1 and 2, cancer including leukaemia, atherosclerosis and/or auto-immune disease."

That recital of diseases is so broad as to encompass a substantial part of the major human diseases—so that the antibody is in effect being presented almost as a "universal panacea"—ie it is not "specific," nor is it "credible." There are no data whatsoever in PD1 [priority date 1] to support any of those medical indications.[42]

Finally, the attorneys differentiated between a discovery and an invention, a distinction that is far clearer in European patent law than U.S. patent law:

The discovery of this new receptor, and identification of the chemokines that bind it, may well be of scientific interest—even importance—but that does not in itself constitute the basis of the grant of a patent.

At the base level, it constitutes a "discovery," which is therefore not patentable "as such" (Art 52(2)(a) and Art 52 (9), which excludes "discoveries … as such").[43]

One day later, on July 27, 2005, Progenics Pharmaceuticals, Inc. of Tarrytown, New York, filed an opposition with the European Patent Office through its attorney, Carol Almond-Martin of Ernest Gutmann-Yves Plasseraud, S.A.S. of Lyon, France.[44] Echoing the previous two oppositions, Progenics' intellectual property attorneys challenged both the novelty of the patent and its inventive step. They too claimed that the patent did not disclose the invention in a sufficient manner and that the subject matter of the patent extended beyond the application's content. Unlike the other two oppositions, however, Progenics did not challenge the entire patent, just claims 25 to 36, which involve using antibodies to bind to HIV.[45] As is shown in chapter 6, Progenics has created a monoclonal antibody, PRO 140, to bind to CCR5. Progenics' lawyers argued that the patent provided no experimental support for patent claim 25, "an antibody which inhibits or reduces the binding of a human immunodeficiency virus type 1 (HIV 1) or the human immunodeficiency virus 2 (HIV 2) to a peptide having an amino acid sequence presenting more than 80% homology to SEQ ID No: 2."[46] There was no mention of the binding between HIV-1 or HIV-2 and CCR5, and the partial blockage of the receptor was not disclosed as being linked to an inability of either virus strain to bind to that receptor.[47] The patent also lacked support for a method to identify any antiligand or antibody.[48] In addition, ten claims added subject matter that extended beyond the content of the patent.[49] The opposition argued that all of these claims failed the priority criterion, citing Jianglin He, Tatjana Dragic, Ghalib Alkhatib, and Hyeryun Choe for priority on the disclosure of the mediation of HIV entry via CCR5 into CD4 cells. And He addressed monoclonal antibodies that were specific to CCR5. Because the amino acid sequence of CCR5 was known, anyone skilled in the art could have produced monoclonal antibodies with a view to halt the infection of HIV-1 or HIV-2 of CD4 cells.[50]

Progenics' lawyers also asserted that some claims lacked novelty: "antibodies to CD4 capable of reducing the binding between HIV and CC-CKR-5 [CCR5] were known, even before the priority dates of the Opposed Patent, and that such antibodies anticipate the subject-matter of claim 25 which thus lacks novelty."[51] Finally, echoing Strawman Ltd. and Hoffmann-La Roche's assertions, they argued that the invention was not disclosed sufficiently clearly and completely in the patent to be carried out by someone who was skilled in the art. This point goes back to the concept of sequence homology. The claims dealt with a class of antibodies that either fully inhibit or reduce HIV's ability to bind to CCR5. Included in that class were all peptides that had an 80% homology to the sequence listed in the patent. Of those peptides, a large number of them would not bind to CCR5:

There is no teaching in the patent as to how to distinguish, amongst the numerous peptides having more than 80% homology with the peptide SEQ ID NO: 2, those which are capable of binding HIV from those which are not capable of binding HIV. The claim requires that the skilled man identify antibodies which have the capacity to block the peptide/virus interaction. However, since the patent does not teach how to first identify peptides which bind the virus, the skilled man cannot, without undue burden identify such antibodies over the whole range of the claim. The invention is thus insufficiently disclosed.

Moreover, there is no teaching that blocking of infection is due to inhibiting the binding between HIV and the CCR5 receptor. There is no correlation between these two concepts in the application as filed. There is therefore an undue burden on those skilled in the art to practice the subject matter as claimed and undue experimentation without any reasonable certainty of success is required.[52]

In response to these three patent oppositions, Euroscreen's intellectual property attorneys—De Clercq Brants & Partners of Brussels, Belgium—decided to amend the patent.[53] First, they limited the claims to the amino acid and nucleic acid sequences that were disclosed in the patent diagrams and did not argue for all those with 80% amino-acid sequence homology. All references to portions of HIV-1 or HIV-2 or sequence homology percentages were deleted, although the entire viruses were still claimed.[54] Claim 1 of the original patent was thus rewritten: "A method for determining whether an anti-ligand is capable of inhibiting the binding of a ligand, said ligand being an HIV virus ~~or a portion thereof~~, to a peptide having an amino acid sequence which is <u>characterized by</u> ~~presents more than 80% homology with~~ SEQ ID NO. 2."[55] Claims 2 through 8 were similarly reworded.[56] Second, several claims were expunged, including a method for determining where an antiligand is capable of binding to an antagonist or agonist; a method for screening drugs for gp120/gp160 (or the glycoproteins that are the outer-coat proteins of HIV-1 and HIV-2);[57] a method for determining if an antiligand is capable of binding HIV; a method for identifying an antagonist or agonist; a method for screening drugs for peptides possessing a 90% and 95% sequence homology with the patented amino acid sequence (although that particular sequence is still a part of the claim);[58] and the antibody elicited by amino-acid sequences of 90% and 95% (although monoclonal antibodies were still enforced by the patent).[59]

Other opposing points De Clercq Brants & Partners deemed as "ridiculous," "without merit," and "absurd" and said that the plaintiffs "misrepresented and mischaracterized" the patent claims.[60] As for the argument that some of the claims were too broad, the lawyers remarked that "the mere fact that a claim would be broad is not in itself a ground for considering the patent not complying with the requirements of sufficiency of disclosure."[61]

They defended their other priority claims, reminding the Opposition Division (OD) of the European Patent Office that "It is well-established jurisprudence that the patent must be construed by a mind willing to understand, not a mind desirous of misunderstanding."[62] As for the industrial application requirement, Euroscreen's lawyers argued that "there is no requirement in the EPC [European Patent Commission] that the claimed subject matter should be 'credible,' 'substantial,' and/or 'specific.'"[63] As for the objections of novelty, Euroscreen's lawyers claimed that "Most of the novelty objections by Opponent 1 [Strawman Ltd.] are based upon a (deliberate or naïve?) mischaracterization and misrepresentation of the interpretation of the claims and terms."[64] They defended their claims by arguing that they are entitled to the first priority date.[65] The same held true for the inventive steps listed in the patent.[66]

In a related process, on August 9, 2006, Progenics Pharmaceuticals filed an opposition to a patent for antibodies binding to chemokine receptor 88C (an earlier name for CCR5, European Patent 0811063B1), originally held by ICOS and then transferred to Euroscreen.[67] The European Patent Office ruled after the oral proceedings of February 19, 2008, that "the patent and the invention to which it relates are found to meet the requirements of the Convention."[68] Euroscreen announced the news of Progenics' defeat on its Web site.[69] That patent is still in effect at the time of writing this book. So things were looking good for Euroscreen's European portofolio of CCR5 patents.

By late summer 2011, however, the fate of one of Euroscreen's patents was to change dramatically. On August 5, the EPO's Oppositions Division (OD), whose opinion is provisional and legally nonbinding, ruled on the three sets of challenges to the patent, as well as Euroscreen's attorneys' responses to them.[70] The OD felt that the patent did indeed suffer from a number of faults and requested oral proceedings for a two-day period, starting on January 19, 2012, at the EPO in Munich.[71] The OD addressed five articles of the EPC's laws that were relevant to the opposition of the patent—articles 132, 83, 87, 54(2, 3), and 56.

Article 132 deals with amending patents, such as when it is and is not permissible. Article 132(2) prohibits the addition of subject matter beyond what is listed in the initial application. Although siding with Euroscreen on its patent application claim that "an anti-ligand is capable of inhibiting the binding of a ligand, said being an HIV virus" and on its method claim for screening drugs for HIV treatment and prevention, the OD was less sympathetic to a number of other claims.[72] It felt that there was no valid basis for the two methods claiming to identify drugs and agonists/antagonists that might be considered to inhibit the actual binding of HIV to the receptor's peptide. The reworded claims 6 and 7 dealt with "a method for determining whether an agonist or antagonist which binds to a peptide comprising the amino acid sequence which is characterized by SEQ ID NO. 2 ... can be used for the treatment and/or prevention of an HIV virus infection ... and determining whether said agonist or antagonist inhibits the binding of HIV virus to said peptide."[73] The OD felt that "the indicated basis by the PP [patent proprietor; Euroscreen, in this case] can therefore not be considered as a [sic] valid for directly and unambiguously deriving the technical feature of 'inhibiting the binding of HIV virus to said peptide.'"[74] In addition, Euroscreen's reworded claim 22 concerning an antibody that inhibits or reduces the binding of HIV-1 or HIV-2 was, according to the OD, invalid. And logically, the related claim 25, which discussed an antibody that decreases the infectivity of a cell by an HIV strain, was also invalid. In a similar fashion, the OD sided with Progenics that two reworded claims 29 and 30 dealing with "a pharmaceutical composition comprising an antibody" and "the use of a pharmaceutical composition for the treatment of an HIV1/HIV2 infection" did not form a valid basis for the subject matter.[75] The OD did, however, side with the Euroscreen on claims for the use of an antibody or antisense oligonulecotide for treatment of HIV infection.[76] In short, the OD found that six of Euroscreen's claims did not fulfill the requirements of article 132(2), which is to say that the company inappropriately added these six claims of subject matter after the granting of the patent.

Article 83 of the European Patent Commission deals with the sufficiency of a patent's disclosure. Progenics argued that some of the claimed methods and products were not enabled by the patent. The Opposition Division disagreed, arguing that the patent application did disclose a sufficiently clear method for the preparation of blood sera against the CCR5. In the OD's view, anyone skilled in the art could carry out such a method; therefore, the claim of an antibody for either inhibiting or reducing the ability of HIV-1 to bind to it was also enabled. Article 83 was upheld by the patent.[77]

Article 87 of the European Patent Commission concerns itself with priority. All three opponents to the patent argued that Euroscreen could not claim a priority date of March 1, 1996, or 365 days prior to the initial patent application EP 96870021, which became patent EP 0883687, for "a ligand being a[n] HIV virus," "treatment and/or prevention of HIV infection," or an "antibody which inhibits or reduce[s] the binding of HIV-1."[78] Although ruling that the date of the initial patent was valid for a particular sequence that refers to the ChemR13 (CCR5) receptor, that application gave no evidence for defining the ligand of that receptor as being HIV.[79] The initial date therefore could not be used for the claimed subject matter. Two scholarly articles published in 1995 have priority over the initial patent.[80] In all other challenges over priority, the OD sided with Euroscreen.

Sections (2) and (3) of European Patent Commission article 54 establish the criteria for novelty. Article 54(2) declares that "[the] state of the art [is] held to comprise everything made available to the public by means of a written or oral description, by use, or in any other way, before the date of filing of the European patent application."[81] Furthermore, article 54(3) extends article 54(2) by adding "the content of European patent applications as filed, the dates of filing of which are prior to the date referred to … and which were published on or after that date."[82] Such an addition assures that not more than one European patent is granted to different inventors for the same invention. Of the numerous challenges to Euroscreen's patent on novelty, the Opposition Division agreed with only one—that other scientists had already described an anti-CCR5 antibody that blocks the binding of HIV to CD4 cells prior to the patent application.[83] The patent's novelty claim of possessing subject matter (an "antibody which inhibits or reduces the binding of a human immunodeficiency virus") was invalid.[84]

Finally, article 56 of the European Patent Commission is the so-called inventive step, which is required by the European Patent Office and which is similar to the nonobvious requirement of the U.S. Patent and Trademark Office. All three opponents to the patent cited numerous examples of prior art. The Opposition Division believed that the articles by Power's and Combadiere's groups could indeed be regarded as prior art that taught that CCR5 acts as the coreceptor for HIV-1 to enter the cell and that MIP-1α, MIP-1β, and RANTES are chemokines that compete with HIV-1 for binding to CCR5, thereby inhibiting HIV-1 infection.[85] In addition, the OD concurred with Strawman Ltd.'s argument that a person skilled in the art would be aware that the blocking of CCR5 would result in reducing the entry of HIV-1 in CD4 cells and would be able to link that knowledge to establishing screening methods created for identifying suitable compounds. There was no inventive step in reworded claim 1 above.[86] The OD requested that the "problem solution approach" be applied in the oral proceedings to see if Euroscreen could claim an inventive step.[87] The "problem solution approach" entails a three-step procedure: identify the closest (or the most relevant) prior art; determine the "objective technical problem" (the technical problem that the claimed invention purportedly addresses and solves); and judge whether the claimed solution to the technical problem is or is not obvious to someone who is skilled in the art.[88]

The OD concluded that it was "of the preliminary and non-binding opinion that the patent cannot be maintained in unamended [sic] form."[89] As a result, it ordered oral proceedings, which in the end never occurred. On December 16, 2011, De Clercq & Partners sent a letter to the European Patent Office stating that Euroscreen "no longer agree[s] to the text of the patent as granted and hence requests revocation of the patent EP 0 883 687, and closure of the opposition procedure."[90] On December 20, the oral proceedings were canceled, and the patent was revoked, nearly seven years and two months after it had been issued.[91] Why did Euroscreen revoke its patent? According to Lannoy, who is responsible for Euroscreen's CCR5 patent portfolio, the company's officials felt that it was simply not worth paying the annual renewal fee. In addition, its patent EP 1482042 is still valid. And ICOS had two CCR5 patents granted by the EPO, both filed on December 20, 1996, with a priority date of December 20, 1995: EP 081106 covers the amino acid sequence of CCR5 (which ICOS called receptor 88C), its DNA vector, a method for producing the peptide in a host cell, an RNA transcript of the polynucleotide, and CCR5 antibodies, and EP 1870465 covers a method for identifying a ligand that interacts with CCR5 (that is, screening claims) and the host cell of that receptor.[92] In January 2008, one year after Eli Lilly bought ICOS, Euroscreen obtained ICOS's patents for CCR5. Euroscreen officials feel that these three patents are sufficient for its financial interests.[93] Moreover, the hope and euphoria of the late 1990s for chemokine-receptor genes and their products turned out to be ephemeral. As is shown in the ensuing chapters, big and small pharma jumped at the chance to synthesize small molecules that could act as inhibitors to the binding of HIV-1 to CCR5. Much money was spent on path-breaking research; however, the treatment of AIDS via CCR5 inhibitors has not been as nearly successful as had been initially hoped.

Big and small pharma undoubtedly defend their interests in Europe. A number of scholars argue that most European governments back gene patents only because they fear that if they did not do so, they would lose their biotech industry to the United States. It is a defensive strategy. It is fair to say, however, that the more stringent patent requirements of the European Patent Office reflect the Europeans' skepticism toward gene patents. A contrast between Europe and the United States is useful because it once again points out that there are alternatives: questions of human value are embedded differently in various legal regimes. The presence of a moral clause in patent law, the considerably higher rejection rate in Europe of gene patents that are based on sequence homology, and Germany and France's decision to limit utility on gene/biotech patents to that described in the specification all demonstrate that the situation in which the United States finds itself is not inevitable.

6 CCR5 and HIV/AIDS Diagnostics and Therapeutics

In the last years of the twentieth century, the *CCR5* gene and its protein product became the objects of state-of-the-art work on diagnostics and drug treatment. The CCR5 patent's lineage is now the subject of biomedical research on chemokine receptors and is entangled in the complex political, social, and biomedical lineages of HIV/AIDS—with big pharma playing the lead role in the story. The gene's genealogy has been humanized and inextricably linked to the lives of the tens of millions infected. After this chapter examines these issues, it returns to intellectual property themes. HIV/AIDS diagnostic tests and medications have been patented by big and small pharma, and the ramifications of those patents have been felt worldwide, particularly in India, where nearly 2.5 million people are HIV+[1] and where attempts are underway to create generic drugs that bind to CCR5 despite patent protection.

Drugs and CCR5

Not surprisingly, the history of HIV/AIDS treatment mirrors the history of the elucidation of the mode of HIV infection. In 1984, biomedical researchers in Robert Gallo's laboratory at the National Institutes of Health and in Luc Montagnier's lab at the Institut Pasteur announced their codiscovery of the retrovirus (a virus with a genome that is comprised of RNA rather than DNA) that is responsible for AIDS; it was later named human immunodeficiency virus.[2] Scientists initially scrambled to find chemicals that could inhibit the process by which a retrovirus replicates, and they took aim at its enzyme, reverse transcriptase, which is present in retroviruses but not in humans (figure 6.1).

On March 19, 1987, the Federal Drug Administration approved azidothymidine (or AZT) as the first drug to inhibit the replication of reverse transcriptase.[3] AZT ushered in the age of nucleoside analog reverse-transcriptase

The HIV Life Cycle

HIV medicines in six drug classes stop 🛑 HIV at different stages in the HIV life cycle.

1 **Binding (also called Attachment):** HIV binds (attaches itself) to receptors on the surface of a CD4 cell.

🛑 **Entry inhibitors**

2 **Fusion:** The HIV envelope and the CD4 cell membrane fuse (join together), which allows HIV to enter the CD4 cell.

🛑 **Fusion inhibitors**

CD4 receptors

CD4 cell membrane

HIV RNA

Reverse transcriptase

HIV DNA

Membrane of CD4 cell nucleus

3 **Reverse Transcription:** Once inside a CD4 cell, HIV releases an HIV enzyme called reverse transcriptase. HIV uses reverse transcriptase to convert its genetic material—HIV RNA—into HIV DNA. The conversion of HIV RNA to HIV DNA is necessary so that the HIV can enter the nucleus (center) of a CD4 cell and combine with the cell's genetic material—cell DNA.

🛑 **Non-nucleoside reverse transcriptase inhibitors (NNRTIs)**

🛑 **Nucleoside reverse transcriptase inhibitors (NRTIs)**

Integrase

4 **Integration:** HIV produces an enzyme called integrase, which allows HIV DNA to enter the CD4 cell nucleus. Once inside the cell nucleus, the HIV DNA is joined (integrated) with the CD4 cell DNA.

🛑 **Integrase inhibitors**

5 **Transcription and Translation:** Once HIV is integrated into CD4 cell DNA, the virus begins to use the machinery of the CD4 cell to create long chains of HIV proteins. The protein chains are the building blocks for more HIV.

Protease

HIV DNA

CD4 cell DNA

6 **Assembly:** An HIV enzyme called protease cuts up the long chains of HIV proteins. The smaller HIV proteins combine with HIV RNA to form a new virus.

🛑 **Protease inhibitors (PIs)**

7 **Budding:** The newly made HIV pushes out ("buds") from the CD4 cell.

inhibitors (NARTIs or NRTIs). Nucleotide analog reverse-transcriptase inhibitors (NtARTIs or NTRTIs) are another group of HIV-1 inhibitors.[4] Both types of drugs are chain terminators, meaning that they interrupt the replication of the reverse transcriptase and thereby halt infection. The second class of drugs used to combat HIV/AIDS are nonnucleoside reserve transcriptase inhibitors (NNRTIs), which do not act as chain terminators but bind to HIV's reverse transcriptase, thereby disabling it from making a DNA copy of its RNA genome.

The third class of drugs used to treat HIV/AIDS are protease inhibitors (PIs), which interrupt the functioning of the HIV-1 protease and which currently constitute the largest and most successful class of drugs used to treat the disease. PI structures are based on the amino acid sequences that are involved in HIV protein cleavage. Most PIs possess an artificial analog of the phenylanine-proline sequence (amino acids 167 and 168) of HIV's gp160. Whereas the protease cuts the viral peptide of the protein to form the two

---

Figure 6.1

The life cycle of HIV

1. Binding/attachment: After infection, HIV travels in the blood and enters into the CD4 cells by binding to the CD4 receptor and the chemokine coreceptor (CCR5 or CXCR4). The entry inhibitor Maraviroc/Selzentry affects this stage of viral infection. *2. Fusion:* The virus then fuses with the host's CD4 cell to inject its genetic material into the cell. Fusin inhibitors are drugs used to thwart this particular process. *3. Reverse transcriptase:* After it is inside the cell, the virus's enzyme, reverse transcriptase, makes a DNA copy of its single-stranded RNA genome to form a double-stranded nucleic acid. Nonnucleotide reverse transcriptase inhibitors and nucleoside reverse transcriptase inhibitors halt this stage of infection. *4. Integration:* HIV then uses integrase, an enzyme that permits HIV to enter into the CD4 cell's nucleus, where the DNA of HIV inserts itself into the host cell's DNA. Integrase inhibitors interfere with HIV's ability to enter into the host's nucleus. *5. Transcription and translation:* The virus is now able to hijack the CD4 cell to produce long viral proteins, which are the building blocks of new HIV viruses. *6. Assembly:* The HIV enzyme protease cuts up those long proteins into smaller ones, which combine with the RNA of HIV to form a new virus. Protease inhibitors intervene at this stage of the life cycle. *7. Budding:* Newly formed HIV viruses push themselves out of the host cell, taking with them the outer proteins of CD4 cell membrane. They then go on to infect other CD4 cells. *Source:* AIDS Info, "The HIV Life Cycle," available at http://www.aidsinfo.nih.gov/education-materials/fact-sheets/19/73/the-hiv-life-cycl, accessed February 6, 2014. See also AIDS.gov, "The Life-Cycle of HIV in Your Cells," revised November 18, 2009, available at http://www.aids.gov/hiv-aids-basics/just-diagnosed-with-hiv-aids/hiv-in-your-body/hiv-lifecycle, accessed February 6, 2014.

envelope glycoproteins, gp41 and gp120, the PI's analog peptide cannot be cleaved.[5] Thus, the ability of the virus to cut nascent proteins is thwarted, and the assembly of new viruses, which would otherwise go on to infect other CD4 cells, is halted.[6] On December 6, 1995, the FDA approved the first protease inhibitor, saquinavir, which Hoffmann-La Roche marketed as Invirase.[7] Big and small pharma still actively creates chemical compounds that can potentially serve as PIs.

Meanwhile, biomedical researchers continued to elucidate the mechanism whereby HIV-1 infects CD4 cells. All stages of infecting the cells, including CD4 binding, CCR5 and CXCR4 (that is, coreceptor) binding, and membrane fusion, are governed by gp120 and gp41 (figure 6.2). The gp120 subunit controls the virus's attachment as well as the CD4 and chemokine-coreceptor binding, and gp41 mediates membrane fusion.[8] The first step in CD4-cell entry is the binding of gp120 with the CD4 receptor. This allows gp120 to undergo critical structural shifts (called confirmational changes), which enable the chemokine coreceptors to bind with gp120.[9] This adhesion brings about subsequent structural shifts that cause the fusion of

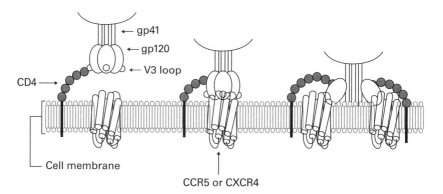

Figure 6.2
The binding of HIV-1 with CD4 and CCR5 during infection. The first step in CD4-cell entry is the binding of gp120 with the CD4 receptor. This leads gp120 to undergo critical structural shifts (called confirmational changes) that enable the chemokine coreceptor (CCR5 or CXCR4) to bind with gp120. This adhesion brings about subsequent structural shifts that cause the fusion of gp41 with the CD4 cell membrane and the glycoprotein's insertion into the host cell plasma membrane via the fusion pore, allowing the viral capsid to enter and infect the host cell. Maraviroc is a CCR5 anatgonist. *Source:* Linos Vandekerckhove, Chris Verhofstede, and Dirk Vogelaers, "Maraviroc: Perspectives for Use in Antiretroviral-Naïve HIV-1-Infected Patients," *Journal of Antimicrobial Chemotherapy* 63, no. 3 (2009): 1087–1096, here 1088.

gp41 with the CD4 cell membrane and the glycoprotein's insertion into the host cell plasma membrane via the fusion pore, allowing the viral capsid to enter and infect the host cell.[10] A fourth class[11] of drugs for HIV/AIDS treatment are entry inhibitors that prevent HIV from entering into CD4 cells. Entry inhibitors are further divided into two subcategories—fusion inhibitors and coreceptor inhibitors. Thus far, only one fusion inhibitor and one coreceptor inhibitor have been approved by the FDA for the treatment of HIV/AIDS.[12]

The first entry inhibitor appeared on the market in 2003—Hoffmann-La Roche's enfuvirtide (Fuzeon), a fusion inhibitor. Approved by the FDA for HIV/AIDS treatment on March 13, 2003, it interferes with the final step in the gp41-fusion of HIV-1 with the CD4 cell membrane. It is a biomimetic peptide that possesses a thirty-four-amino acid sequence that is identical to a portion of HIV-1 gp41.[13] The drug blocks the region of gp41 that is responsible for drilling a hole into the cell membrane so that the virus cannot invade the host cell.[14]

After CCR5 and CXCR4 were shown to be chemokine coreceptors for HIV-1, pharmaceutical companies around the globe searched for chemicals that could potentially bind to the coreceptor, thereby creating a new type of entry inhibitor that binds to the coreceptors rather than to HIV-1. CXCR4 (or fusin) is important to numerous physiological processes. Mice in which the *CXCR4* gene is knocked out die in the embryonic phase as a result of numerous defects of the vascular system, heart, and brain. Humans with truncated mutations of CXCR4 suffer from WHIM syndrome, an immunodeficiency syndrome that involve warts, hypogammaglobulinemia (a primary immune deficiency), and various infections.[15] Since the late 1990s, a number of small-molecule inhibitors that bind to CXCR4 have been produced, but they did not significantly reduce viral loads of HIV.[16] Currently, there are no CXCR4 antagonists in active clinic trial due to their toxicity.[17] CCR5 is less critical for well-being than CXCR4; those homozygous for the *CCR5-Δ32* mutation lead, as far as we call tell, normal lives.[18] As a result, CCR5 inhibitors have progressed further in development than CXCR4 inhibitors.

The techniques that biomedical researchers of big pharma employ to identify small molecules that could bind to CCR5 are high-throughput screening (HTS) and structure-activity relationships (SARs). HTS, the brainchild of pharmaceutical giant Pfizer in the 1980s, is a process by which large numbers of compounds are tested for their ability to bind to and elicit biological activity against target molecules. HTS is used to test molecules that can inhibit enzymatic activity, compete for binding of a ligand to its receptor, or act as agonists or antagonists for receptor-mediated processes—precisely what the Human Genome Sciences patent application for CCR5 claimed. With HTS, robotics, liquid handling, sensors, and data processing are used to investigate hundreds of thousands of molecules and to identify chemicals, antibodies, or other proteins that interact with biological targets that control biochemical pathways. HTS assays are composed of wells, each of which is filled with a chemical compound or antibody and the substance to which it should bind. After allowing time for incubation, an automated machine can measure certain properties, such as the reflectivity of polarized light, thereby determining (for example) if a chemical has bound to a receptor.[19] Pharmaceutical companies often use HTS as the first step toward drug design.

After a target molecule has been pinpointed, medicinal chemists alter certain aspects of molecules via chemical synthesis to test their efficacies as drugs. SAR is the relationship between the three-dimensional structure of a molecule and its biological or pharmaceutical activity, based on the assumption that molecules with similar structures possess similar functions.[20] Introduced in 1972, it now represents the fine-tuning that is done after HTS has identified a target molecule. The two main goals of SAR analysis are to determine the limits of variation in the structure of a chemical that give rise to a specific effect and to define the ways in which changes in structure elicit different properties.[21] Through SAR, medicinal chemists can establish precise correlations between chemical functional groups and biological effects.[22]

There is only one FDA-approved chemokine receptor antagonist that is an entry inhibitor, and it is the first drug to target a component of the human immune system rather than HIV itself. This is Pfizer's Maraviroc, also known as Selzentry outside of the United States, and formerly known as UK-427,857 (figure 6.3). Unlike Hoffmann-La Roche's Fuzeon, which is an injection drug, Maraviroc is an oral drug that inhibits an earlier step in the HIV-1 infection of CD4 cells by binding to CCR5. Its creation was the result of medicinal chemistry optimization based on HTS.

In 1996, a small group of scientists—led by Manos Perros, Anthony Wood, and Elna van der Ryst (all based at Pfizer in Sandwich, United Kingdom)—began work on what would become Maraviroc.[23] Wood was a young chemist who had just completed his postdoctoral training and was hired by Pfizer to replace a retiring scientist as head of its antiviral chemical group. Perros received his Ph.D. in biochemistry two years earlier and had subsequently worked as a postdoc at Yale University before being hired by Pfizer. Van der Ryst is a medical doctor from South Africa who saw firsthand

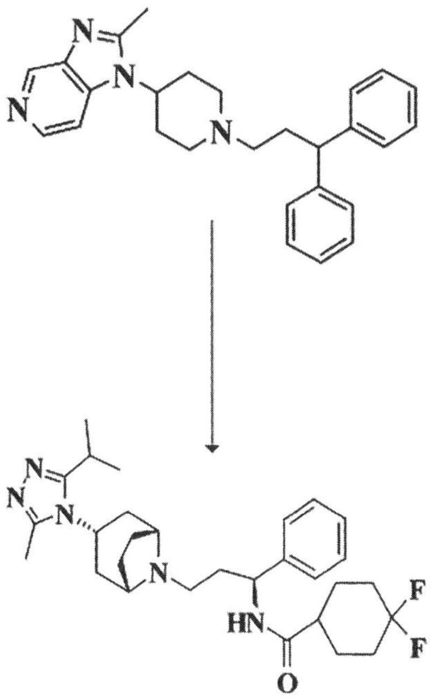

UK-107,543

Maraviroc
(UK-427,857)

Figure 6.3
Pfizer's Maraviroc (UK-427,857) and its precursor (UK-107,543) discovered by high-throughput screening and structure-activity relationship analysis. *Source:* Patrick Dorr, Mike Westby, S. Dobbs, et al., "Maraviroc (UK-427,857): A Potent, Orally Bioavailable, and Selective Small-Molecule Inhibitor of Chemokine Receptor CCR5 with Broad-Spectrum Anti-Human Immunodeficiency Virus Type 1 Activity," *Antimicrobial Agents and Chemotherapy* 49, no. 11 (2005): 4721–4732, here 4724.

the devastation that the epidemic wrought on her homeland. "Every single South African," she noted, "has been touched by HIV, and even as a young doctor I lost friends and patients to the disease. Seeing patients die early in the epidemic shaped my career. For me, it was personal."[24] She jointed Wood and Perros at Pfizer in 1999.

The team commenced the analysis by screening for inhibition of MIP-1β to CCR5 expressed in HEK (human embryonic kidney)-293 cells, the idea being that substances that were similar in structure to the natural ligand would be more likely to bind the receptor.[25] Although there is no guarantee that binding to the chemokine will necessarily mean that the selected molecule will bind to the portion of CCR5 that recognizes HIV-1's gp120, it was a logical place to start. After HTS revealed a number of potential targets, the group filtered out those that did not follow Lipinski's rule of five,[26] those with a low target affinity and ligand efficiency, and those associated with toxicity.[27] In 1997, two compounds from Pfizer's Sandwich library of around 500,000 survived the cut: UK-107,543 and UK-179,645.[28] The next phase, referred to as the "hit-to-lead phase post HTS," tested the viability of hits through SAR studies.[29] Ultimately, UK-107,543 served as the starting point of Pfizer's medicinal chemistry SAR studies that would eventually yield Maraviroc.[30]

Over a two-and-a-half-year-period from 1997 to 1999, nearly a thousand compounds were synthesized and screened based on the structure of UK-107,543 and UK-179,645.[31] For months, team members found numerous synthesized compounds that bound to CCR5, but they did not hinder the replication of the virus. They then found a small molecule that did indeed halt HIV-1's replication. Unfortunately, this molecule also was bound to a protein product of the *hERG* gene (KCNH2) that was involved in the potassium voltage-gated channel, the ion channel that contributes to the electrical activity of the heart coordinating its beats.[32] This could lead to a fatal condition referred to as "long QT syndrome." As a result, parallel screening of the remaining compounds was subsequently implemented for optimal binding potency against CCR5, antiviral activity, absorption, pharmacokinetics, and unwanted selectivity against key human targets, such as cytochrome P4502D6 (CYP2D6), an important enzyme that is involved in metabolizing xenobiotics in the body, and KCNH2.[33] The group also developed two assays—one to measure envelope binding to the cell surface receptors and one to model the subsequent membrane fusion events.[34]

The biomedical researchers produced related compounds to the lead molecule, modifying certain chemical groups and therefore properties of the compounds.[35] After they linked specific chemical groups with specific chemical properties, the group synthesized a compound that showed sufficient potential to merit further clinical exploration, UK-427,857, in late 1999.[36] This compound inhibited MIP-1α, MIP-1β, and RANTES from binding to the CCR5 ligand of HEK-293 cells. It also inhibited virus attachment to CCR5 by competing against the soluble subunit of HIV-1 envelope glycoprotein gp120.[37] In early in vivo trials, the chemical exhibited antiviral activity against lab-adapted HIV-1 strains, primary HIV-1 isolates, and clinically derived HIV-1 envelopes from patients who were resistant to retroviral drugs.[38] The chemical compound would later be called Maraviroc/Selzentry. Pfizer applied for the basic patent in December 1999. It was subsequently awarded by the U.S. Patent and Trademark Office and will expire in December 2019. Pfizer also owns patents for a derivative and for crystalline Maraviroc expiring in 2022 and 2021 respectively. Maraviroc is currently manufactured by ViiV Healthcare, an independent company that was founded by Glaxo-SmithKline and Pfizer in November 2009 and that focused all of its research and development on HIV/AIDS, "combining the power and expertise in the management of HIV from both GSK [GlaxoSmithKline] and Pfizer."[39]

CCR5 again appeared in scientific headlines as the successful target of HTS for drug development during a period when the assay's efficacy was being questioned.[40] Critics argued that HTS undermined the creativity of the pharmaceutical industry, was of poor quality, produced too many false negatives, was too expensive and time consuming, was "anti-intellectual" and "irrational," and failed to locate a sufficient number of lead target molecules.[41] CCR5 became the poster protein for HTS's success. Supporters of HTS, such as Ricardo Macarron, who was vice president of sample management technologies at GlaxoSmithKline, proclaimed in 2011 that it

has matured to become an integral part of pharmaceutical research and a cornerstone in the expansion of biomedical knowledge, following the completion of the Human Genome Project. HTS has provided tool compounds to enhance basic scientific research and lead compounds that have fueled drug discovery projects, resulting in marketed pharmaceutical products. Furthermore many side benefits have arisen from the development and HTS technologies [for example, a clearer understanding of the biology of key target classes such as receptor changes, RNA interference screening, and crystallography].[42]

Such statements serve their purposes and can be misleading at times. Maraviroc was indeed a success story, but despite the enthusiasm and optimism that were generated with the initial success, no other chemical compound binding to CCR5 has been approved by the FDA.

Pfizer was not the only pharmaceutical company to seek CCR5-entry inhibitors. Other companies also turned to HTS and SAR analysis to comb through known chemical compounds as well as synthesize new ones that could target the G protein-couple receptor (GPCR) superfamily.[43] Because antiviral assays had a limited throughput in the mid-1990s, creating a high-throughput strategy that was capable of screening hundreds of thousands of compounds and that provided short turnaround times for SAR generation seemed to be the best way forward in discovering these small-molecule antagonists.[44] The hunt was on.

As was discussed in chapter 2, many of the blockbuster drugs on the market today regulate GPCR activity. Prior to 1996, big pharma had built up substantial libraries of chemical compounds that targeted GPCRs, but two problems quickly became apparent. First, unlike most aminergic GPCRs (ones that are activated by one of the biogenic amines whose ligand domains are limited to the recognition of small basic druglike compounds),

CCR5 recognizes only short polypeptides that bind the receptor in a series of complex processes.[45] Second, it is difficult to synthesize low-molecular-weight inhibitors based on analogy to the natural receptor ligands; therefore, lead chemicals needed to come from random HTS hits.[46] These obstacles notwithstanding, Merck, Schering-Plough, AstraZeneca, GlaxoSmithKline/ONO, Novartis, and Takeda all initiated small-molecule discovery programs that searched for candidates among the known GPCR pharmacophores (the molecular characteristics that are required for recognition of a ligand by a biological molecule).[47] Less than three years after the announcement that CCR5 was the coreceptor for HIV-1, biomedical researchers from the Japanese big pharmaceutical company Takeda synthesized a small-molecule CCR5 antagonist, TAK-779, which was identified via HTS and SARs from lead compounds.[48] Its development was subsequently halted. Another small molecule, TAK-220, was shown to inhibit the binding of MIP-1α to CCR5 and to elicit impressive antiviral properties in vitro. Most recently, these scientists demonstrated that Takeda's TAK-652 competes with MIP-1α, MIP-1ß, and RANTES for binding to CCR5.[49] In addition to Takeda, Merck also published detailed SARs of a series of its chemical compounds that possess CCR5 antagonist activity.[50] Merck's CMPD-167 (MRK-167) was licensed to the International Partnership for Microbiocides, which was developing it as an intravaginal gel to protect women from HIV infection.[51]

The first CCR5 antagonist to advance to human efficacy trials was Schering-Plough's Ancriviroc, which also is known as SCH-C and SCH-351125. Discovered in 2001, it possessed a clear antiviral effect; however, cardiac side effects were detected, particularly interference with the aforementioned hERG potassium ion channel.[52] Another small molecular compound that bound to a hydrophobic pocket of the transmembrane helices of CCR5 was Vicriviroc (SCH 417690/SCH-D), also developed by Schering-Plough in 2003 via HTS and SAR analysis focusing on GPCR pharmacophores.[53] By binding to a small hydrophilic section of CCR5, the receptor underwent a conformational change thereby preventing its binding to HIV-1's gp120.[54] In September 2007, Schering-Plough initiated phase 3 trials[55]—referred to as VICTOR (Vicriviroc in Combination Treatment with an Optimized Antiretroviral Therapy Regimen in HIV-Infected Treatment-Experienced Subjects)-E3 and VICTOR-E4—of the drug; however, the results were not as successful in decreasing viral loads as had been hoped, and it also was associated with interference with the potassium ion channel.[56] As a result, in January 2010, Merck, which had purchased the rights to Vicriviroc from Schering-Plough, decided against seeking FDA approval for the drug.[57]

In October 2005, GlaxoSmithKline and ONO Pharmaceuticals of Japan, which has a licensing agreement with Euroscreen for its CCR5 patent, halted its development of Aplaviroc (GSK873140), a potential CCR5 inhibitor, due to phase 2b reports of idiosyncratic hepatotoxicity (damage to the liver).[58] This molecule had also been developed based on HTS and SAR.[59] In 2005, Incyte started phase 1 trials with INCB-9471, a pipeazinylpiperdine derivative, the exact structure of which remained a secret until after the patent had been granted. Incyte turned to Schering-Plough's Sch-D as a lead compound to create INCB-9471 via rational design.[60]

In addition to synthetic small-molecule antagonists, monoclonal antibodies (mABs)—molecules that bind to the same site, or epitome, of an antigen—are also being investigated as potential HIV therapy. In May 2007, Progenics Pharmaceuticals released the results of phase 1b of the clinical trial of their PRO 140, a mouse anti-CCR5 monoclonal antibody that binds to CCR5, reporting that the drug demonstrated "potent and prolonged antiviral activity."[61] PRO 140 produced highly significant reductions in viral replication for two to three weeks. Nine months later, the FDA designated PRO 140 for fast-track approval, and the drug entered into phase 2 clinical trials.[62] Phase 2 trials further indicated that PRO 140 lowered HIV-1 viral loads in the blood.[63] Because Progenics played a role in the identification of CCR5 as an HIV-1 coreceptor,[64] it is easy to appreciate its displeasure (discussed in chapter 5) over needing to pay a licensing fee to Euroscreen and HGS.[65] PRO 140 has still not entered phase 3 testing.

Human Genome Sciences also decided to develop monoclonal antibodies to CCR5. In September 2006, HGS announced that a phase 1 clinical trial of HGS004 inhibited antiviral activity and could be well tolerated by patients who were infected with HIV-1.[66] Two years later, the mAB once again was shown to elicit antiviral activity and could be tolerated by patients.[67] During the writing of this book, HGS004 remained at phase 1 clinical trial.[68]

In short, the success of therapies that aimed at binding to CCR5 has been limited at best. Perros, one of the Pfizer scientists who developed Maraviroc, expressed the disappointment of biomedical researchers:

But the path leading to potential new therapies has been unexpectedly treacherous. From a number of molecules that once held promise as future therapeutics only a handful remain in development today [2007]. Early chemical lead matter has been relatively easy to find (most chemical files being rich in GPCR pharmacophores) but development of orally bioavailable, selective clinical candidates has proved more challenging.[69]

Medically speaking, these drugs have not been successful.

Intellectual Property, Again

In May 2002, Pfizer completed a licensing agreement with Euroscreen for use of CCR5 to produce Maraviroc as an oral medication.[70] In February 2007, the executive director of the National AIDS Treatment Advocacy Project, Jules Levin, reported the findings of a twenty-four-week study of two randomized, placebo-controlled phase- 2b/3 studies called MOTIVATE (Maraviroc Plus Optimized Therapy in Viremic Antiretroviral Treatment-Experienced Patients)-1, which illustrated the efficacy of the drug.[71] A second, parallel study involving 1,049 patients, MOTIVATE 2, reported that patients who were treated with Maraviroc for forty-eight weeks had "significantly greater suppression of HIV-1 and greater increases in CD4 cell counts" when compared with subjects treated with a placebo.[72] As a result, Maraviroc received accelerated approval from the FDA on August 6, 2007, and traditional approval on November 25, 2008.[73] The FDA's Steven Galson, who later became the acting Surgeon General of the United States and Assistant Secretary for Health, declared, "This is an important new product for many HIV-infected patients who have not responded to other treatments and have few options."[74] It was initially approved for use in adults with R5-tropic HIV-1 infection who were infected with multiple drug-resistant strains and who were treatment-experienced with other antiretroviral therapies. After reviewing a forty-eight- and ninety-six-week efficacy and safety study of phase-3 MERIT (Maraviroc versus Efavirenz Regimens as Initial Therapy), which was a study involving 721 patients beginning antiretroviral therapy for the first time, the FDA advisory committee approved Maraviroc for initial treatment of HIV/AIDS patients trial by a vote of ten to four on October 9, 2009.[75]

The FDA's decision was met with some protests. Several FDA reviewers pointed out that higher viral roads were present in patients treated with Maraviroc than those treated with the NNRTI Sustiva (efavirenz). In addition, 32% of the patients in the MERIT study did not respond to Maraviroc, whereas only 24% did not respond to Sustiva.[76] And many members of the public balked at the cost of Maraviroc, which was "poised to be the most expensive first-line AIDS drug."[77] In 2009, Maraviroc cost $13,767 per patient per annum, after increasing by nearly 10% over a two-year period.[78] Michael Weinstein, president of AIDS Healthcare Foundation, strongly criticized Pfizer's pricing:

In this time of growing national concern over ballooning healthcare costs, it is simply criminal for Pfizer to continue to price Selzentry [Maraviroc] at the salvage therapy rate, especially now that the market for the drug will be vastly expanded by the FDA's likely upcoming approval of the drug for first-line use. Government programs such as AIDS Drug Assistance Programs and Medicaid are likely to be the largest purchaser of Selzentry. Where exactly does the burden of Pfizer's price-gouging fall? On the taxpayers. And for what reason? So that the largest pharmaceutical company in the world, Pfizer, can make just a little more profit—while bankrupting government programs already hurting for funds as they work to ensure that Americans living with HIV/AIDS receive the lifesaving treatment they need. While any new HIV/AIDS drug on the market is welcome, we urge Pfizer to use restraint and to lower the price of Selzentry immediately upon FDA approval for this expanded use.[79]

When the FDA approved Maraviroc for treatment-experienced patients in August 2007, Pfizer optimistically predicted sales of $500 million by 2012. In January 2008, their prediction for 2012 was increased to $650 million.[80]

Such optimism seemed to be substantiated on September 24, 2008, when Maraviroc garnered Pfizer the Prix Galien USA for the "Best Pharmaceutical Agent (Small Molecule)" as a medicine that symbolized "what the biopharmaceutical industry can do to improve the human condition."[81] It went on to win the best new drug award at the 2008 Scrip Awards ("which recognize innovation and excellence across the international biopharmaceutical industry") in London some six weeks later. Maraviroc was described as a "brilliant new approach to anti-HIV therapy by blocking the penetration of the virus, after attachment, into host cells."[82] And in 2010, Perros, Wood, and van der Ryst were recipients of the Discoverers Award presented by the Pharmaceutical Research and Manufacturers of America for "new medicines [that] have greatly benefited humankind" for their work.[83]

The euphoria, however, was ephemeral. Maraviroc sales barely reached $46 million in 2008 and $80 million in 2009, while Sustiva earned $1.15 billion for Bristol-Myers Squibb.[84] Maraviroc sales improved to $124 million in 2010, $177 million in 2011, $204 million in 2012, or less than a third of what Pfizer had predicted in 2008, and $225 million in 2013.[85] And in response to Weinstein's criticism that Selzentry was too expensive, Pfizer did create a patient assistance program (PAP) for HIV/AIDS sufferers who did not possess and could not afford public or private health insurance.[86]

Intellectual property affects the treatment of HIV/AIDS, and it also plays a central role in diagnostics. The FDA requires an assay test before a physician may prescribe Maraviroc. HIV-1 possesses distinct tropisms, as was discussed in chapter 1.[87] When gp120 binds to the primary CD4 receptor, it undergoes a confirmational change that exposes its V3 loop segment and enables it to bind to a secondary coreceptor.[88] Tropism refers to the type of receptor that HIV-1 recognizes on CD4 cells. M-tropic HIV-1 (now more commonly referred to as R5-tropic virus) uses CCR5 as a coreceptor, and T-tropic HIV-1 (now more commonly referred to as X4-tropic virus) uses CXCR4 as a coreceptor. Dual-tropic (or mixed-tropic) HIV-1, which uses both CCR5 and CXCR4 as coreceptors, has also been observed.

Viral isolates during the early stages of HIV-1 infection, before the onset of AIDS, consist predominantly of R5-tropic virus, and after symptoms appear, X4 tropic or dual-tropic strains are isolated from most patients.[89] X4-tropic virus appears in approximately 50% to 60% of the patients on average five years after the initial infection.[90] As David Hardy, researcher and clinician at the Division of Infectious Diseases at Cedars-Sinai Medical Center in Los Angeles, conceded early on: "We don't know exactly what causes this to happen. We don't know whether it's the virus that changes and causes the T cells to fall or whether it's perhaps the falling T cells that have some effect on the virus. But we do know that about half the people who do go on to die from HIV will have an R5 to X4 virus switch sometime during their decline in T cells."[91] Biomedical scientists have recently argued that the shift from R5 to X4 most likely results from the saturation of CCR5 molecules. During the initial phases of infection, R5-tropic virus vastly outnumbers the X4-tropic strains, although small amounts of X4-tropic virus are present. After all of the CCR5 molecules are totally saturated by R5-tropic strains, X4-tropic virus is selected for and enters the hosts' cells via CXCR4.[92] The increase of X4-tropic virus over R5-tropic over time and its correlation with the progression of AIDS strongly suggest that the ability of the viral envelope to interact with CXCR4 signals an important step in HIV's pathogenesis.[93] Because combination antiretroviral therapy (cART), which previously was referred to as highly active retroviral therapy (HAART), preferentially suppresses the replication of X4 strains in vivo, a shift in coreceptor use may contribute to the efficacy of the treatment.[94]

Because Maraviroc binds to the CCR5 receptor, the drug is efficacious in treating only the R5 virus. A tropism assay is needed to see whether the patient is R5 tropic, X4 tropic, or dual (or mixed) tropic. HIV tropism may be assayed either genotypically or phenotypically.[95] The V3 loop of gp120 is the major factor for tropism determination, so the patient's receptor protein can be sequenced. One rule of thumb, referred to as the 11/25 rule, states that if the amino acids at positions 11 and 25 of the gp120 V3 loop have a basic sidechain (arginine or lysine), then it more likely will be an X4 virus.[96] Rules of thumb tend to be imprecise, and the stakes are simply too high for imprecision. The 11/25 rule has less than a 60% sensitivity for detecting X4 virus use.[97]

One tropism blood test, known as the Trofile Assay, is offered by Monogram Biosciences Laboratory, which is now a subsidiary of LabCorp, an international medical biotech company that is headquartered in Burlington, North Carolina. This single-cycle recombinant DNA virus assay involves the construction of a pseudovirus by using recombinant DNA technology with the *gag* and *pol* genes (both necessary for the replication of the virus) taken from HIV-1 to which a light-emitting luciferase gene used as a marker is annealed. This recombinant vector is added to a packing cell, HEK-293, with another recombinant vector, the envelope (*env*) expression vector, which contains the envelope gene taken from the virus found in the patient's blood. The *env* gene codes for gp120, including its V3 loop. The resulting HIV-1 cells then are expressed as cell lines. If all of the lines emit light, then the patient has the R5-tropic virus. If no lines emit light, the patient is X4-tropic. If some lines emit light and some do not, then the patient is dual or mixed tropic.[98] Monogram Biosciences enjoys an out-licensing partnership with Euroscreen/HGS (now GlaxoSmithKline) for the rights to use the *CCR5* gene product.[99] Out-licensing is a type of collaboration in which an inventor takes the initial steps of creating a new product or process but then hands over the work to a third party that markets the product. Both the inventor and the third party profit from the venture.

Health Research Incorporated (HRI) also has developed a coreceptor assay to test for HIV-1 tropism. HRI is a not-for-profit corporation affiliated with the New York State Department of Health (DOH) and the Roswell Park Cancer Institute (RPCI) in Buffalo, New York. HRI's mission is to assist the DOH and RPCI by soliciting and administering financial support for their projects and disseminating scientific expertise through technology transfer.[100] Whereas Monogram Biosciences' test cost $2,800 in 2010, HRI's assay was offered at approximately $1,200.

HRI's heteroduplex tracking assay (HTA) originated in the early 1990s as a method to detect and estimate genetic divergence between HIV strains based on DNA heteroduplexes that form between related but not identical nucleic acid sequences.[101] A heteroduplex is a double-stranded DNA molecule that possesses nearly complementary strands: one strand contains one or more mismatched or unpaired nucleotides. PCR-amplified V3 sequences from a patient are hybridized to the V3 sequences of known R5 or X4 virus. The resulting heteroduplexes will have a reduced mobility during gel electrophoresis, a process by which macromolecules are separated.[102] Whereas the Trofile ES (extrasensitive) test is a cell-based phenotypic assay that tests the entire HIV-1 envelope protein sequence, the HTA test is a nucleic acid–based genotypic test that is based solely on examination of the V3 loop of gp120, coded for by a portion of the *env* gene.

Health Research Incorporated either has patented or has patents pending for a number of methods that are relevant to HTA, including amplifying via PCR of the *env* gene's V3 region that determines the coreceptor binding, generating a population of heteroduplex molecules, separating those heteroduplex molecules via gel electrophoresis, and determining from those molecules whether the coreceptor is CCR5, CXCR4, or both.[103] On November 15, 2007, the U.S. Patent and Trademark Office awarded U.S. Patent 7,294,458 for "Analysis of HIV-1 Co-receptor Use in the Clinical Care of HIV-1 Infected Patients" to HRI, which licensed its test to the California-based company Pathway Diagnostics, which was permitted to sublicense it.[104] Pathway Diagnostics entered into a nonexclusive license agreement with Quest Diagnostics of Madison, New Jersey, on October 26, 2007, for the heteroduplexing technology underlying Pathway Diagnostics' SensiTrop™ HIV Co-Receptor tropism test.[105] Pathway Diagnostics was subsequently acquired by Quest Diagnostics in 2008. A more sensitive assay, SensiTrop II™, was created. Quest Diagnostics currently markets CE-HAD assay, the newest one used for tropism testing. It employs capillary, rather than agar-based, electrophoresis.[106] The nonexclusive license helps enormously to prevent a high cost for the test. Because more than one party may use the product, the cost is lowered.

Intellectual property is relevant to diagnostics and therapeutics not only at the national level. The international conflict between the World Trade Organization and World Health Organization over the protection of intellectual property covering AIDS medications in the face of piracy by Indian companies has been well documented.[107] As a result of intensive negotiations during the first decade of the new millennium, the then secretary general of the United Nations, Kofi Annan, convinced big pharma to offer drugs at cost to developing countries.

In December 2007, the Mumbai Patent Office granted Pfizer a patent on Selzentry. *The Body* reported, "This is the latest development in a series of struggles between multinationals, who want patent protection in the Indian market, and patients' advocates, who say millions of poor people will be affected by decisions that determine the drugs' pricing and availability."[108] Pfizer-India quickly countered, "We are committed to bringing meaningful improvement to the lives of people living with and those at risk of HIV/AIDS through outreach programs that will enable access to innovative medicines to patients."[109]

In November 2010, the Indian drug maker Natco Pharma informed Pfizer that it intended to make and sell a low-cost generic version of Selzentry for the treatment of HIV infection under a compulsory license, which permits another party to produce a patented item or process without the consent of the patent owner. Indian patent law grants compulsory licenses three years after a patent is granted for the remainder of the patent's life if it can be demonstrated that the patented product is not affordable to the public.[110] This generic version would cost Indians $330 a month, as opposed to $1,430 a month for Selzentry. The patent holder has six months to respond after receiving a notice for a voluntary license. In June 2011, ViiV Healthcare, which markets Selzentry, queried Natco's ability to create and market a generic of its drug.[111] In the fall of 2011, Pfizer and Natco were negotiating terms, and as this book was being written, the issue still had not been resolved. Most expect Pfizer to decline the license, citing that research and development for the drug were too expensive, and Natco will most likely reapply.[112] The *Dow Jones Newswires/Smart Money* reported that "Natco Pharma's move is significant because, if successful, the Indian generic drug maker will set a precedent for other Indian companies to override multinational drug makers' patents for the treatments of diseases ranging from cancer to hypertension."[113] According to *Economic Times*, "The fate of the case this year and the government's response could shake up foreign drugmakers' ability to sell high priced patented products in India."[114] They continue by reporting that "this will be the acid test and set a precedent for the use for C[ompulsory] L[icensing] to make medicines affordable for masses in India."[115] Once again, CCR5 is involved in a controversy whose ramifications are far-reaching. Tapan Ray, director general of Organisation of Pharmaceutical Producers of India, argues that "Proposals to promote the use of CL could inhibit technological development in the sector in India and thereby undermine efforts to make medicines and other products widely available to patients."[116]

In March 2012, the Indian government granted Natco a compulsory license to produce its generic version of Nexavar, Bayer's drug that is used to combat liver and kidney cancer. Natco is selling the generic for $170 per month, and the cost of Nexavar is $5,000 per month.[117] In April 2013, the Supreme Court in India ruled that Novartis should not be granted a patent for a cancer drug, Gleevac, because it was too similar to an early drug that the company produced.[118] India law requires that the new drug be demonstrably more effective than the one it is replacing. As a result, Indian companies may now produce generic versions of Gleevac throughout India. In short, the Supreme Court of India seems to favor the issuance of compulsory licenses and a tougher stance on expensive drugs from Western pharmaceutical companies.

This chapter has offered a glimpse into the world of big pharma and its attempt to treat HIV/AIDS patients with a new class of drugs—CCR5 entry inhibitors. But small pharma (such as Progenics and Agouron) is interested in HIV/AIDS treatment as well. The *CCR5* gene's genealogy in this chapter fits squarely under the rubric of biocapitalism. Maraviroc was the product of private research and development. How much did Pfizer spend on that research and development? That is not public knowledge. Big pharma points out that patent protection and the drug's high price are necessary to recoup research and development costs. As Angell has demonstrated, those arguments are commonplace and can be misleading.[119] Intellectual property protection of drugs can result in the exclusion of many people from treatment, given how expensive many of these drugs are. This is where governments need to intervene to support the general welfare. Compulsory licensing might be the way forward.

7   Race, Place, and Pathogens

The *CCR5-Δ32* allele provides some of the most fascinating stories of the *CCR5* gene. It has become a focal point in the debate about allele frequencies and natural selection. Could those who are immune to AIDS have ancestors who were immune to the bubonic plague, smallpox, or staphylococcus infection? How can historians collaborate with population geneticists and demographers to provide a richer history of medicine and biology and a clearer picture of the forces of natural selection? A history of the *CCR5-Δ32* allele is informative because it typifies how molecular biologists, population geneticists, biomedical researchers, and evolutionary biologists study alleles and mutations[1] and determine which ones are present in various human populations. In cases where large differences in allele frequencies are present, population geneticists and evolutionary biologists attempt to determine which (if any) environmental factors are selecting certain alleles over others. As discussed below, soon after the physiological role of CCR5 was elucidated in late spring and summer 1996, the *Δ32* allele was defined, in large part, in terms of race and ethnicity. Biomedical researchers often study populations and genetic diversity by using racial and ethnic categories, despite the fact that there are innumerable ways to analyze human differences.

This chapter offers a genealogy of the gene in the classical sense. After biomedical researchers identified the allele, they immediately sought out its possessors and their ancestors. A map that traces both place and time slowly emerged—a complex family tree of *CCR5-Δ32*. Whereas previous chapters of this book discuss how the federal government (the U.S. Patent and Trademark Office and at times the lower courts) has greatly assisted the biotech sector, this facet of the gene's genealogy owes much to another agency of the federal government—the National Institutes of Health. The USPTO and lower courts passively deferred or acquiesced to the various interests of that sector, but the NIH played an active role in conducting the research and framing the allele in terms of race and ethnicity.

Identifying *Δ32*

In January 1995, five months before Human Genome Sciences filed its patent application for the gene coding for what would become known as CCR5, Rich Koup and his colleagues at the Aaron Diamond AIDS Research Center and an international team from the University of Ancona (Italy), NIH, the University of California at Los Angeles, Duke University, George Washington University, the Public Health Office of San Francisco, and Johns Hopkins University published two articles in the *New England Journal of Medicine* that discussed high-risk men who had been HIV+ for over a decade without any symptoms of the secondary infections that are associated with the onset of AIDS.[2] HIV possesses an unusually long latency period: in most HIV+ subjects, symptoms appear within the first ten years after infection. A handful of individuals, however, remain healthy and immunologically normal (they possess a steady and normal level of CD4 T cells) for longer periods of time. Most of these long-term nonprogressors (LTNPs) possess some plasma viral load (sometimes it can be a substantial amount) of HIV, but some LTNPs possess no viral load. Often the virus cannot be isolated from their plasma; however, the virus can at times be obtained in minute quantities from lymph-node mononuclear cells, or peripheral-blood mononuclear cells (PMBCs).[3] The CD4 T cells of some of these LTNPs can resist high dosages of virus in vitro.[4] This latter group is known as viral controllers.[5]

This phenomenon of individuals who are AIDS negative despite long-term exposure to the virus was related to another, earlier mystery. Biomedical researchers wondered why around 10% to 25% of the 12,000 hemophiliacs who received HIV+ blood between 1978 and 1984, which was before blood could be screened for the virus, evaded infection. More astonishing, approximately 1% of those with HIV in their blood had not progressed to AIDS after fifteen years or more.[6] The geneticist Stephen O'Brien, formerly the chief of the Laboratory of Genomic Diversity at the National Cancer Institute (NCI) (and featured in the PBS documentary discussed in chapter 1), was determined to find the answers.

The origins of O'Brien's research date to 1984. To find HIV-resistant alleles in humans, he and his colleagues turned to the fields of AIDS epidemiology, human molecular genetics, and population genetics.[7] They enrolled public health epidemiologists who were enlisting cohorts in a massive study of HIV/AIDS. These AIDS cohort studies, which commenced in the 1980s and now are conducted globally, offer an ongoing study of HIV infection in thousands of homosexual and bisexual men.[8] Physicians have monitored these groups over the years, taking blood and tissue samples and providing case reports to biomedical researchers.

Scientists drew on the science of retroviruses that previously had been gleaned throughout the twentieth century, particularly David Baltimore and Howard Temin's discovery in 1970 of reverse transcriptase, the enzyme of retroviruses that create a DNA copy from its RNA genome. Knowing that these viruses recognize receptors on host cells and hijack host cell enzymes to insert their viral genes into the host's chromosomes, O'Brien and his colleagues focused on roughly fifty genes whose proteins could in principle influence the life cycle of HIV. They screened individuals within the cohort who possessed different DNA sequences for segments near these genes. Those genetic markers might indicate that alleles of nearby genes differ among the various individuals. The biomedical researchers then divided each cohort into two groups—for example, HIV+ versus HIV– after prolonged exposure or those who rapidly developed AIDS after exposure versus those who either developed AIDS symptoms more slowly or not at all. Finally, they compared how often each allele appeared in each group.[9] As the years went by, more and more data were accrued. By 1997, researchers had over 10,000 samples.[10]

As was noted in chapter 1, during the late spring and summer of 1996, five articles published by a number of U.S. laboratories and one from Belgium appeared in major scientific journals and identified the seven transmembrane G protein, CCR5, as the coreceptor of the HIV-1.[11] Approximately a month later, Nathaniel R. Landau, Bill Paxton, and Richard Koup,[12] of the Aaron Diamond AIDS Research Center of Rockefeller University, and other researchers from Berlex Biosciences of Richmond (California), Massachusetts General Hospital, and the Mount Sinai School of Medicine were among the first to determine that the *CCR5-Δ32* allele conveyed virtually total resistance to HIV-1 infection. Paxton had been sought out by Steve Crohn, a self-described homosexual of European descent who was featured in the PBS documentary, whose partners had died of AIDS, and yet who himself remained HIV-1 negative. Paxton and Koup had been researching individuals who remained HIV-1 negative despite lifestyles that would put them at high risk for the disease. They hypothesized that since these subjects were not closely related, the mutation must have originated in a common ancestor some point in history.[13] When Paxton infected a sample of Crohn's blood with three thousand times the amount of virus needed for HIV-1 infection, the virus failed to enter into Crohn's CD4 cells. Crohn seemed to be immuned to HIV-1 infection. After subsequent tests, Paxton discovered that Crohn was homozygous for the *Δ32* allele.[14]

Landau and Koup's lab then estimated the allele frequency of the *Δ32* mutation, testing 122 unrelated individuals from Western Europe. Twenty-four of them were heterozygous ($24/(122 \times 2$ alleles per person), or an allele frequency of 9.8%). The remaining were homozygous for the wild type. None was homozygous for the mutant allele.[15] As a comparison, forty-six genomic DNAs from Venezuela were tested, and the *Δ32* mutation allele was not found in any of them. They concluded that "the allele is common in some human populations but much rarer in others. These findings suggest a rather recent evolutionary origin of this mutation."[16] Although the article did not mention of race or ethnicity, it mentioned "general population of persons with western European heritage."[17] The allele's genealogy was pointing to a European origin.

Samson's Belgian group and Doms's laboratory at the University of Pennsylvania School of Medicine came up with similar results, and the article was published shortly after Landau, Paxton, and Kroup's study.[18] Whereas Landau, Paxton, and Koup spoke of "human populations," the paper coauthored by the Belgians and the Penn scientists spoke of the "caucasian [sic] populations" and "black populations from Western and Central Africa and Japanese populations."[19] Unsurprisingly, both groups sought to find individuals who might be naturally resistant to AIDS. That is standard procedure when trying to determine how a disease functions and how the spread of infection might be stopped.

Several months later, Mary Carrington of O'Brien's group discovered that *Δ32* appeared in approximately one out of five individuals.[20] Returning to the cohort data, O'Brien's group immediately divided the nearly two thousand high-risk patients into HIV+ and HIV– and compared their *CCR5* genotypes. Three percent of the noninfected individuals were homozygous for *Δ32*, and none of the 1,343 HIV+ group was.[21]

Some U.S. scientists now turned to the aforementioned AIDS cohort studies to gather as much data as possible on the *Δ32* allele.[22] Michael Dean of the National Cancer Institute and Carrington analyzed the DNA of 1,955 individuals, all of whom were in high-risk groups—hemophiliacs, sexually active gay men, and intravenous drug users.[23] The participants were either HIV-1 exposed seronegative, HIV-1 infected AIDS patients, or HIV-1 infected individuals who had not progressed to AIDS over a long period of time. Among the Caucasian cohort (n = 1,250), the *Δ32* allele possessed a frequency of 11.5%, whereas the frequency among African Americans (n = 620) was 1.7%.[24] Such a difference in allele frequency is significant. A pattern began to emerge. Dean postulated that

A large difference in the frequency of the *CKR5Δ32* [*CCR5-Δ32*] allele was observed between Caucasians and African Americans. If widespread screens of African racial groups affirm the absence of the *CKR5Δ32* allele as has been reported in a survey of 124 Africans, it may be that *CKR5Δ32* is a recent mutation that occurred on the

Caucasian lineage subsequent to divergence from the African-Caucasian ancestor estimated to have occurred 150,000 to 200,000 years ago. The frequency observed in African Americans could be entirely due to admixture from Caucasian gene flow in the New World, estimated to be as high as 30%. The relatively high prevalence of the inactivating *CKR5Δ32* allele is suggestive of an historic selective pressure among Caucasians, perhaps by another pathogenic virus or parasite, that also used the CKR5 [CCR5] receptor as an entry point. Such historic increases in recessive disease mutations due to epidemiologic agents have been suggested for other hereditary diseases, including sickle cell anemia, thalassemia, and lysosomal storage diseases.[25]

A similar study was conducted to investigate the frequency of the *Δ32* allele from a random population of platelet donors from the New York Blood Center. About 95% of the samples were from self-identified Caucasians and the remaining 5% from self-reported populations of Asian or African ancestry. Researchers found that the frequency of the mutant allele was skewed toward Caucasians, with an allele frequency of 8.08%—13.3% heterozygous and 1.4% homozygous. Among the much smaller cohorts of those with Asian or African ancestry, they did not detect the allele.[26] The study then investigated the role of the *Δ32* allele in HIV-1 transmission sampling 1,252 participants, all of whom were gay men, 72% (or 907) of whom were Caucasian from the Chicago group of the Multicenter AIDS Cohort Study. Of those from the Chicago study, 461 Caucasian subjects were HIV+, and 446 remained uninfected. Not a single individual who was HIV+ was homozygous for the *Δ32* allele, whereas 3.6% of Caucasians who were at high risk but HIV– were homozygous.[27]

A third study used 1,222 samples obtained from random blood donors at the American Red Cross and the National Laboratory of Parasitic Diseases of the National Institute of Allergy and Infection Diseases. The samples reflected the general racial distribution of North America.[28] As was generally the case, all donors were classified by self-identified racial groups and were mostly homosexual men infected by sexual activity. These included LTNPs who were HIV+, who were asymptomatic for AIDS, who had not had antiretroviral therapy, and who had a CD4 T-cell count of >500/μl for the previous seven years.[29] The study concluded that the *Δ32* allele is common among Caucasian North Americans, is significantly less common in other North American racial groups (African Americans, Native Americans, and Hispanic Americans), and could not be found among samples of Tamil Indians and West African blacks.[30]

In a study involving 3,342 individuals worldwide, the *Δ32* allele seemed to be present with a frequency of around 10% of those of "European descent" and was not found in the "black population," with the exception of African

Americans, in whom admixture "with people of European descent has been considerable."[31] Some researchers did warn that although over four thousand "European and Caucasian-American samples" had been assayed, only 747 samples from indigenous non-Europeans had been analyzed.[32]

Scores of articles appearing in biomedical journals generated a more refined and detailed allele distribution global map for *CCR5-Δ32*.[33] One now began to read about studying geographic populations as a way to sharpen the focus of allele-frequency analysis (figure 7.1). For example, over 2,500 individuals from eighteen "European populations" were genotyped, confirming that the highest percentage of the *Δ32* allele was found in northeastern Europe.[34] One study listed the distribution of the allele in terms of geography (nations); however, it also included ethnicities such

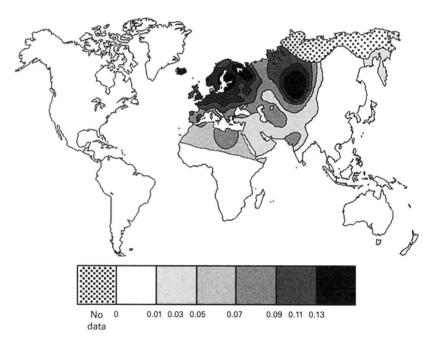

No   0   0.01 0.03 0.05   0.07   0.09 0.11 0.13
data

Figure 7.1
Worldwide frequency distribution of *CCR5-Δ32*. The allele is found with the greatest frequency (the darkest shaded areas) in the Scandinavian and Baltic countries and parts of Russia. The claim is that the "[o]nly frequencies of Native populations have been evidenced in Americas, Asia, Africa and Oceania." *Source:* Eric Faure and Manuela Royer-Carenzi, "Is the European Spatial Distribution of the HIV-1 Resistant *CCR5-Δ32* Allele Formed by a Breakdown of the Pathocenosis Due to the Historical Roman Expansion?," *Infection, Genetics and Evolution* 8 (2008): 864–874, here 865.

as "Caucasian American," "Hispanic American," "Israel, Ashkenazim," and "Israel, "Sephardim."[35] Another study also analyzed the frequency in terms of nations and ethnicities. For example, sampling 4,166 individuals from "thirty-eight ethnic groups," National Cancer Institute scientists found that the allele occurred with the highest frequency of over 13% of the populations in Slovakia, Poland, Estonia, Russia, and Sweden and was not present at all in among Georgians, Lebanese, Saudis, several tribes of Native Americans (Cheyenne, Pima, and Pueblo), Koreans, and Chinese.[36]

Racial and ethnic categories, however, still dominated the literature.[37] In addition to *Δ32*, seven other *CCR5* alleles were identified, five of which were detected in a population of Hispanic Americans, two among Chinese Americans, and two among Japanese Americans. None of these seven mutations was found in the Caucasian Americans screened.[38] One study concluded "that the mutations in *CCR5* are relatively specific to different ethnicities."[39] The terms *race* and *ethnicities* were never precisely defined in these multiple studies. Indeed, the terms seem to be used interchangeably (figures 7.2, 7.3, 7.4).

Genetic Variants of the CCR5 Gene

VARIANT[a]	NUCLEIC ACID SUBSTITUTION	No. of Alleles Observed/Total No. of Chromosomes (Frequency)[b]	
		Caucasians	African Americans
I12L	A25C	1/382 (.003)	0/664 (.0)
C20S	T58A	2/698 (.003)	0/664 (.0)
A29S	G85T	NT	1/64 (.015)
I42F	A124T	1/170 (.001)	NT
L55Q	T164A	29/708 (.041)	5/664 (.007)
R60S	G180T	NT	1/76 (.013)
A73V	C218T	3/462 (.002)	0/664 (.0)
S75S	T215C[c]	0/212 (.0)	9/664 (.013)
C101X	T303A	NT	1/70 (.014)
I164I	C492A[c]	1/98 (.010)	NT
Δ32(185)	Δ32	520/5,210 (.10)	38/2,030 (.019)
R223Q	G668A	1/64 (.016)	NT
228delK	680del3	1/490 (.002)	0/494 (.0)
V300V[c,d]	C900A	1/242 (.0)	0/100 (.0)
G301V	G902T	1/90 (.011)	0/268 (.0)
A335V	C1004T	1/174 (.006)	12/484 (.025)
Y339F	A1016T	0/242 (.0)	3/116 (.026)

[a] Except in the case of 228delK, the first letter in each entry denotes the wild-type amino acid; the number denotes the position; and the letter following the number denotes the mutated amino acid; 228delK is a triplet deletion of lysine (K) at position 228. In the case of I12L, A29S, and Y339F, the substitutions are conservative, based on net charge; all other substitutions are nonconservative, resulting in alteration of amino acid charge.

[b] "NT" denotes that controls for the variants were not included on gels representing that particular region; thus, it is not certain that the variant would have been identifiable if it indeed had been present on that gel.

Figure 7.2
Genetic variants of the *CCR5* gene found in Caucasians and African Americans. *Source:* Mary Carrington, Terri Kissner, Bernard Gerrard, et al., "Novel Alleles of the Chemokine-Receptor Gene *CCR5*," *American Journal of Human Genetics* 61 (1997): 1261–1267, here 1264.

Clinical Description of Individuals with CCR5 Alleles Altering Amino Acid Sequences

Variant (Patient)	Risk Group	Race	HIV-1 Status	AIDS Status[a]	No. of Years HIV-1 Positive and AIDS Negative[b]	CCR5-Δ32 Genotype[c]
I12L	Hemophilia	Caucasian	Positive	Negative	13.6	+/CCR5-Δ32
C20S(1)	Homosexual	Caucasian	Positive	Negative	15.1	+/+
C20S(2)	Homosexual	Caucasian	Positive	Positive	12.2	+/+
A29S	IV drug user	African American	Positive	Negative	5.7	+/+
I42F	Homosexual	Caucasian	Negative	Negative	NA	+/CCR5-Δ32
L55Q(1)[d]	Hemophilia	African American	Positive	Negative	8	+/+
L55Q(2)	IV drug user	African American	Positive	Negative	7.4	+/+
L55Q(3)	IV drug user	African American	Positive	Negative	8.5	+/+
L55Q(4)	IV drug user	African American	Negative	Negative	NA	+/+
L55Q(5)	IV drug user	African American	Negative	Negative	NA	+/+
R60S	IV drug user	African American	Negative	Negative	NA	+/+
A73V(1)	Hemophilia	Caucasian	Positive	Positive	11.9	+/CCR5-Δ32
A73V(2)	IV drug user	Caucasian	Negative	Negative	NA	+/+
A73V(3)	Homosexual	Caucasian	Positive	Positive	7.8	+/CCR5-Δ32
C101X	IV drug user	African American	Positive	Negative	6.3	+/+
R223Q	Homosexual	Caucasian	Positive	Positive	13.1	+/+
228delK	IV drug user	Caucasian	Positive	Negative	11.3	+/+
G301V	Homosexual	Caucasian	Positive	Negative	15.2	+/+
A335V[x]	Hemophilia	Caucasian	Positive	Negative	14.9	+/+
Y339F(1)	Hemophilia	African American	Positive	Positive	10.5	+/+
Y339F(2)	IV drug user	African American	Positive	Negative	7.3	+/+
Y339F(3)	IV drug user	African American	Positive	Negative	2.8	+/+

[a] According to 1987 CDC definition.

Figure 7.3
Individuals categorized by race with CCR5 alleles, which result in different amino acid sequences. Source: Mary Carrington Terri Kissner, Bernard Gerrard, et al., "Novel Alleles of the Chemokine-Receptor Gene CCR5," American Journal of Human Genetics 61 (1997): 1261–1267, here 1264.

NCI scientists screened Caucasian Americans and African Americans to seek out the frequency of various CCR5 alleles.[40] They reported sixteen new CCR5 alleles of which "eight … were identified only in Caucasians, five were found exclusively among African Americans, one was found only in a Hispanic, and two mutations, L55Q and A355V, were present in both Caucasian and African Americans."[41] The higher frequency of the L55Q mutations among Caucasian Americans when compared to African Americans suggested that the mutation was relatively new and added to the African American population after admixture with Caucasian Americans. On the other hand, the A335V mutation was found at higher levels among African Americans than Caucasian Americans and therefore was either old, before the split between the two groups, or of recent African origin.[42] Not just Δ32 but a number of other CCR5 alleles and haplotypes (or allele combinations at adjacent loci or chromosomes) seemed to have "race-specific HIV-1 disease-modifying effects."[43] Enrique Gonzalez of the University of Texas Health Science Center of San Antonio and Michael Bamshad of the University of Utah (now at the University of Washington) demonstrated that amined the phenotypic effects of several *CCR5* alleles that share some mutations but are diverse for others.

Racial distribution of evolutionarily-related *CCR5* alleles
If *CCR5* alleles have a hierarchical, history-dependent structure, then their racial distribution may reflect the specific evolutionary relationships and selective pressures among the observed alleles. To this end, we found that the genotype frequencies of each of the polymorphisms studied were in Hardy-Weinberg equilibrium ($P > 0.05$), and that the allelic frequencies in the different racial groups of the *CCR2-64I* and *CCR5-Δ32* alleles mir-

mozygous for the *CCR5-927C* allele. These trends were significant for prolongation of survival in the cohort as a whole (Relative hazard (RH) = 0.76; 95% confidence interval (CI) = 0.60–0.97; $P = 0.03$) and for AIDS-free survival in seroconverters (RH = 0.62; 95% CI = 0.39–0.98; $P = 0.039$), and approached significance for survival in seroconverters (RH = 0.56; 95% CI = 0.31–1.0; $P = 0.058$) and AIDS-free survival in the whole cohort (RH = 0.80; 95% CI = 0.64–1.0; $P = 0.056$).

We next examined the disease-modifying effects of the two haplotypes associated with the *CCR5-927T* allele. Inspection of the KM curves showed that, relative to the *CCR5-927T* alleles

Table 2 Racial distribution of different *CCR2*, *CCR5* and *SDF* genotypes

Race	CCR2-64			CCR5+29			CCR5+927			CCR5		SDF-1-3'A		
	V/V	V/I	I/I	A/A	A/G	G/G	C/C	C/T	T/T	wt/wt	wt/Δ32	G/G	G/A	A/A
Caucasian	479 (82.7)	95 (16.4)	5 (0.86)	459 (79)	113 (19.5)	9 (1.6)	471 (81.4)	103 (17.8)	5 (0.86)	490 (84.5)	90 (15.5)	354 (61.1)	197 (34)	28 (4.8)
Afr. Amer.	288 (72.5)	96 (24.2)	13 (3.3)	353 (88.5)	46 (11.5)	0	261 (65.6)	116 (29.2)	21 (5.3)	380 (95.5)	18 (4.5)	45 (64.3)	22 (31.4)	3 (4.3)
Hispanic	52 (74.3)	16 (22.9)	2 (2.9)	64 (91.4)	6 (8.6)	0	48 (68.6)	20 (28.6)	2 (2.9)	66 (94.3)	4 (5.7)	45 (64.3)	22 (31.4)	3 (4.3)
Other	20 (62.5)	12 (37.5)	0	25 (78.1)	7 (21.9)	0	18 (56.3)	14 (43.8)	0	28 (87.5)	4 (12.5)	17 (53.1)	13 (40.6)	2 (6.25)

Numbers in parenthesis denote the frequency of the indicated genotypes in different racial groups. 'Other' indicates Asians, American Indians, and other racial groups. *SDF-1-3'A* denotes the *SDF1-G801A* polymorphism.

Figure 7.4
Racial distribution of different *CCR2* (chemokine receptor 2), *CCR5*, and *SDF* (stromal cell-derived factor) genotypes. *Source:* Srinivas Mummidi, Seema S. Ahuja, Enrique Gonzalez, et al., "Genealogy of the *CCR5* Locus and Chemokine System Gene Variants Associated with Altered Rates of HIV-1 Disease Progression," *Nature Medicine* 4, no. 7 (1998): 786–793, here 788.

This varied distribution of *CCR5* haplotypes results in an uneven distribution of *CCR5* haplotype pairs in global populations.... For example, 75% of the *CCR5* haplotype pairs in Europeans or Asian Indians can be accounted by only eight or six *CCR5* haplotype pairs, respectively, and six of these haplotype pairs are common to both populations. In contrast, in individuals of African descent (e.g., in African Americans), the eight most common *CCR5* haplotype pairs account for less than 50% of the haplotype pairs and, of these, only three are among the most common haplotype pairs found in Europeans or Asian Indians.[44]

Jianming "James" Tang of the University of Alabama–Birmingham School of Medicine concurred, arguing for a "racial distribution" of chemokine-receptor genes: "Thorough documentation of the extended *CCR2* and *CCR5* haplotypes has suggested that stable CCR haplotypes, alone or paired as genotypes, may influence the course of HIV-1 infection differentially according to their racial distribution" (figure 7.5).[45]

Other research showed that the range of *CCR5* haplotype pairs associated with different rates of disease progression in HIV-1 infection differs between Caucasian and African Americans. For example, two haplotypes,

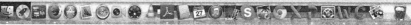

Table 1. CCR5 haplogroup frequencies in different racial and ethnic groups

	African		African American		Asian	Caucasian		Hispanic American
Haplogroup	Pygmies	Non-pygmies	Uninfected	HIV-1 infected	Uninfected	Uninfected	HIV-1 infected	HIV-1 infected
HHA	70.6 (34)	26.5 (49)	22 (209)	20.1 (410)	16.8 (158)	10.7 (248)	9.3 (618)	9.5 (74)
HHC	2.0 (25)	10.6 (71)	15.6 (212)	14.8 (410)	36.5 (163)	37.1 (206)	36.3 (618)	34.5 (74)
HHD	0 (37)	20.1 (82)	18.4 (212)	20.1 (410)	4.4 (34)	0 (429)	1.0 (618)	3.4 (74)
HHE	11.8 (38)	20.7 (58)	18.4 (193)	18.7 (410)	25 (376)	31.8 (140)	31.9 (618)	30.4 (74)
HHF*1	6.3 (40)	11.8 (68)	4.1 (195)	5.0 (410)	1.6 (478)	2.0 (154)	0.8 (618)	2.7 (74)
HHF*2	6.3 (40)	14.7 (68)	14.1 (195)	14.9 (410)	12.8 (478)	5.5 (154)	8.6 (618)	14.2 (74)
HHG*1	2.5 (40)	0.7 (71)	4.5 (210)	3.7 (410)	0.8 (518)	3.3 (151)	4.4 (618)	2.0 (74)
HHG*2	0 (40)	0 (71)	2.6 (210)	2.3 (410)	0.1 (518)	5.6 (151)	7.7 (618)	3.4 (74)

The number in parentheses denotes the number of individuals from whom the haplotype frequency (%) was derived. HHB haplotypes are rare, and their frequencies are not shown. Also, because of failure to amplify by PCR all CCR5 polymorphisms and/or limited DNA quantities, the number of noninfected individuals for whom complete haplotype frequency data are available varies. Hence, for these two reasons the frequencies approximate but do not total to 100%. Individuals in whom a CCR5 haplotype appeared to be a product of a recombination event were excluded from analysis.

strable in African Americans (Fig. 3 a and b) but not Caucasians   are no demonstrable differences between various combinations

Figure 7.5

Comparison of CCR5 haplotype frequencies found in different racial and ethnic groups. *Source:* Enrique Gonzalez, Michael Bamshad, Naoko Sato, et al., "Race-Specific HIV-1 Disease-Modifying Effects Associated with CCR5 Haplotypes," *Proceedings of the National Academy of Sciences (PNAS) USA* 96, no. 21 (1999): 12,004–12,009, here 12,006. Copyright 1999, National Academy of Sciences, USA.

HHA and HHF*2, are present in significantly higher frequencies in African Americans than in Caucasian Americans. Their phenotypic effect, however, was present only in African Americans. The haplotype HHC, on the other hand, is found in a disproportionately higher frequency in Caucasians: when present in African American populations, it increased the rate of HIV progression to AIDS unless it was paired with an HHA or HHF*2 allele.[46] CCR5 haplogroup frequencies (or an aggregate of a number of distinct haplotypes, which possess a common ancestry) "varied substantially among races and ethnic groups."[47] Such interactive effects among CCR5 haplotypes can be explained not by simply looking at DNA mutations but also by gathering information about the various populations' evolutionary histories. The relationship between allele variants of the CCR5 gene and disease progression is germane for the design, implementation, and testing for HIV-1 as well as for the efficacious treatment and prevention of AIDS.[48]

Attention was then turned to the various CCR5 alleles in Africa, where the HIV/AIDS epidemic had reached epic proportions. In 2000, Δ32 was found with a frequency of merely 0.1% in South African Africans (SAAs), and 9.4% in South Africans of Caucasian descent (SACs).[49] The allele frequency of the *SDF1'3A* allele of the *CCR5* gene was 1.0% among SAAs and 20.3% among SACs, and the allele *CCR5m303* had a frequency of 0.7% among SACs and was not found in SAAs.[50] In 2001, South African geneticists identified seven novel alleles to the *CCR5* gene locus, all of which occurred in non-Caucasians, hinting at an African origin of those mutations. In addition, a 24-base pair deletion in the *CCR5* gene was found only in a central African population.[51] Investigators also found that the *Δ32* allele was absent in all 134 Africans studied but possessed a 3% allele frequency among "the Coloured population," most likely due to admixture with SACs.[52] A high frequency for a mutation at codon 35 of *CCR5* was found among SAAs and the "Coloured" population and was absent in all SAC members of the study, indicating "a definite African origin."[53] Similarly, one study suggested that the *codon-335* allele was present in nearly the same frequency among SAA and "Coloured" population at circa 2%. A subsequent study had the SAA frequency over 7% and found the allele in one of 35 SACs.[54] In short, South African investigators found sixty- and thirty-seven polymorphisms in the SAA and SAC populations, respectively.[55]

The *Δ32* allele is not only rare in South African blacks and absent in Central and Western African populations, but it is also extremely rare among other non-European populations. In 2000, an article in *Clinical Infectious Diseases* declared that *CCR5-Δ32* "do[es] not exist in Chinese people."[56] Despite this pronouncement, one year earlier groups at Mount Sinai School of Medicine in New York and in China had reported the "first case of *ccr5-Δ32* mutation in the Chinese population" from a sample of 407 individuals from mainland China.[57] The frequency in that sample was 0.00123, significantly lower than in Caucasians. In 2001, a study confirmed the frequency of *CCR5-Δ32* to be 0.00119 (or 0.12%) in China.[58] A 2003 study of seventy Chinese adults, ten each from seven different ethnicities (Han, Meng, Zang, Weiwuer, Zhuang, Yi, and Dai), found only one heterozygote *CCR5-Δ32* in an individual of Weiwuer ethnicity.[59] The Weiwuer Chinese live near the Russian border; hence, gene flow from Russia seemed to be the likely cause of the presence of that allele. The likelihood of finding someone in China who is homozygous for *Δ32* is around one in a million.

U.S. biomedical researchers also investigated alleles in the *CCR5* promoter region (the portion of the DNA that initiates the gene's transcription into mRNA) to see if there was a link to race there as well.[60] One mutation in the promoter region of *CCR5* (*CCR5P1*) accelerates the rate of infection and progression to AIDS in both African Americans and Caucasian Americans;

however, it has a dominant effect in African Americans and a recessive one in Caucasian Americans.[61] The reason for this counterintuitive result may be the presence of modulating genes or an as yet unknown polymorphism that differs between the two groups.[62]

The key point of these studies that link various populations with differing alleles of *CCR5* and its promoter and regulatory sequences is the link between race, genetics, and medical treatment: "to predict possible clinical responses to the AIDS epidemic and thus develop proper preventive and treatment measures in advance."[63] Other studies underscore the fact that "[t]he *CCR5* variants exhibit distinct patterns of ethnic distribution, with *CCR5 Δ32*, for example, being most prevalent in white populations (moderately so among inhabitants of Europe, the Middle East, and the Indian subcontinent) but exceedingly rare among Africans and most Asians."[64] Once again, one hears that "[i]t is well known that genetic polymorphisms and haplotype structures can vary among ethnic groups."[65] An "Asian-specific *CCR5 893(-)* allele" was discovered as a single-nucleotide deletion in the *CCR5* coding region (figure 7.6).[66]

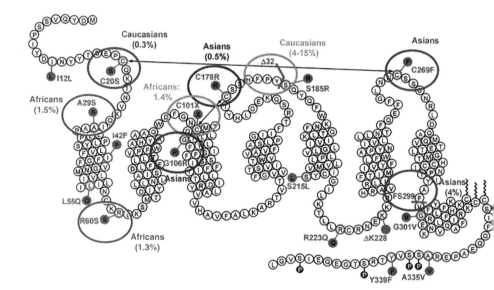

Figure 7.6
CCR5 mutants and variants: frequency of mutations giving rise to different amino acid sequences in Africans, Asians, and Caucasians. *Source:* Fernando Arenzana-Seidedos and Marc Parmentier, "Genetics of Resistance to HIV Infection: Role of Co-receptors and Co-receptor Ligands," *Seminars in Immunology* 18, no. 6 (2006): 387–403, here 391.

By the millennium's end, scientists concluded with relative confidence that the *CCR5-Δ32* allele has the highest frequency in northern Europe, particularly in the Baltic region (around 16% overall, which a high of 18% observed on the isolated Estonian Island of Dagö, or Hiiumaa[67]), and decreases in frequency in a southeast cline, with Portugal and Greece having a frequency between 4% and 6%.[68] Allele frequencies in northern Africa are around 2%, and the allele is not found in central or western Africa. The Middle East and India both have low frequencies, as do Japan and China. In the United States, as mentioned in chapter 1, the frequency among Caucasians is about 10%, and the frequency among African Americans is merely 2% based on admixture.[69] Given those frequencies, approximately three in a hundred persons from the Baltic are homozygous for *Δ32*, about one in 100 Caucasian Americans is homozygous, and about one in 2,500 African Americans is. Everyone seemed to agree with the worldwide distribution percentages of the *Δ32* allele, and most seemed happy to argue that given those frequencies, there must have been some selective advantage to possessing the mutation.

Dating *Δ32* or Picking Your Parasite

If the variation in allele frequency is indeed an example of natural selection, what in nature was (and perhaps still is) selecting for it? Could it be a pathogen? Did the allele render lucky homozygous owners immune to an epidemic, as O'Brien originally claimed in the PBS documentary of 2002? HIV itself seemed an unlikely candidate because the virus's origin dates back to the 1920s or 1930s: it is too recent to account for such a range in global frequencies. The case might be similar to the story of malaria. Those who are heterozygous for sickle-cell allele are immune to malaria infection. A relatively high percentage of the sickle-cell allele is found in regions of the world where malaria is present. It is not a so-called black disease, as was thought in the early twentieth century, but rather a disease that is selected for by a pathogen in a particular environment. Another gene that gives rise to a disease and that is selected for is *ΔF508*. It is associated with cystic fibrosis and is present in approximately one in thirty Caucasians. Scientists believe that this mutation conveys a selection advantage by reducing water loss during cholera infection. And the so-called thrifty genes, proposed by the geneticist James V. Neel in 1962 to explain the prevalence of diabetes, enable individuals to turn food efficiently into fat during times of abundance. During periods of food scarcity throughout history, they survive by drawing on their stored fat.[70] In short, *CCR5-Δ32* could become another example of an allele that is associated with protection from a disease selected for by natural selection or "a case study in the co-evolution of a parasite-host system."[71]

Geneticists needed to determine the age of the allele to see which historical diseases might have selected for Δ32. They already had mapped the space (or geographic distribution) of the allele; they now needed to map its history. The leaves of the genealogical tree were located, so now it was time to date its trunk. The date, spatial distribution, and frequency of the allele are all related. The greater the age of the mutation, the greater the time for genetic drift to act on a neutral polymorphism. If the mutation is relatively young and the frequencies are high, then chances are that some selection must be occurring. Recall from chapter 1 that Goldstein and O'Brien dated Δ32 by analyzing genetic markers in the vicinity of the allele. Mathematical models yielded an approximate age of seven hundred years for the origin of the mutation, which corresponded to the time of the outbreak of Black Death in mid-fourteenth-century Europe. Most, but not all, early studies corroborated that date.[72] These biomedical researchers suggested that the Black Death from 1346 to 1352 provided that selective pressure. It fell within their time frame of the mutation's origin, and it was an extremely lethal plague that, in principle, would strongly select for the relevant allele.[73]

In 2001, William Klitz of the University of California at Berkeley, with the assistance of colleagues from UC at San Francisco and Israel, studied the Δ32 mutation in Jewish and northern European population samples, suggesting that Δ32 was indeed between seven hundred and a thousand years old and that it was favored by a relatively recent selection, corroborating earlier studies that suggested that a selection process took place on the allele in northern Europe within the past thousand years.[74] Their evidence for this conclusion was the discrepancy between allele frequencies of Ashkenazi and Sephardic Jews, the former of whom separated from the latter and moved to northern Europe some thousand years ago. It turns out that the allele frequency of Δ32 is about 13% to 14% among Ashkenazi Jews and 4.5% among Sephardic Jews.[75] The high percentage among Ashkenazi Jews is attributed to admixture with northeastern European populations. More important to my story than the support of the allele dating was Klitz and his colleagues' suggestion of a different epidemic—smallpox.[76] With a fatality rate of 25%, the variola virus that causes smallpox could provide a strong selection pressure on the Δ32 allele because the first known outbreak of the virus in Europe occurred during the eighth century A.D. And it turns out that the myxoma virus of the poxvirus family, which includes the variola virus, recognizes chemokine receptors—specifically, CCR1, CCR5, and CXCR4.[77] In addition, the crystal structure of cowpox virus, which possesses a 95% genetic similarity to smallpox, reveals a site of conserved amino acid residues, which are likely candidates for the binding of CC-chemokines, such as CCR5.[78]

The allele's genealogical account took an interesting turn later that year when Gérard Lucotte of the Center of Molecular Neurogenetics in Paris proffered an explanation for the distribution of the $\Delta 32$ allele.[79] He and his colleague Géraldine Mercier had suggested in 1998 that the Vikings might be crucial to the allele's dissemination across Europe because $\Delta 32$ occurred in the largest frequencies among the Nordic populations.[80] In 2002, he revisited that hypothesis.[81] The Vikings conquered territories along the northern coasts of what are now Germany, France, Spain, and the United Kingdom. The Varangians in Russia migrated to the east, where they established the Russian state. The high frequency of $\Delta 32$ in Finland, Estonia, and Russia can be explained by this hypothesis.[82] Lucotte added that if the variola virus did result in a selective force for the $\Delta 32$ allele, this would explain the rapid increase of the allele throughout Europe.[83] In 2003, Lucotte and his colleague Florent Dieterlen continued to flesh out the Viking hypothesis by tracing the allele distribution against the Viking raids throughout the eighth, ninth, and tenth centuries:

So, it could be considered that the Viking theory of the origin of the $\Delta 32$ mutation fits well historical (estimated date of origin) and geographical (deduced allele map) data. During the Viking age (the eighth-tenth centuries), the Scandinavian Vikings dominated much of the northern [sic] of Europe and elsewhere. They raided during this period in various European countries: Normans on the coasts of France and Spain, Danes in Britain, Varangians in Finland and Russia. That sort of distribution in $\Delta 32$ frequencies indicates the existence in the past of a Scandinavian center of origin, and further dissemination of the mutation from this center.[84]

By December 2003, biologists were becoming unconvinced that the Black Death could be the selective agent for $\Delta 32$; perhaps the early studies had been premature.[85] The Black Death was indeed as widespread as it was lethal, killing 25% to 40% of Europeans of all ages from 1346 to 1352. Subsequent plagues, however, were less severe, and sporadically affected individual cities. The Great Plague of 1665 and 1666 wiped out between 15% and 20% of London's population. Afterwards, the bubonic plague wrecked far less havoc: the last recorded outbreak in France was in 1720 and 1721, and England was free from the pest after 1667. After 1750, the bubonic plague had by and large vanished.[86] Whereas the bubonic plague is transmitted via flea bites, smallpox is transmitted directly from person to person, and children are most susceptible because they are, immunologically speaking, the weakest. As a result, smallpox infected most Europeans up to the age of ten, and it possessed a mortality rate of about 30%.[87] In addition, the mortality gradient that was wrought by the Black Death sloped in the opposite direction of present-day genotypes. According to the population geneticist Montgomery Slatkin and epidemiologist Alison Galvani, "the Black Death and Great Plague pandemics in Europe represent strong bouts of episodic selection, whereas ongoing smallpox epidemics represent weaker, but more continuous selection."[88] Finally, historians have placed the origins of the Black Plague in or near China and hypothesized that it traveled to Europe via infected fleas on rats hitching a ride on the Silk Road. Why, then, is the allele frequency of $\Delta 32$ low in China?

Galvani and Slatkin's mathematical model of a population found that the bubonic plague could not generate the necessary allele frequencies that were observed across Europe, even assuming that the $\Delta 32$ allele was dominant over seven hundred years. The model demonstrated that the plague would not have pushed up the allele frequency to 1% during the three centuries that it infected Europe. Smallpox, however, given its ability to kill more children than the plague over a much longer span of time, could have provided the sufficient selective pressures to generate the observed allele frequencies.[89] Although their model assumed the age of allele to be seven hundred years, it turns out that an older date would favor the smallpox theory because it would allow more generations to generate higher frequencies. Historical evidence suggests that smallpox epidemics have existed for over two thousand years.[90] Scandinavian countries were hit much harder by smallpox than other European countries, whereas central Europe suffered more under the bubonic plague. Finally, experiments were performed to test the *Y. pestis* hypothesis, and clinical studies suggested that *Y. pestis* does not interact with CCR5.[91] A study published in *Nature* detailed the experiments on the susceptibility of two groups of mice to *Y. pestis*, one group possessed CCR5 and the other did not.[92] The researchers found that that there was not a significant difference between the bacterial load or of the survival rate of the two groups. They concluded "that CCR5 deficiency in mice does not protect against infection or death caused by experimental *Yersinia* infection, making it unlikely that the *CCR5Δ32* allele protects against plague."[93] Colleagues at Imperial College in London concurred, concluding that "[t]he plague connection was an excellent story to tell, but the analysis indicates that the temporal correlation between the estimated allele age and the historical plague epidemic was probably coincidental."[94] Smallpox had emerged as the new leader in the CCR5 saga.

The speculation continued, as is commonplace when theories are con-cocted to account for limited data. Three British scholars—S. R. Duncan from the University of Oxford's Department of Engineering Science and Susan Scott and Christopher J. Duncan from the University of Liverpool's School of Biological Sciences—decided to add a new twist. They supported yet another candidate pathogen.[95] At the time, Scott and C. J. Duncan had just completed their book, *Biology of Plagues: Evidence from Historical Popula-tions*,[96] which drew on techniques provided by molecular biologists, his-torians and sociologists of epidemics, and computer scientists working on disease modeling. They purported that the Black Death of the 1340s and 1350s and the Great Plague of the 1660s were not caused by *Y. pestis* but by some other microbes, probably filoviruses, which cause hemorrhagic fevers such as the Ebola fever.[97] Not surprisingly, they postulated that these filovi-ruses—and neither *Y. pestis* nor the variola virus—caused these plagues and served as the selective force of the *Δ32* allele. They disputed the younger age of seven hundred years and supported an older age of a few thousand years. The allele reached its fourteenth-century frequency "by sporadic epidem-ics of haemorrhagic plague which occurred widely over the eastern Medi-terranean area during a very long time span."[98] They pointed to evidence that hemorrhagic plague continued in Scandinavia, Poland, Russia, and the European-Asian borders throughout the eighteenth century.[99] Downplay-ing the importance of reoccurring smallpox epidemics every five years in Europe from the 1340s to 1970 as a selective factor, they insisted that a lethal form of smallpox first appeared in England in the 1620s, resulting in an annual smallpox death rate in London that consistently exceeded a thousand only after 1710.[100] The number of deaths brought about by small-pox declined rapidly in Europe after 1900. Hence, "smallpox could have acted effectively only during the period from 1700 to 1830, whereas the modeling shows that over 600 years of epidemics would be required to raise the frequency to 10%."[101] During that period, the *Δ32* allele might have provided some partial protection from smallpox.

One form of evidence that Duncan, Scott, and Duncan enrolled to attack the date of seven hundred years for the allele was a solid, experimental one—the astonishing announcement at an international conference at the University of Queensland on ancient DNA that the *Δ32* mutation had been found in four of seventeen Bronze Age skeletons dating back 2,900 years from the Lichtenstein Cave in the Harz Mountains in central Germany.[102] So the allele is much older than seven hundred years. The German scientists from the University of Göttingen who made the announcement also tested for the allele in two mass graves from the city of Lübeck near Hamburg—the grave of fourteen people who died from the fourteenth-century plague and the grave of twenty people who died in the famine of 1316. They also tested the remains of nineteen individuals buried from 1750 to 1810 in Goslar in central Germany as well as nineteen Sicilians from the village of Alia who died during a cholera outbreak in 1837.[103] In addition to the four Bronze Age individuals who tested positive for the *CCR5-Δ32* allele, their analysis showed that seven of nineteen individuals from the Goslar group and one of nineteen from Sicily had the allele.[104] Their data revealed the *Δ32* allele frequencies in populations, which to this point had only been estimated by means of mathematical modeling. The allele frequency of 14.2% in the skeletal remains in the fourteenth-century mass grave of plague victims in Lübeck did not differ significantly from the frequency of those who died during that time of famine, 12.5%. If *Y. pestis* were a strong selective force for *Δ32*, then the allele should have been found in a much lower frequency in the mass grave of plague victims. They concluded "that bubonic plague most probably did not exert major selective pressure on this mutation."[105] Finally, DNA collected from archeological sites in Poland from the eleventh through fourteenth centuries also indicated that past plagues did not affect the allele's frequency.[106]

In November 2005, when most scientists were convinced that *Δ32* had undergone strong selection throughout history even if they could not agree on the specific selecting agent, the story once again was about to take an unexpected turn.[107] An article in *PLoS Biology* fundamentally challenged all the previous work on the role of selective pressure on *CCR5-Δ32*.[108] One of the authors of the paper was O'Brien himself, who had been one of the key original actors in this story when he proposed *Y. pestis* as the selective agent for *CCR5-Δ32*. He had now changed his mind.

Pardis Sabeti and her colleagues at the Broad Institute at the Massachusetts Institute of Technology and Harvard University referred to *CCR5* as "one of the most prominent reported cases of recent natural selection in the human genome."[109] They reevaluated the evidence with much denser genetic maps and extensive control data, which had not been available some seven years earlier. With much more comprehensive information about patterns of allelic diversity in the human genome, they were able to perform high-density single-nucleotide polymorphism (SNP) genotyping around the *CCR5* gene locus in many different populations. They then compared their results with large genomic databases and refined physical and genetic maps. They concluded that "*CCR5-Δ32* does *not* clearly stand out in terms of genetic diversity or long-range haplotypes relative to other variants at the locus or throughout the genome."[110]

Drawing on the data that were generated by the International Haplotype Map (HapMap) (discussed in detail in chapter 8), they studied 340 chromosomes from three populations—European Americans, Chinese, and the Yoruba from Nigeria. Eight of the European Americans were heterozygous for the Δ32, and twelve were homozygous, thereby providing the biomedical researchers with thirty-two Δ32 alleles (8 × 1 + 12 × 2). The allele was absent from the other two populations. They examined the allele frequencies at SNPs around CCR5 in all three populations and then determined the derived allele frequency (DAF) distribution, which indicates the possibility of selection. They observed no evidence for selection.[111]

Next, they tested whether it was significant that the Δ32 allele possessed a frequency of about 8% in the European Americans and 0% in the Chinese and Yoruba populations. It turns out that such a distribution is not as rare as originally thought. Of the other SNPs that were present at similar frequencies (7% to 9%) found in European Americans, about 7% are not found in the other two populations for 168 genes studied, and 6% are absent from the same populations in the HapMap data.[112] Hence, CCR5-Δ32 is not unique in terms of allele frequency distribution, differentiation between the populations, or linkage disequilibrium.

Finally, Sabeti and her colleagues discussed the age of the Δ32 allele. Recall that the early dating was based on two microsatellites that were associated with each other more frequently than one would expect based on a random distribution, despite the large separation along the chromosome. Seven years later, however, the genetic map had become much more refined, and the microsatellites were found to be not nearly as far apart as O'Brien, Goldstein, and their colleagues had originally thought. And the microsatellites were actually found on either side of the allele, rather than both being centromere-distal to it. With this new map, they calculated an age of Δ32 to be seven thousand years, differing from the earlier study by an order of magnitude, with a 95% confidence interval of 2,900 to 15,750 years. When they extended their study to include thirty-two genetic markers that are genotyped to the Δ32+ chromosomes, the estimated age became 5,075 years, with a 95% confidence interval of 3,150 to 7,800 years.[113] They therefore claimed that the observed frequency of CCR5-Δ32 allele cannot be solely attributed to a strong selective event within the past thousand years. Although they did not rule out the possibility of selective pressure, if it existed at all, it must have occurred over a thousand years ago. Their work was used to provide an example of the importance of the HapMap Project:

Although much of the interest in HapMap focuses on disease genetics, its data are equally powerful in uncovering potential sites of natural selection in the human genome. Pardis Sabeti, Eric Lander and their colleagues at the Broad Institute, together with Stephen O'Brien and his colleagues at the National Cancer Institute, used the HapMap to re-examine earlier work on natural selection on *CCR5-Δ32*, a genetic variation in a T-cell receptor that confers strong resistance to infection by HIV and that has been implicated in resistance to bubonic plague. "With the benefit of greater genotyping and empirical comparisons from the HapMap, we were able to show that the pattern of genetic variation seen at *CCR5-Δ32* does not stand out as exceptional relative to other loci across the genome and is consistent with natural evolution," said Sabeti, a student at Harvard Medical School and a postdoctoral fellow at the Broad Institute. "In fact, the *CCR5-Δ32* allele is likely to have arisen more than 5000 years ago, rather than during the last 1000 years as was previously thought." They report their findings in the November issue of *PLoS Biology*, and show that the HapMap also gives scientists unprecedented ability to identify novel candidates for natural selection.[114]

Just when it seemed that closure on this issue had been reached, Eric Faure and Manuela Royer-Carenzi reopened the case for selection in 2008.[115] They postulated that the allele frequencies that are present today are not the product of mere gene spreading but rather are due to a negative selection resulting from the spread of various pathogens (the precise nature of which remains unknown) during the Roman expansion. The spread of the Roman legions maps nicely onto the allele distribution.

Recently, scientists at the New York University School of Medicine have proposed that CCR5 is a receptor for *Staphylococcus aureus* luekotoxin (Luk) ED.[116] They demonstrated that LukED-dependent cell toxicity is inhibited by the CCR5 antagonists, such as Maraviroc. And mice that did not possess CCR5 were mostly resistant to *S. aureus* infection. Could *Δ32* be selected for by the bacteria responsible for staph infection?

However the controversy will be settled in the future, perhaps the most interesting moral was the one drawn by the University of Glasgow medieval historian S. K. Cohn Jr. and his colleague, the pediatrician L. T. Weaver:

The exciting correlations discovered by geneticists and epidemiologists between present-day genotypes in human populations, and varying levels of resistance to diseases, now demand a new cooperation between scientists and historians. Together, they can explore the connections between events, environment, biological change, and possible selective pressures that have occurred in the historical (and not just the pre-historical) past.[117]

Similarly, Faure and Royer-Carenzi concluded that "Our analyses also suggest that only a holistic approach which combinates [sic] various fields of investigation (molecular biology, parasitology including virology, evolutionary and population genetics, paleoepidemology including pathocenosis aspects) has enabled us to understand the interrelations between parasites and the *CCR5-Δ32* resistance allele."[118]

In conclusion, the Human Genome Project and Haplotype Map have given geneticists a treasure trove of data for studying genes under present or past adaptive selection. The *CCR5-Δ32* had been seen as "one of the most-celebrated examples of adaptive selection."[119] Indeed, the *CCR5* alleles in general were the test cases for procedures determining neutrality and selection tests. The instability of claims based on limited data generated before the HapMap led to some fascinating, albeit incorrect, prognostications about the gene's genealogy. None of the biomedical investigators publishing the *CCR5* studies of the 1990s seem to have given much thought to what constituted race or ethnicity, despite the importance of those categories to their analysis. For example, the samples used were mostly from Caucasians (as the scientists themselves conceded), with race being defined by donors themselves. A number of the molecular biologists who were the first to determine the function of CCR5 and whom I interviewed were adamant that they were not giving much thought to race. They often spoke about how difficult it was to speak about race because it was a loaded term, and they expressed the fear that thinking in terms of race would have resulted in being labeled racist.

The moral of interdisciplinarity is an important one but perhaps for a reason other than the one offered by the scientists. From the beginning, studies on *Δ32* were inextricably linked to the themes of race and ethnicity. Historians, anthropologists, and sociologists have their own views on those topics. Serious dialogue and exchanges with them might have led scientists to give more thought to those categories or perhaps to choose other ways to account for human variation, such as geographic ancestry and local environmental adaptation. Using the various alleles of *CCR5*, a number of scientists, as is shown in chapter 8, are claiming the gene's alleles are linked to race. This portion of the *CCR5*'s genealogy is not one that displays scientific folly but rather one that shows how allele frequencies are used by contemporary evolutionary biologists to work back in establishing the historical forces of natural selection.

8   Race, Difference, and Genes

After having his DNA tested in 2008, Henry Louis Gates Jr., a Harvard University scholar and director of the W.E.B. DuBois Institute [now the Hutchins Center] for African and African American Research, was told that he was approximately half Irish, which means that about 50% of the genetic markers tested descended from Irish stock. Apparently he shares ten of eleven DNA matches with the descendants of Niall of the Nine Hostages, a fourth-century Irish warlord. Ironically, he is related to the Cambridge, Massachusetts, police officer who arrested him for disorderly conduct after a neighbor reported that two men had broken into the house that Gates was living in.[1] Gates's 2010 PBS series, *Faces of America*, which introduced the nation to the use of genome sequencing for both ancestral mapping and personal health, served as an advertisement for personal genomics companies, such as 23andMe, Knome, deCODE Genetics, and Navigenics. These companies invite people to play an active role in understanding their personal health: "Knowing how your genes may impact your health can help you plan for the future and personalize your healthcare with your doctor."[2]

In addition to the relevance to health, these tests offer a glimpse into ancestry. The company 23andMe.com advertises that "You can even connect with relatives through our Relative Finder feature"[3] and encourages its customers to "uncover the heritage in your genes" by asking "Where in Africa or Europe did your ancestors live?" In addition, it says that "If you're African-American, 23andMe can tell you approximately what fraction of your ancestors were African, and what fraction were European. If you're of European descent, we can pinpoint what populations your DNA is most similar to."[4] Or "Using a technique called Ancestry Painting, 23andMe can determine whether you have any Native American ancestors within the past five generations."[5] All this for $99.

This chapter situates the *CCR5* gene, specifically the *Δ32* allele, in the contexts of four distinct yet related enterprises—race and genomics, big

and small pharma, personalized medicine, and personal genomics companies. Biocapitalism is not restricted to intellectual property: it also is fueled
by the hopes of personalized medicine (pharmacogenomics), race-based
medicine, and Americans' fascination with their genealogies.[6] As Nikolas
Rose remarks: "The new molecular knowledges of human difference are
being mapped out, developed, and exploited by a range of commercial
enterprises, sometimes in alliance with states, sometimes autonomous from
them, establishing constitutive links between human differentiation and
biovalue."[7]

Genetic Markers: A Modern Version of Finding No Racial Overlap

With the rise of molecular genetics and the cornucopia of techniques that
it provides, biomedical researchers in both the public and private sectors
have turned to the human genome to search for variations between the
world's populations to trace human evolution and migration patterns, predict genetic disorders, and offer insights into an individual's genealogy.
Whereas eighteenth- and nineteenth-century scholars fetishized external
characteristics to classify humans, late twentieth- and early twenty-first-
century scholars turn to the internal sequence of the genome.

In the 1970s, the field of molecular biology was beginning to make
important inroads into the elucidation of molecular processes. One important project of those early years was genetic mapping, or the determination of the precise location of genes and other DNA sequences in various
genomes. In 1975, Terri Grodzicker's lab at Cold Spring Harbor was working
with restriction fragment length polymorphisms (RFLPs), or differences of
samples of homologous DNA, which are derived from locations in the DNA
where restriction endonucleases cut, and demonstrated that they could
be used to detect genetic differences among viruses.[8] Five years later, Alec
(now Sir Alec) Jeffrey of the University of Leicester analyzed human globin
gene clusters by means of RFLPs.[9] He famously applied RFLP technology to
forensic science. In 1980, Massachusetts Institute of Technology biologist
David Botstein (now at Princeton University) and his colleagues published
a critical article detailing a method for creating a genetic linkage map using
RFLPs.[10] By the late 1980s and into the early 1990s, more markers uncovered by Botstein's technique, known as second-generation genetic markers,
became critical to the early success of the Human Genome Project. These
techniques included analyses that were based on polymerase chain reactions (PCRs) for microsatellite markers, which are comprised of two, three,
or four repeated nucleotide sequences. Most recently, single-nucleotide

polymorphisms (SNPs), short tandem repeat polymorphisms (STPs),[11] and *Alu* insertion polymorphisms,[12] which represent a third generation of genetic markers developed in the mid-1990s, have become the genetic markers of choice.[13]

Genetic markers are critical for the mapping of genomes and also for studying the genetic causes of inherited diseases. Either by themselves or in combination with others, they are associated with a specific disease pheno-type and therefore enable physicians and biomedical researchers to identify patients who are at high risk for multifactorial diseases, such as cardiovas-cular disorders, asthma, and hypertension. These markers might alter the expression or function of a gene, which is directly related to the disease. Or they may be located in the vicinity of a functional variant: because of their close proximity on the chromosome, a marker and its functional variant tend to be inherited together. Before the use of advanced genetic-marker techniques, only rare, single-gene disorders could be investigated.[14] So how do markers assist in the diagnosis and risk assessment of disease susceptibility or drug response? Generally, two approaches are used to find genetic markers: candidate gene studies are employed for single genes, and genomic studies examine the entire human genome. In the case of monogenic studies, clinical diagnosis is simple. A marker is found that is associated with the candidate gene that is responsible for a disease, such as Huntington's disease.

Unfortunately, most diseases are not straightforward. Polygenic diseases, such as hypertension and heart disease, involve numerous genes as well as complex interactions with environmental and physiological factors. The genomic approach is the way forward in these cases. Researchers use an array of techniques of whole genome scans and microarray gene profiling, or the measurement of the expression of thousands of genes at one time, with reverse-transcriptase PCRs to identify relevant gene clusters.[15] New genetic markers are then identified. The key is to show that a particular allele or SNP indicates a significant risk factor for a particular phenotype. The problem is that studies that indicate a positive correlation between SNP and disease are difficult to replicate due to inconsistently defined phenotypes, small sampling sizes, false-positive and false-negative associa-tions, population stratification, and "studies conducted in different ethnic groups (SNP allele frequencies can differ widely in different populations)."[16] Certain genetic makers are passed down from generation to generation. They become the target of intensive research with a view to use them in family-based linkage analysis.[17] In researching alleles that might lead to certain diseases, race and ethnicity are used (often interchangeably) as analytical categories of choice for describing populations, as was shown in chapter 7.

In 2002—before the passing of the Genetic Information Nondiscrimination Act (GINA) in May 2008—investigators at the National Institute for Occupational Safety and Health were interested in cases where preemployment testing for susceptibility to chronic beryllium disease might be informative to employers.[18] The malady results in a debilitating granulomatous lung disease in workers who are exposed to beryllium. It turns out that a marker is linked to that disease—*HLA-DPβ1*. Researchers tested four different racial populations to determine the allele frequencies among African Americans, Caucasians and Hispanics from the United States, and Chinese from mainland China. The phenotype that they wished to link with this marker was race. Although the frequency was essentially the same for African Americans, Caucasians, and Hispanics, the allele was found at a significantly higher level among the Chinese studied. Does that mean that those who identify themselves as having an ancestry from mainland China need to take the genetic test to determine if they have the allele? Before GINA came into effect, companies in several states demanded such tests to deny employment or workers' compensation. In this particular case, the point was rendered moot because the investigators subsequently determined that the test for the marker had a relatively low specificity, meaning that many individuals who tested positive for the allele did not develop the disease. And the negative predictive valve was high.

The interleukin-4 (*IL-4*) gene on chromosome 5 has been affiliated with asthma. Biomedical researchers sought to determine if a particular SNP in the gene's promoter region was associated with severe asthma in whites and African Americans. Counterintuitively, 4% of whites who possessed this SNP (a replacement of a cytosine with two thymines) suffered from severe asthma, and 30% of African Americans having that same SNP were asthmatic but not severely so.[19] Similar studies looked at the frequency of genetic markers of various loci of drug-metabolizing enzymes among Africans, Caucasians, Pacific Islanders, and East Asians (defined as Chinese plus Papua New Guineans for these studies).[20] Studies also purportedly linked certain SNPs to type 2 diabetes in Mexican American populations.[21] And there have been numerous studies of hundreds of microsatellites linked to hypertension, cancer, and diabetes scrutinizing which of those markers, if any, are found disproportionately between the various races.

Genetic markers are also crucial to the study of human variation with a view to determine the differences between humans at the level of DNA.[22] Differences between groups point to human migration patterns and to the history of natural selection on populations. Some think that differences at the group level are best understood in terms of and categorized by race. In the eighteenth and nineteenth centuries, race was associated with skull volumes, and in the early twentieth century, people were classified in terms of intelligence quotient score, which also was linked to race in sinister ways. However, there were always overlaps between the races. Not even the most ardent eugenicist could argue that the lowest Caucasian IQ was higher than the highest Negro IQ. Similarly, the smallest Caucasian skulls were smaller than the largest Negro skulls. Molecular biologists see genetic markers as being more precise and lacking the pernicious baggage. Indeed, most view them as being neutral. Therein lie the origins of the debate. Could there be genetic markers that are free of overlap and that therefore could be used to characterize human differences at the level of race? The United States of the early twenty-first century is not the nation of the early twentieth century. Much of the debate on the biology of race today is a result of the desire to include, rather than exclude, populations when it comes to medical care and treatment.[23] The formation of groups or populations, however, always necessarily and simultaneously involves processes of inclusion and exclusion. That tension lies at the heart of this chapter.

In the aftermath of the horrors of the sterilizations in the United States of those who were deemed by eugenicists to be not worthy to procreate and the Nazi atrocities committed in the name of racial purity, many postwar scholars—historians, sociologists, anthropologists, and biologists—have argued that races do not comprise genetically distinct groups.[24] In the last twenty years, however, research in molecular biology, genetics, and genomics has led some scientists to reintroduce the biology of race, this time at the level of DNA. And numerous projects have been dedicated to investigating the biological differences between populations, leading some to question whether there is scientific credibility in the genetics of race. How is the word *population* defined? How can scientists best infer genetic groups and individual ancestry? How do groups defined by genetic data correspond with groups that are differentiated by using ethnic and racial labels? What is the overlap between groups and genetic polymorphisms? Are their polymorphisms unique to a particular population? Can that population be accurately described as a race?[25]

I do not seek to answer those questions. Rather, as a historian of science, I am interested in illustrating how the *CCR5-Δ32* gene has been a major player in the debate and a clear example for those who wish to argue for a genetic basis of race. I am also interested in noting that the ways in which biomedical scientists group humans are both biological activities and also political processes that involve sociocultural, historical, and economic considerations. Finally, as a historian, I need to show that there are always alternatives. Arguing that dividing up humankind as races is natural misses a key historical lesson and renders analysis, debate, and intervention irrelevant.

The HapMap

The genetic markers and techniques for finding and analyzing human genes played a critical role in the elucidation of the International Haplotype Map (HapMap). By 1998, when scientists were mapping and sequencing the human genome, it was time to compare and contrast sequences between various peoples to explore human genetic variation and develop novel medical treatment options. The National Institutes of Health human genome programs established numerous goals for the identification and subsequent mapping of single-nucleotide polymorphisms (SNPs). The DNA of any two individuals is about 99.5% similar, unless they are identical twins or are members of triplets, etc.[26] Although many feel that this high percentage underscores our similarities as humans rather than our differences, for some that 0.5% difference is important because it is comprised of SNPs: one person might possess an adenine at a certain nucleotide position, and someone else might have a guanine. Biomedical researchers reckon that such differences are critical to understanding why one individual might respond to a certain medication and another might not. This is the underlying premise of pharmacogenomics, the branch of pharmacology that deals with the role of genetic variation on drug response and that has played an important role in so-called race-based medicine. Genetic markers are therefore critical investigative tools in pharmacogenomics.

SNPs occur randomly throughout the human genome. They occur about one out of every three hundred nucleotides and comprise about 10% of human genetic variation. They are therefore informative when mapping diversity. For a variation to qualify as an SNP, it must be present in at least 1% of the population. Many sets of SNPs are passed down intact from generation to generation, creating associations of alleles in various regions of the chromosomes. These sets of associated SNP alleles are known as haplotypes.[27] Numerous studies have shown highly significant levels of linkage disequilibrium, or the nonrandom association of two alleles among human populations. The strong associations of SNPs in the human genome mean that there are relatively few haplotypes that account for the variation among people in particular regions.[28] Hence, only about 260,000 to 470,000 of the more than 10 million SNPs in the human genome generate most of the information on variation patterns in a particular region.[29] Ancestry-informative markers (AIMs) are SNPs, which exhibit markedly different frequencies among various populations. A migration out of Africa occurred some 60,000 to 125,000 years ago,[30] and mutations, genetic recombination in combination with bottlenecking[31], founder effects[32], and natural selection due to differing environments all influence the allele variants and their frequencies.

In April 1999, the SNP Consortium was created. It included ten major pharmaceutical companies and was headed up by Britain's Wellcome Trust philanthropy, which contributed $14 million to the effort. The Consortium comprised AP Biotech, Astra Zeneca Groups PLC, Aventis, Bayer Group AG, Bristol-Myers Squibb Co., Hoffmann-La Roche, Glaxo Wellcome OLC, IBM, Motorola, Novartis, Pfizer, and SmithKline Beecham PLC. The Wellcome Trust made it clear that it would patent all SNPs that it uncovered and would make the information publicly available at no cost. Such a move ensured that other companies could not have exclusive rights to the genetic information. That sentiment was echoed by the scientists of the HapMap Project, which "adopted an interim protective strategy to try to ensure that no restrictive patents are filed by researchers who use the HapMap Project data…. Project researchers will not seek patents on the data that they generate for which they have not demonstrated a specific use (such as relating a particular haplotype to a disease)."[33]

The initial meeting to discuss the creation of the HapMap Project was held in Washington, D.C., on July 18–19, 2001. By that time, about 2.4 million SNPs had already been identified.[34] In October 2002, the HapMap Project was established to map those SNPs. It was a worldwide collaboration among scientists from the United States, the United Kingdom, Canada, China, Japan, and Nigeria that was funded by both not-for-profit and for-profit organizations.[35] The goal of the HapMap Project was "to determine the common patterns of DNA sequence variation in the human genome, by characterizing sequence variants, their frequencies, and correlations between them, in DNA samples from populations with ancestry from parts of Africa, Asia and Europe."[36] A year later, the number of SNPs located in the human genome and filed in the database had risen to 5.7 million.[37]

Scientists view the HapMap Project as "a natural extension of the Human Genome Project. Where the reference sequence constructed by the Human Genome Project is informative about the vast majority of bases that are invariant across individuals, the HapMap focuses on DNA sequence differences among individuals."[38] The HapMap Project is about the science of difference—how it is defined, categorized, and classified. The genetics of population differences, rather than the genetics of individual differences, has generated much controversy.[39] Finding genetic differences among humans is predicated on selecting the groups. But how should they be selected? How should they be characterized?[40] For the original HapMap, 269 individuals from four major populations with African, Asian, and European ancestry offered their DNA for analysis—thirty sample sets of two parents and child (a so-called trio set) from the Yoruba of Nigeria, forty-four unrelated Japanese living in Tokyo, forty-five unrelated Han Chinese living in Beijing, and thirty U.S. trio samples from residents with northern and western European ancestry.[41] Only a small subset of the SNPs is polymorphic in any given population, suggesting that both common and rare haplotypes are shared across the various major populations.[42]

After the initial three-year period was complete, scientists who were working on the project concluded that "Our understanding of SNP variation and LD [linkage disequilibrium] around common variants in the sampled populations is reasonably complete; the current picture is unlikely to change with additional data."[43] Despite such success, a more detailed SNP map was deemed to be necessary, and the HapMap was prolonged with an additional funding of $3.3 million, increasing the density of the HapMap from one SNP per three thousand bases to one SNP every six hundred bases.[44] For phase 2 of the HapMap Project, 270 individuals were sampled, the same 269 from phase 1 plus one extra sample from the Japanese population. By the end of phase 2 of the HapMap, a further 2.1 million SNPs were genotyped on the same individuals.[45]

Why were these populations chosen for the HapMap Project? As the sociologist of science Troy Duster has argued, these populations were chosen because of "convenience and accessibility. Cell and tissue repositories are created to decrease the cost and difficulty of obtaining samples, and the archived samples will be extensively characterized and frequently utilized."[46] Cells and tissues had previously been taken from these groups for collecting data on populations. As the sociologist of medicine Steven Epstein points out, there is a seemingly infinite number of ways in which populations can be studied: "Out of all of the ways by which people differ from one another, why should it be assumed that sex and gender, race and ethnicity, and age are the attributes of identity that are most *medically meaningful*? Why these markers of identity and not others?"[47] He goes on to show that the answer is sociopolitical, economic, and cultural. Just as important, when biomedical researchers discuss their findings on human differences, they often do so by reducing variation to biology, thereby potentially counteracting policy interventions, which could redress the sociocultural, political, and economic forces leading to health disparities.[48] Consider Duster's point:

It is possible to make arbitrary groupings of populations (geographic, linguistic, self-identified by faith, identified by others by physiognomy, etc.) and still find statistically significant allelic variations between those groupings. For example, we could examine all the people in Chicago, and all those in Los Angeles, and find statistically significant differences in allele frequency at *some* loci.[49]

Similarly, as Fujimura and Rajagopalan point out, *population* can be defined in a myriad of ways, and its meaning is predicated on the particular study, discipline, and time frame, to name just a few options.[50] Why race and ethnicity? Why not weight-height distribution? Why not age? Or perhaps most important: why not social class? After all, many scholars have argued that genetic differences among humans pale in comparison to the differences between the social classes and their respective access to healthcare.[51]

Because defining a population is crucial, what exactly were the criteria for choosing these particular individuals for the HapMap? The Yoruba donors were required to have all four grandparents be Yoruba. For the Han Chinese, three out of the four grandparents needed to be Han Chinese. The samples were collected from a residential community at Beijing Normal University. A university community was chosen because it comprised all fifty-six officially recognized ethnicities in China. The Japanese samples were taken from the Tokyo metropolitan area to ensure a diverse selection of Japanese genotypes: "Thus, this set of samples can be viewed as representative of the majority population in Japan. It is considered culturally insensitive in Japan to inquire about ancestral origins."[52] All four of the donors' grandparents, however, needed to be from Japan. The U.S. samples were perhaps most interesting. They all were collected from Utah residents by the 1980s and were originally classified as being American with northern and western European ancestry. As "The Guidelines for Referring to the HapMap Population in Publications and Presentations" explains:

Because the importance of precision in assigning group membership to prospective donors based on ancestral geography was not well appreciated in 1980, it is unclear how accurately these samples reflect the patterns of genetic variation in people with northern and western European ancestry. These samples should not be described as "European," nor seen as representing people with ancestry from other parts of Europe (e.g., southern or eastern Europe). The samples also should not be described as "Caucasian," a term that carries racial overtones, and that technically refers only to people from the area between the Black and Caspian Seas.[53]

At the initial July 2001 HapMap meeting, fears of reifying race were passionately expressed. A lively exchange ensued between the geneticist Ara-
vinda Chakravarti (who later became president of the American Society of
Human Genetics) and a number of senior molecular biologists. Chakravarti
insisted that ethnic and racial makers should be kept off samples and suggested that only SNP patterns should be used as the basis for analyzing,
grouping, and categorizing. The opposing molecular biologists countered
that unless the samples were identified in terms of races and ethnicities,
HapMap researchers would be seen as mindlessly ignoring important
aspects of human genetic variation.[54] Two years later the scientists working
on the HapMap project noted that

Careful and sustained attention must also be paid to the ethical issues that will be
raised by the HapMap and the studies that will use it. By consulting members of
donor populations about the consent process and the implications of population-
specific findings before sample collection, the project has helped to advance the
ethical standard for the international population genetics research. Future population genetics projects will continue to refine this approach. It will be an ongoing
challenge to avoid misinterpretations or misuses of results from studies that use
the HapMap. Researchers using the HapMap should present their findings in ways
that avoid stigmatizing groups, conveying an impression of genetic determinism, or
attaching incorrect levels of biological significance to largely social constructs such
as race.[55]

Two years later, in 2005, other scientists echoed this warning. David Altshuler of the Broad Institute insisted that

Given the potential for confusion if associations of uncertain validity are widely
reported (and a persistent tendency towards genetic determinism in public dis-
course), we urge conservatism and restraint in the public dissemination and interpretation of such studies, especially if non-medical phenotypes are explored. It is
time to create mechanisms by which all results of association studies, positive and
negative, are reported and discussed without bias.[56]

The HapMap scientists wanted to make their purpose and procedure
clear from the outset. The ethicists and biologists in the Population and
ELSI (Ethical, Legal, and Social Issues) Group needed to deal with "two
interrelated scientific and ethical questions": how should human variation
be sampled to find common haplotypes, and should the donors' populations be named?[57] This group made recommendations to the Steering Committee, and a number of the ELSI Group members also served on HapMap's
communication group. The scientists immediately identified a problem
in defining a population—"a group of people with a shared ancestry and

therefore a shared history and pattern of geographical migration."[58] The medical anthropologist and ethnohistorian Morris W. Foster and his colleagues conceded parenthetically, "It is important to note, however, that on the basis of this definition, many individuals can claim membership of more than one population, while some of those who claim a particular population identity do not share the same biological ancestry; this situation makes doing genetic variation research with identified populations both scientifically and ethically complex."[59]

From the start, biomedical researchers realized that they would be damned for using ethical and racial categories in their research and damned if they did not. In the end, naming the populations from where the samples were taken was chosen. This did have a slight advantage, some argued, over keeping them protected and anonymous and allowing their identity to be inferred by researchers, who might otherwise impose their own interpretations of how such identity relates to genetic variation. This self-identification allowed donors input into how they thought their population should be named. And naming the population would permit biomedical researchers, geneticists, and ethicists a clearer context for interpreting the biological significance of particular genetic constellations present in certain populations. Yet not all problems were remedied. For some groups, such as Native Americans, precise ancestry has sociocultural, religious, and economic ramifications that are related to origin stories, land rights, and items of cultural patrimony.[60] No samples from Native American tribes were included in the initial phases of the HapMap Project.[61] In 2003, the National Human Genome Research Institute (NHGRI) met with a number of leaders of the Native American health-research community to inquire about participation in the Project. Most were not interested in having tribal participation, "citing concerns that the HapMap will facilitate population-history studies and comparisons among populations."[62]

HapMap scientists and bioethicists surely were thinking of the problems that had been experienced by the ill-fated Human Genome Diversity Project (HGDP) a decade earlier. The ghosts of the HGDP haunted the HapMap scientists. Conceived in 1991, the HGDP originally was proposed by leading geneticists and evolutionary biologists to investigate human diversity at the level of the DNA. They had made it clear from the start that they were particularly interested in genetic material "of isolated indigenous people."[63] Problems arose, however.[64] In 1993, the Rural Advancement Foundation International accused the organizers of the HGDP of, among other things, desiring to profit from the patenting of the genes of indigenous peoples.[65] As the sociologist of science Jenny Reardon argues, some saw the HGDP as arising "out of Western economic interests that sought to transform the genetic differences of indigenous peoples into dollars (a process that critics would soon label biocolonialism)."[66] Despite attempts by two of the HGDP leaders, the lawyer Henry T. Greely and geneticist Luigi Luca Cavalli-Sforza, to assuage such concerns by insisting that the HGDP was not a commercial venture, no one could guarantee that pharmaceutical companies somewhere down the line would not attempt to patent the protein products of those genes. Big pharma could even go to the country where the gene initially was located and enter into nefarious financial deals.[67] In the end, the fear of racial and ethnic typing trumped the good intentions of the geneticists and evolutionary biologists.

The HapMap pressed on despite the failure of its distant, older cousin. Data from phase 3 were made public in spring 2009. Phase 3 provided a much denser map of about 1.5 million SNPs from 1,397 individuals comprising eleven populations, including 250 of the original 269/270 from phases 1 and 2 and an additional 1,147 individuals. These eleven populations included the original four from phases 1 and 2 and added those of African ancestry living in the Southwest United States; Chinese in metropolitan Denver, Colorado; Gujarati (an Indian ethnicity) in Houston, Texas; Luhya in Webuye, Kenya; Mexican ancestry in Los Angeles; Maasai in Kinyawa, Kenya; and the Tuscans of Italy.[68]

The Genetic Debate

In a recent work, sociologist of medicine Ann Morning demonstrates that, despite the common belief expressed in the social-science literature that race is no longer a legitimate category, no such consensus has been reached in the biomedical sciences.[69] According to Lundy Braun, professor of pathology and laboratory medicine and Africana studies at Brown University:

Multiple, frequently conflicting, and generally implicit understandings of the concepts of race and ethnicity circulate in biomedical circles, with some researchers proposing that race has no genetic meaning, others arguing that the estimated 5 to 6 percent [sic] genetic difference is sufficiently meaningful biologically to justify an intensive research program, and still others arguing that the whole controversy can be circumvented by substituting ethnicity for race.[70]

The spectrum is wide: some argue for a essentialist view (that race can be found at the level of DNA), others assert that it is "a social construction" with no basis found in nature for such a view, and others maintain a position somewhere in between (that race is simultaneously biological and sociocultural). To portray the debate as merely between the constructivist (race is simply ideology) versus essentialist (race is genetic) is too simplistic to represent accurately the debate's complexity because such a dichotomy ignores the various positions of what Morning calls the antiessentialists.[71] Antiessentialists use biological evidence to attack biological notions of race: they stress both the overwhelming similarity of the DNA sequences among humans and the arbitrariness and inaccuracy of drawing racial boundaries based on phenotypic characteristics. Although they do not deny biological variation among humans and many support personalized medicine in the form of pharmacogenomics, they oppose the claim that race is an accurate measure of such diversity. Geographic variation and local adaptation to environments are often mentioned as being more helpful alternative categories for investigating biological difference.[72]

In 2001, James F. Wilson of Edinburgh's Centre for Population Health Sciences[73] and Robert S. Schwartz, then deputy editor of the *New England Journal of Medicine*,[74] questioned the legitimacy of using racial categories in medical research. Schwartz, a physician, argues passionately that "Race is a social construct, not a scientific classification" and that "'race' is biologically meaningless" and a "pseudoscience."[75] Schwartz does not deny that the "frequencies of certain allelic variants or mutant genes among people who share a geographic origin or culture have medical value."[76] Sharing geographic origin or culture, which are important analytical alternatives, should not be conflated with sharing the same race. He concluded his article with the hope that the lesson learned from the Human Genome Project was that "there is only one race—the human race."[77] Along similar lines, Wilson and his colleagues from University College, London and Oxford, argued against the use of ethnic categories in biomedical research, concluding that "commonly used ethnic labels are both insufficient and inaccurate representations of the inferred genetic clusters."[78] By analyzing microsatellite markers in eight populations—South African Bantu speakers, Amharic- and Oromo-speaking Ethiopians from Shewa and Wollo provinces collected in Addis Ababa, Ashkenazi Jews, Armenians, Norwegian speakers from Oslo, Chinese from Sichuan, Papua New Guineans from Madang, and Afro-Caribbeans from London—their results indicated that black, Caucasian, and Asian "are insufficient and inaccurate descriptions of human genetic structure."[79]

Another group of geneticists, biomedical researchers, and statisticians, however, maintains the opposite and claims that "from both an objective and scientific (genetic and epidemiologic) perspective there is great validity in racial/ethnic self-categorizations, both from the research and public policy points of view."[80] Although they agree that racial categories cannot be based on skin pigment, they claim that racial groups are readily distinguishable based on a number of random genetic markers.[81] Geneticist Neil J. Risch, who was at Stanford University at the time and is now at the University of California at San Francisco, is interested in SNPs, which are associated with various diseases and their frequencies in Caucasians, Asians, African Americans, and Hispanics.[82] He is adamant about refuting the claim that "'Genetic data ... show that any two individuals within a particular population are as different genetically as any two people selected from any two populations in the world.'"[83] Such a claim is both "counter-intuitive and factually incorrect."[84] For example, "Two Caucasians are more similar to each other genetically than a Caucasian and an Asian."[85] And unlike arguments that clusters identified by genotyping are far more informative than those identifying geographic and ethnic labels, Risch asserts that "self-defined race, ethnicity or ancestry are [sic] actually more genetically informative than clusters based on analysis of random genetic markers."[86] According to Risch, molecular genetics should embrace the diversity of races because "Ignoring our differences, even if with the best of intentions, will ultimately lead to the disservice of those who are in the minority."[87] That was the message of Esteban González Burchard, currently professor of biopharmaceutical sciences and medicine and director of the Center for Genes, Environment, and Health of the University of California at San Francisco.[88] Burchard's group fears that if biomedical investigators ignore racial and ethnic backgrounds and if persons are sampled randomly, then most clinical samples in the United States would still be from white participants. As shown in chapter 7, several biomedical researchers cautioned against the premature use of race as a category of analysis in understanding *CCR5-Δ32* allele frequencies because an overwhelming majority of the samples were from self-identified Caucasian Americans. According to Burchard, nothing would change. Those of color again would be discriminated against; diseases that exhibit racial patterns would never be discovered, and thus diagnostics and therapeutics would never be developed. Whereas the Tuskegee syphilis study represented the pernicious and racist past of U.S. medicine, ignoring race would be a form of modern-day racism.[89]

Burchard argues that there are three instances of genetic variation between the five major populations in the United States: "black or African American, white, Asian, native Hawaiian or other Pacific Islander, and American Indian or Alaska native."[90] First, studies of indigenous groups show that the human population has major branches that correspond to the major racial groups, with subbranches of each group representing each indigenous group. Second, analyses of genetic clusters result in the charting of major clusters that are associated with racial categories. Third, studies of allele frequencies at both microsatellite and SNP markers indicate that a certain percentage of them are most likely race specific. Race-specific alleles are more common among Africans because they possess the greatest genetic diversity and have more low-frequency alleles.[91] Burchard is convinced that "There are racial and ethnic differences in the causes, expression, and prevalence of various diseases."[92] He concludes, like Risch, with a call for embracing the genetic studies of racial diversity:

Ignoring racial and ethnic differences in medicine and biomedical research will not make them disappear. Rather than ignoring these differences, scientists should continue to use them as starting points for further research. Only by focusing attention on these issues can we hope to understand better the variations among racial and ethnic groups in the prevalence and severity of diseases and in responses to treatment. Such understanding provides the opportunity to develop strategies for the improvement of health outcomes for everyone.[93]

A number of these researchers, Burchard included, are people of color.[94] They wish to redress the sins of the past that were committed by the American medical establishment; the memories of eugenics and Tuskegee have indelibly been cast on our collective national memory. And they have won the support of a number of leading African American organizations and research groups that stress that race-blind genomic medicine ignores racial variation in disease susceptibility and death and fails to address the ethnic and racial divisions in morbidity and mortality.[95]

So how can biomedical researchers have diametrically opposed views on the matter of race? Perhaps the best example of the confusion is reflected by the shift of opinion of the former director of the Human Genome Project, Francis Collins, from initially denying that race was a biological category in 2000 to admitting in 2003 that "All this study of genotypes will have profound consequences on our understanding of race and ethnicity."[96] A year later, he conceded that "it is not strictly true that race or ethnicity has no biological connection."[97] In late August 2005, the Race, Ethnicity, and Genetics Working Group (REGWG) of the National Human Genome Research Institute of Bethesda, Maryland, addressed that issue. The key to this apparent contradiction is the sampling design. Genetic clustering studies have often been taken from widely separated and socially defined populations. They can be used accurately only to separate out individuals whose ancestors diverged many millennia ago. Substantial genetic difference among these individuals is necessary for a genetic cluster analysis to

be accurate.[98] When individuals who are more evenly distributed geographically are sampled, the clustering is far less clear.[99]

African populations possess the greatest genetic diversity because they
are the oldest: humankind originated on that continent.[100] About 85% to
90% of the total human genetic variation is found within populations from
one of the three continents—Africa, Asia, and Europe.[101] An additional 10%
to 15% of variation is found between them.[102] In other words, the average
proportion of genetic differences between two individuals from two different major populations only slightly exceeds that between two unrelated
individuals from the same major population.[103]

Wishing to provide a finer analysis of groups than the three major continents, Noah A. Rosenberg, who runs a mathematical, theoretical, and
computational laboratory in genetics and evolution at Stanford University,
analyzed fifty-two populations from Africa, Europe, the Middle East, Cen-
tral/South Asia, East Asia, Oceania, and America and was able to divide
1,056 individuals into five major gene clusters based on 377 autosomal
microsatellite loci (a type of genetic marker). Without knowing the origins
of these individuals, Rosenberg's lab was able to identify six main genetic
clusters (five of which corresponded to major geographic regions) and sub-
clusters that are associated with individual populations.

How do these figures help researchers create groupings? Michael Bamshad, at the time at the University of Utah and now professor of pediatrics and adjunct professor of genome sciences at University of Washington,
conducted an interesting experiment to test these clusters. If the ancestry information of individuals from different continents is removed, how
many markers do biomedical researchers need to differentiate between
groups and accurately assign individuals to these groups? Given about two
hundred samples from twenty ethnic groups in sub-Saharan Africa, Europe,
and East Asia, Bamshad demonstrated that researchers needed only approximately sixty *Alu* insertion polymorphisms and tetranucleotide microsatellites (both being types of genetic markers) to assign an individual to the
correct continent 90% of the time. Using 160 such markers, the accuracy
increased to between 99% and 100%, a very small percentage of overlap
indeed.[104]

Whether these populations correspond to races turns out to be a trickier
question. Both Rosenberg's and Bamshad's studies were based on populations in which the degree of genetic variation between them was maxi-
mized, meaning that these populations are far apart from each other and
there is minimal admixture between them. In populations with much more
admixture, it was impossible to link a genetic cluster with a particular race.

As Bamshad underscores: "Importantly, the inclusion of such samples [of the Middle East and Central Asia, which are regions geographically inter-mediate between the regions studied] demonstrates geographic continuity in the distribution of genetic variation and thus undermines traditional concepts of race."[105] At this point, we cannot definitively infer race from genetic markers. Some scientists, however, hold out hope that in the future, with enough informative genetic markers, we may indeed be able to link genetic clusters with race even in very heterogeneous populations.

In 2004, Bamshad and his colleagues analyzed 63,724 SNPs that were located in the regulatory and coding regions of 3,931 genes. When they compared 50,736 SNPs that are polymorphic in African Americans and European Americans and defined a common SNP as one with a minor allele frequency of 10% in either one or both populations, Bamshad found 20,409 common SNPs, of which 7,779 were common only in African Amer-icans and 2,802 common only in European Americans. Of those 20,409 SNPs, 4,704 were specific to African Americans and 585 were found only in European Americans. Only 9,831 were common in both populations, of which 4,015 had significantly different allele frequencies. If one changes the definition of *common* from 10% to 20%, then 12,641 common SNPs were found, of which 4,322 were common only in African Americans and 2,902 common only in European Americans. Of these 12,641 SNPs, 1,220 were found only in African Americans and 117 were found only in Euro-pean Americans. Bamshad argues:

Whether these findings can be generalized to the entire genome and all main human populations is unclear, but they do indicate that more data are needed before we can conclude that common variants are typically shared by all main human populations. If they are not, it might be necessary to develop initiatives to identify additional alleles that are common specifically in each population to be studied.[106]

In short, although the genetic differences among humans are relatively small, some claim that the differences can be used to divide them within "broad, geographically based groupings."[107] According to Rosenberg, "The challenge of genetic studies of human history is to use the small amount of genetic differentiation among populations to infer the history of human migrations. Because most alleles are widespread, genetic differences among human populations derive mainly from gradations in allelic frequencies rather than from distinctive 'diagnostic' genotypes."[108] As we have seen, some argue that these allele frequency patterns provide biological evidence of race because the continental clusters map roughly onto the classifica-tions of humans—sub-Saharan Africans; Europeans, western Asians, and northern Africans; eastern Asians; Polynesians and other inhabitants of Oceania; and Native Americans. Others claim that the same data subvert such an interpretation of racial groupings: major populations considered to be races do not form their own genetic clusters.[109] Not surprisingly, categories used by the U.S. Census Bureau for administrative, political, and socioeconomic purposes do not seem to have precise DNA correlates. The Race, Ethnicity, and Genetics Working Group saw an opportunity for geneticists

> to reduce at least some of the confusion and controversy surrounding the issues of race, ethnicity, ancestry, and health. They can demonstrate the irrelevance of racial and ethnic labels for pursuing many research questions and health improvement objectives—for example, by clarifying the many ways in which environmental factors that extend across groups interact with biological processes to produce common diseases.... By emphasizing the close genetic affinities between members of different groups, researchers can reduce the widespread misconception that substantial genetic differences separate groups.[110]

Major biomedical journals recognize the politically explosive topic of studying the relationship between genetics and race. *Nature Genetics*, *Archives of Pediatrics and Adolescent Medicine*, and *British Medical Journal* requested that their authors define *race* when they use the term.[111] Unfortunately, despite the hope for clarity and the opportunity to educate, ambiguity remained. In 2007, bioethicists surveyed 330 randomly chosen articles on genetic research published between 2001 and 2004 and found that less than 10% of the articles using the term race or ethnicity explained the basis for using it to study populations.[112] That was certainly the case with the articles on *CCR5* and its so-called racial and ethnic alleles.

By 2009, things had not improved. After analyzing 204 biomedical research journal publications, the sociologist Catherine Lee concluded that it was "unclear what researchers *do* and *mean* when they use race or ethnicity in their investigations."[113] Once again, despite invoking the terms *race* or *ethnicity*, authors rarely defined what they meant: "No author explicitly articulated a definition of race—that is, the investigators did not explain if they conceived and utilized race as a biological construct, a socio-political identity, or social proxy for cultural and behavioral practices."[114] In thirty-five of the thirty-nine cases where a definition was given, the researchers merely stated that race or ethnicity was "self-reported." Of the remaining cases, authors either defined *ethnicity* as the birthplace of the subject's father or grandfather or defined *ethnicity* as "ancestry."[115] The reader is never sure if *race* and *ethnicity* refer to biological or sociocultural categories or if there is a distinction between those terms.[116] Lee concludes her article by concluding that "a growing faith in biomedicine and genomics and an uncritical acceptance of scientific studies of race or ethnicity may foster essentialized and biologically reductionist approaches to not only addressing health disparities but also other racial or ethnic inequalities."[117] The result might be the opposite of what Burchard and his colleagues desire—that "This biomedical and genetic focus may lead to biomedical solutions and the withdrawal of social, political, or economic approaches to easing social and economic inequalities."[118]

The Federal Government, the Private Sector, and Patient Advocacy Groups

So why do biomedical scientists view human variation through the lenses of race and ethnicity? As a result, in part, of the initial abundance of research data on white men with HIV/AIDS and the corresponding paucity of information on women and people of color, the U.S. Congress passed the National Institutes of Health Revitalization Act, which required the inclusion of women and people of color in NIH-funded research. In the 1980s, Congresswomen Patricia Schroeder and Olympia Snowe, cochairs of the Congressional Caucus for women's issues, picked up on the growing sentiment in Washington, D.C., that women were underrepresented in medical research. Congress subsequently required the NIH to include more women in NIH-funded studies. As legislators crafted new NIH guidelines, the African American members of Congress insisted on an extension of the mandate to include people of color. As a result, *minorities* was added to the wording.[119] Congress passed the act in 1990, but it was vetoed by President George H. W. Bush because he did not approve of the reversal of the ban on fetal tissue research, which was tied to the act. In 1993, President Bill Clinton issued an executive order that removed the ban on fetal research. The act quickly went through Congress, and Clinton signed it into law in June 1993. Women and members of minority groups needed to be included in NIH-funded studies starting in fiscal year 1995.[120] The act reads:

The inclusion of women and members of minority groups and their subpopulations must be addressed in developing a research design or contract proposal appropriate to the scientific objectives of the study/contract. The research plan/proposal should describe the composition of the proposed study population in terms of sex/gender and racial/ethnic group, and provide a rationale for selection of such subjects. Such a plan/proposal should contain a description of the proposed outreach programs for recruiting women and minorities as participants.[121]

As anthropologist of science Duana Fullwiley suggests, the NIH Revital-
ization Act serves as the historical context for the NIH's Pharmacogenomics
Research Network (PGNR) founded in 2000 and the subsequent HapMap
Project.[122] Biological differences have become the objects of investigation:

[F]or many working in this field race as an organizing principle emerges as a natural
choice and referent for categorizing human individuals not because of any explicit
commitment to a political agenda or racism, but because the hopeful curiosity that
often spurs contemporary research into raced groups is set within institutional for-
mal structures that give human variation its sense on multiple registers.... [B]ack-
and-forth between DNA and its seemingly natural organization by societal descrip-
tors of race works to *molecularize* race itself.[123]

She demonstrates that the methodology that Burchard and some of his
colleagues use "is itself *designed* to bring about a *correspondence* of these
two domains: (1) body traits made meaningful through conceptions of
race (given certain social and political contexts) *and* (2) supposedly politically and socially neutral DNA."[124] She studies biomedical researchers who
wish to link propensity to disease and racial differences based on ancestry
informative markers (AIMs), which are a type of SNP that is used to identify genetic markers that allegedly distinguish one continental group from
another.[125] Her research is a microanalysis of how molecular biologists who
are interested in genetic markers relevant to race construct their laboratory experiments and theories. The AIMs that the biomedical researchers
used are associated with genes that have some ecological or evolutionary
function, such as protection from malaria, vitamin D regulation, and mel-
anin concentration.[126] As Fullwiley points out, although the laboratories
grouped these SNPs along ancestral lines or shared continental origin, they
could have as easily grouped the SNPs based on similar historical environmental exposure. The two are not necessarily the same.[127] The key, again,
is that there are alternatives to the groupings. Assignment based on ancestral lineage is not inevitable. It is a product of the emphasis of race in late
twentieth- and twenty-first-century biomedicine.[128] She insists that "if the
American cultural context was one that was less interested in 'race' and
more interested in 'ecology,' then the few AIMs that dramatically differ in
selected Africans, Europeans, and Native Americans might be renamed, or
at least rethought, as possible 'environmental exposure markers,' with the
'exposure' bearing the broad-ranging effects of human history."[129] Again,
sickle-cell anemia is better understood as conveying immunity to heterozygous individuals in geographic areas where malaria is present than being
seen as a disease affecting a specific race.

The U.S. Food and Drug Administration also began to embrace the inclusion of underrepresented subgroups: the white male no longer stood as the universal representative of the species.[130] Starting in 1988, the FDA required additional information on new drug applications, including "the number, age range, and sex distribution of subjects."[131] It was a start. By 1993, the governmental agency permitted the participation of women of child-bearing age in clinical trials of new drugs.[132] The FDA had in the past ruled that these women were not permitted to take part in experimental drug trials for fear of harm to the fetus.[133] The thalidomide fetal malformations, experienced widely in Europe, weighed heavily on those at the FDA. In 1997, the Food and Drug Modernization Act, emerging in the context of drug development, directed that "the Secretary [of Health and Human Services] shall, in consultation with the director of the National Institutes of Health and with representatives of the drug manufacturing industry, review and develop guidance, as appropriate, on the inclusion of women and minorities in clinical trials."[134] One year later, the FDA issued a rule requiring pharmaceutical companies to generate safety and efficacy data for "important demographic subgroups, specifically gender, age, and racial subgroups."[135] In 1999, the FDA's guidelines on "Population Pharmacokinetics" recommended the use of this subfield of pharmacology[136] for developing drugs with a view to establish any differences in drug safety and efficacy among subgroups, including race and ethnicity.[137] And in 2005, the FDA announced a guideline ("Collection of Race and Ethnicity Data in Clinical Trials") that recommended that there be a standardized procedure for collecting and reporting information on race and ethnicity that could be used in clinical trials for drug approval.[138]

In a real sense, the federal government strongly encouraged the defining of *CCR5-Δ32* and other genes and their alleles in terms of race and ethnicity. Much of the research at U.S. nonprofit institutions on the *CCR5* gene and its various alleles was either partially or fully funded by the NIH. We can begin to see why race and ethnicity were chosen over the other innumerable alternatives of comparing and contrasting humans. And the FDA requirements were certainly applicable to any entity (either public or private) that wished to have its drug approved for binding to CCR5.

Initially, the pharmaceutical industry balked at the FDA's requirements, viewing them as unwarranted meddling of the government in private industrial affairs.[139] Big pharma, however, quickly changed its tune when it realized the potential new market that would be created. The anthropologist Michael Montoya has written on the multicultural pharmaceutical marketing conferences where participants hear about strategies for products that target ethnic groups. Such was the case at the meeting that he attended of the American Diabetes Association, where Aventis Pharmaceuticals marketed Amaryl®, which is used to treat diabetes, with an advertisement depicting a Latin American or Caribbean farmer. Similarly in November 2000, Aventis's press release declared that "Amaryl® tablets provide significant reductions of HbA1c and fasting plasma glucose (blood sugars) in Mexican Americans with Type 2 diabetes." It continued by asserting that "10.6 percent of Mexican Americans are diabetic, that Mexican Americans are twice as likely to develop diabetes than whites and that since 1990 there has been an alarming 38 percent increase in the prevalence of diabetes among this population."[140] As Montoya points out, although Amaryl® might lower the blood sugar levels among Mexican American diabetics, "the implication that it is more effective than when used by other ethnic groups is a specious one."[141] Another conference included sessions on "Zeroing In on Special Market Segments to Accelerate Your Multicultural Growth Strategies."[142] Those "special market segments" were people of color.

AutoGenomics, a California company, claimed that different races have different responses to the anticoagulant Coumadin (warfarin), or as one of the company's PowerPoint presentations of 2008 stated: "Infiniti Warfarin XP: Because Ethnic Diversity Matters When Dosing with Warfarin."[143] Similarly, the brochure of the Sixth Annual Multicultural Pharmaceutical Market Development and Outreach Conference proclaimed, "The unprecedented growth in ethnic populations across various regions in the United States opens doors to a wide array of new market opportunities for healthcare and pharmaceutical companies.... With the onslaught of generics, pricing battles and DTC [direct-to-consumer] competition, reaching out effectively to America's emerging majority is a clear road to brand building and market growth for U.S. pharmaceutical and healthcare companies."[144] A session at the September 2007 meeting of the Pharmaceutical Marketing Research Group was entitled "When the Ivory Tower Goes to the Ebony Hood."[145]

Drug makers can now narrow down the population of research subjects to include only those whose genomes indicate that they will most likely benefit from a certain drug. As the legal scholar Dorothy Roberts argues, race "provides a large, identifiable group of consumers for drugs developed using genetic research.... [I]t does make market sense to sell their products to vastly larger patient pools of blacks, Asians, whites, or Hispanics. Instead of developing small batches of designer drugs, companies can develop drugs for entire racial groups."[146] In short, race enables personalized medicine to generate marketable products.[147] Pharmaceutical companies also realized that they could legitimately resist pressure to cut the enormous costs of pre-scription drugs because one size does not fit all (as the government insists): no single generic drug would work.[148] In addition, these companies also can thwart attempts to turn their drugs into generics by extending intellectual property protection. They simply need to show that the drug is more effica-cious in certain races or ethnicities. There is an interesting contradiction: pharmacogenomics, which is supported by big pharma, is about the indi-vidual. I cannot imagine that pharmaceutical companies will develop drugs that are specifically tailored to each individual: that would clearly not be in their financial interest. Rather, dividing humanity into racial groupings, pharmaceutical companies come across as caring about specific characteris-tics to which a group of individuals can relate and with which they closely identify.

Race has indeed become a biomedical commodity, as the BiDil story has made clear. BiDil serves as a classic example of how the private sector embraces the use of racial and ethnic categories in the analysis of drug safety and efficacy. On June 23, 2005, the FDA approved a race-based drug for the first time. Some have heralded BiDil as the atonement for the sins of the U.S. medical community's past, and others argue that it is not personalized medicine but the exploitation of race in the market place.[149] Such a move, Sankar and Kahn argue, "reifies and biologizes racial groups" and sets a dan-gerous precedent of stopping pharmaceuticals from becoming generics by searching for reasons to renew their patents in the name of alleviating the disparities that plague people of color in the United States.[150] In the 1980s, cardiologist Jay Cohn and his colleagues found that the combination of two vasodilators, hydralazine and isosorbide dinitrate (H/I), was efficacious in treating heart disease. Cohn applied for a methods patent on H/I, which is now called BiDil, and the application was approved, giving him exclusive rights for twenty years to use the drug to treat heart failure. No mention of race was given in the patent application. Cohn then licensed BiDil to the North Carolina pharmaceutical company Medco, which filed a new drug application (NDA) for FDA approval. Again, race was not mentioned. In 1997, the Cardiovascular and Renal Drug Advisory Committee of the FDA rejected Medco's application on the grounds that although BiDil might work, the company's statistical analysis did not meet FDA standards.

Medco quickly lost interest, and the intellectual property rights reverted back to Cohn. He and his colleague Peter Carson, another cardiologist, culled the fifteen-year-old data and decided to analyze them by race. As Sankar and Kahn argue, "Race apparently became relevant only when it offered a means to revive the commercial prospects of BiDil."[151] In 1999, Carson and Cohn coauthored a paper in which they purportedly demonstrated racial

differences in response to BiDil based on forty-nine African American subjects. Cohn then relicensed the drug to the Massachusetts biotech company
NitroMed. In 2000, both Cohn and Carson applied for a race-specific methods patent to use BiDil to treat heart failure in African American patients.
The FDA informed them that the drug could in principle be patented as
a race-based drug, provided that it could be confirmed in a trial on African American subjects. As a result of such a promising outcome, NitroMed
was able to raise $34 million in private venture-capital funding from
which it would fund the FDA trial, A-HeFT (African American Heart Failure
Trial). In November 2003, NitroMed went public and raised $66 million in
shares.

   A-HeFT enrolled 1,050 African Americans with either class III or IV heart
failure.[152] The results were so impressive that the study was cut short in July
2004, and the FDA granted approval. A week later, NitroMed's stock more
than tripled. In November 2004, when the results were published, it rose
sharply again. After announcing that it was submitting an NDA to the FDA,
NitroMed held another public offering, raising nearly $80 million to fund
the launching of BiDil. The revised patent extends to 2020.[153] As Sankar
and Kahn point out: "By testing BiDil in doses that are not available for
its generic components (hydralazine and isosorbide dinitrate), NitroMed
has discouraged doctors from easily devising ways for patients to get the
same benefits from the long available, and much less expensive, generics.
Additionally, NitroMed's race-specific methods patent will also prevent
insurers from recommending to doctors that they use generic substitutes
to save money."[154] A week after FDA approval, NitroMed announced that
BiDil would cost $1.80 per pill, or $10.80 a day, based on a dosage of six
pills daily. The estimated cost of the generic is a mere twenty-five cents a
pill, or $1.50 per day.

   The story becomes more interesting. The A-HeFT studied the effects of
BiDil on African Americans and demonstrated that African American subjects who were given BiDil in conjunction with their standard heart medication did better than those who were given a placebo in addition to their
regular medication. It did not contrast this group with Caucasian Americans, Hispanic Americans, or Native Americans. Some twenty years earlier,
it was established that H/I combined with the standard heart medication
improves the health of those taking. As Sankar and Kahn conclude,

   The great irony here is that NitroMed admits that BiDil might work in people who
   aren't African American, and many of the A-HeFT investigators themselves have
   expressed the hope that the drug is prescribed to anyone who might benefit from
   it, regardless of race.... With the FDA approval of BiDil's NDA based on race-specific

indication, only NitroMed will be able to publicly market it as a therapy for heart failure. Generic manufacturers will still be able to sell hydrazaline and isosorbide dinitrate separately, but they will not be able to advertise them as treatments for heart failure....

Thus, in addition to considering how BiDil's approval reifies race, it is essential also to examine its emergence at the intersection of commerce and health disparities. The problem with BiDil is not only that it biologizes race but also that it uses race as biology to create the impression that the best way to address health disparities is through commercial drug development. By exploiting race in the service of product promotion, it distorts public understanding of health disparities and of efforts to address them.[155]

Ironically, despite the emphasis on the genomic in pharmacogenomics, there are as yet no definitive genetic data or explanations supporting BiDil's efficacy in African American patients. Steven Nissen, chair of the FDA advisory committee that reviewed BiDil, wrote in 2005 that "we're using self-identified race as a surrogate for genetic markers."[156]

In a similar fashion, the biotech company VaxGen used race-based marketing for its AIDSVAX, a failed vaccine for AIDS. In 2003, VaxGen reported that 5.8% of those receiving a placebo had become infected over the course of the trial, while 5.7% of those using the vaccine became HIV+. In essence, the vaccine failed to have any effect. However, VaxGen reported that the vaccine worked better in "blacks, Asians, and other minorities enrolled in the trial."[157] It turns out that officials from the NIH and Emory University's School of Medicine subsequently found the data likely to be spurious. Both BiDil and VaxGen, it was hoped, would bolster the argument and support for pharmacogenomics. Supporters still point to the significant differences between Caucasians and Asians in the activity levels of enzymes critical to drug metabolism, for example Cytochrome P4502D6 (CYP2D6). Another example often cited is the drug Travatan, which is used as eye drops for controlling elevated intraocular pressure in black people.[158]

In addition to public and private institutions, patient advocacy groups have seized on the chance of having their interests heard and agendas implemented. In the spirit of inclusion and civil rights, various groups of people who suffer from genetic ailments have mobilized and have played an active and critical role in the diagnosis and treatment of diseases. In the 1970s, for example, prominent members of the African American community convinced the medical community and governmental officials that more money should be given to assist African Americans who were suffering from sickle-cell anemia. The idea was to empower African Americans to take a more active and responsible role in their healthcare.[159] More recently, Howard University, a historically black private university, joined forces with First Genetic Trust, a company that was interested in creating a "biobank" of the genomes of 25,000 individuals comprising the African diaspora. The goal of this bank, called the GRAD (Genomic Research in the African Diaspora) Biobank, is "to provide the biomedical research community with the clinical resources to better understand the genetic, biological, and environmental basis for differential disease risk, disease progression and drug response in persons of African descent."[160] There are now personal genomics companies that target the African American community.[161]

African Americans are not alone in relying on patient advocacy groups to address genetic disorders. A number of American organizations, such as the Center for Jewish Genetic Disorders of Mount Sinai Hospital and the Chicago Center for Jewish Genetic Disorders, are committed to diagnosing and treating Jewish genetic diseases, such as Tay-Sachs and Canavan disease. And patient advocacy groups are not limited to racial and ethnic interests. These grassroots organizations have played a huge role in diagnosing and treating HIV/AIDS and breast cancer over the past three decades.[162] As Epstein has demonstrated, the recent trend to speak of race at the level of the DNA is based on the desire to include (rather than exclude, as had been the case with eugenics) groups that historically have been marginalized. Regardless of the intent, the fear of essentializing race is real.

Reenter *CCR5*

It should come as no surprise that biomedical researchers have studied the responses of numerous subgroups to Maraviroc for HIV/AIDS treatment. One of the subgroups was based on race and ethnicity. Using subgroup analyses of data from the MOTIVATE 1 and 2 studies discussed in chapter 6, a team of scientists concluded that there was no difference in the efficacy and safety of Maraviroc based on race or ethnicity. Another subgroup was gender, and again no difference was detected.[163]

There are commercial tests available for the *Δ32* mutation. Apparently, it is one of the most commonly tested alleles by personal genomics companies. The company 23andMe encourages individuals to be tested for the allele.[164] These companies discuss how the allele arose in Europe and the debate about the allele's role in disease resistance.[165] Similarly, the sequence company XY Gene, which offered genetic tests for "man," labeled *CCR5-Δ32* "the HIV gene" and explained why it is important that people take the test.[166] The company also informed readers that the allele "is most prominent in individuals of European descent" and offered a breakdown of the percentages based on ethnicities—"European descent: 16%, African Americans: 2%, Ashkenazi Jew: 13%, Middle Eastern: 2–6%."[167] Many direct-to-consumer genetic-testing companies often include race in their marketing.[168] FamilyTreeDNA prominently displayed its advanced test for *CCR5-Δ32* on its Web site.[169] In March 2009, the test was featured as the company's "advanced test of the month."[170] It discussed the relevance of geography to the allele and offered outdated information about conveying resistance to the plague: "The deletion is believed to be associated with plague immunity. The deletion is found in up to 20% of Europeans, and is rare among Africans and Asians. The deletion in CCR5 is widely dispersed throughout Northern Europe and in those of European descent."[171] The Canadian company PALFIR HumanGenetic also advertises its test for *Δ32*: "Find Out If You Are Resistant to HIV—NOW ONLY $199.00."[172] People do not need to rely solely on their physicians: they can be their own expert and listen to the genetic-testing companies.

Biomedical researchers at nonprofit institutions, such as universities and federal agencies, have also defined *CCR5-Δ32* in part in terms of race and ethnicity. As was shown in chapter 7, many scientists (Burchard included) illustrate the biological basis of race by pointing to certain allele frequencies that vary between the races and by citing *CCR5-Δ32*:

Another important gene that affects a complex trait is *CCR5*—a receptor used by the human immunodeficiency virus (HIV) to enter cells. As many as 25 percent of white people (especially in northern Europe) are heterozygous for the *CCR5-delta 32* variant, which is protective against HIV infection and progression, whereas this variant is virtually absent in other groups, thus suggesting racial and ethnic differences in protection against HIV.[173]

In their 2003 *Scientific American* article, Michael J. Bamshad and Steve E. Olson posed the critical question "Does Race Exist?"[174] They concluded that genetic information can be used to distinguish groups possessing a common ancestry; however, a person might fit into one grouping according to one characteristic and another grouping according to a second characteristic. Bamshad and Olson conceded: "Human populations are very similar, but they often can be distinguished."[175] These groupings do not correspond very well with our older notions of race, such as those based on skin color, but new groupings based on genetic similarities can be useful in understanding how different populations experience disease or respond to drug treatment.

To find an example of an allele present in certain populations and not in others, they too turn to the *CCR5* gene locus:

This polymorphism [$\Delta 32$] in the *CCR5* receptor gene is found almost exclusively in groups from northeastern Europe.

Several [other] polymorphisms in *CCR5* do not prevent infection but instead influence the rate at which HIV-1 infection leads to AIDS and death. Some of these polymorphisms have similar effects in different populations; others only alter the speed of disease progression in selected groups. One polymorphism, for example, is associated with delayed disease progression in European Americans but accelerated disease in African-Americans. Researchers can only study such population-specific effects—and use that knowledge to direct therapy—if they can sort people into groups.[176]

Bamshad was the second author of an article analyzing the race-specific HIV-1 disease-modifying effects of certain *CCR5* haplotypes mentioned in the previous chapter.[177]

In 2005, Bamshad wrote an article for the *Journal of the American Medical Association* dealing with genes, race, and health asserting that geographic ancestry and explicit genetic information are more useful and accurate alternatives to antiquated notions of race:[178] "Making accurate ancestry inferences is crucial because common diseases and drug responses are sometimes influenced by gene variants that vary in frequency or differ altogether among racial groups. Thus, operationalizing alternatives to race for clinicians will be an important step toward providing more personalized health care."[179] To make his point, Bamshad needed to differentiate between ancestry (which he defined as "objective genetic relationships between individuals and among populations") and race (which "has always been a somewhat arbitrary definition of population boundaries").[180] Although there is an overlap between the two concepts, they are distinct. According to Bamshad, geographic ancestry does generate accurate but not perfect predictions of genetic ancestry. Geographic ancestry is less accurate when dealing with peoples who have experienced admixture throughout their histories, such as Hispanics and South Asians.[181]

Race, on the other hand, is far more imprecise. Recent studies suggest that the percentage of West African ancestry in African Americans averages around 80%; however, the range is from 20% to nearly 100%.[182] Likewise, Americans claiming European ancestry varies considerably, with 30% having less than 90% European lineage.[183] Worldwide, the notion of race is even less informative, and although a clearer picture of human ancestry is being uncovered, much is still being extrapolated from rather limited data sets.

CCR5, once again, plays a role, this time in Bamshad's argument as an example of the variation in gene copy number influencing disease risk in different populations based on geographic ancestry, rather than race. The *CCL3L1* gene, which codes for one of CCR5's natural ligands—MIP-1αP—varies in copy number from about two in Europeans to six in Africans, with most Asians having between three to four copies.[184] Because MIP-1αP competes with HIV-1 in binding with CCR5, a lower gene copy number is associated with lower concentrations of MIP-1αP, and therefore HIV-1 has better access to the receptor. As a result, a more rapid decline in the number of CD4 T cells results. It is not the absolute gene copy number that is critical, however, but the copy number standardized by the mean population number: "Therefore, *CCL3L1* gene dose can be interpreted as a risk factor only when considered along with an individual's group membership or geographic ancestry, possibly because mean copy number is associated with other genetic factors that influence risk."[185]

Bamshad's shift from using "race" to speaking of "geographic ancestry" or "genetic ancestry" is both informative and typical.[186] Over the past ten years or so, in response to people who advocate for a genetics of race, a growing number of biomedical researchers and medical geneticists have expressed their desire to avoid using race as a population category altogether for two reasons:[187] it carries with it excessive sociocultural baggage, and most biomedical researchers find the category unhelpful.[188] The problem with substituting ancestry for race is that genetic ancestry can be vague and imprecise, as well.[189] How is ancestry defined? Why are specific geographic divisions more important for variation studies than others? What time frame is the relevant one? And like race, geographic ancestry, when defined, is usually done so with respect to politics and culture.[190]

As has been shown, biomedical researchers are obsessed with differences. There are alternatives of differentiation, and those alternatives might be more informative. The analytical and experimental tools that some medical geneticists are employing are based on overall population rather than racial or ethnic differences. Developed in 2005, genome wide-association studies (GWAS) analyze millions of genetic variants (based on SNPs) found in hundreds of thousands of individuals to see if any are associated with a specific trait, such as a disease. Researchers compare the genetic information of two groups of people—one that suffers from a particular disease and another that does not. If an SNP allele is present in one group more than another, then that SNP is deemed to be associated with the disease. The technique, however, cannot determine if the association is causal or not.

In 2006, a group comprising medical and population geneticists and mathematicians from Harvard Medical School's Department of Genetics, Broad Institute's Program in Medical and Population Genetics, and

Brigham and Women's Hospital's Division of Rheumatology, Immunology, and Allergy invented an algorithm called EIGENSTRAT, which seeks out genetic markers for disease based on ancestry without the reliance on racial or ethnic categories.[191] Although the data that medical geneticists using EIGENSTRAT and GWAS might have been culled in terms of race or ethnicity, researchers claim that they do not use those categories while analyzing SNPs in relation to disease. EIGENSTRAT enables biomedical researchers "to account for genetic differences in their analyses, while race categories—which they viewed as socio-cultural concepts—were inappropriate for their genetic analyses."[192] Just as was the case with Bamshad, these researchers wished to use genetic ancestry or genetic history rather than race as an analytical tool. They spoke of EIGENSTRAT as "adjusting for ancestry."[193] They are embracing the gene's genealogy.

But is *genetic ancestry* or *genetic history* just another term for *race*? As Fujimura and Rajagopalan argue, some biomedical researchers using GWAS and EIGENSTRAT still speak of race and genetic ancestry interchangeably. In addition, "even though some researchers believe that race categories are socio-historical concepts and that race is an incorrect concept for use in genetics, the notion of shared ancestry is often read as race by the media, the public, or other researchers."[194] In recent *Δ32* studies, EIGENSTRAT was used; however, the researchers still analyzed groups based on race. For example, in 2009, Swiss biomedical researcher Jacques Fellay's lab performed GWAS and EIGENSTRAT in a group of 2,554 HIV-1-infected Caucasians and claimed that their study "represents a comprehensive assessment of common human genetic variation in HIV-1 control in Caucasians."[195] They concluded: "All variants securely identified in this study together explain 13% of the observed variability in HIV-1 viremia in a population of mostly male Caucasian adults.... Comparable studies are certainly needed in additional populations, notably in other ethnic groups, in women and in children to fully access the impact of common human genetic variation in HIV-1 control."[196] Fellay and others are interested in the role of human genetic variation in combatting infection agents, such as HIV-1.[197]

Similarly, Fellay's colleagues at Duke University School of Medicine performed a GWAS using EIGENSTRAT of 515 African Americans who are HIV-1+.[198] This study, which the authors believed was the first genome-wide association study on HIV-1 outcomes carried out in an African American cohort, found that a particular SNP was associated with viral load set point, or the amount of virus that stabilizes after a period of acute infection. The higher the viral load set point, the faster the appearance of AIDS symptoms. Their analyses confirmed that a member of the histocompatibility leukocyte antigen (HLA)-B*57 group of alleles is the most important common variant that influences viral load variation in African Americans, which is consistent with what has been observed for individuals of European ancestry, among whom the most important common variant is HLA-B*5701.[199] Here HIV-1 allele differences were categorized, at least partially, by race or ethnicity using GWAS and EIGENSTRAT.

In conclusion, questions about scientifically analyzing the differences among humans were and still are politically charged. To ask what is scientific and what is political would be to ask the wrong questions. It is not that the boundary between the scientific and the political for human classification has simply eroded: it never existed. The *CCR5-Δ32* allele was identified by the biomedical researchers as having distinct frequencies in difference races immediately on its discovery. Well-meaning decisions made by the National Institutes of Health (as reflected by the Revitalization Act of 1993 to include people of color and women in clinical research) as well as the FDA's subsequent rulings that pharmaceutical companies need to study the safety and efficacy of drugs for numerous subgroups, including racial subgroups, culminated in attempts to define *race* and *ethnicity* in terms of genetic alleles to improve the health care of all Americans. Once again, *CCR5* took center stage.

The racial and ethnic lens of analysis was reinforced by personal genomics companies and big pharma, both of which want patients to take control of their health and identity. "Be your own expert" seems wonderfully liberating and enlightened. In reality, such a mentality plays into the hands of private companies, which are happy to advertise their products to an educated public. As Gregg Bloche argues in the *New England Journal of Medicine*, "the emergence of the combination treatment as a race-specific drug was driven in large measure by regulatory and market incentives."[200] Personal genomics companies are eager to capture the imagination of an American market of people who are hungry to know where their ancestors hailed from and what might await them in their medical future. Those advocating the molecular basis of race are not doing so with racism in mind; rather, they see it as an opportunity for science to serve those who have historically been marginalized by the medical community in the United States. So while advocating for the individuality of pharmacogenomics, many are simultaneously seeking the legitimation of collective categories, such as race. In the case of race, the desires of the federal government to address sins of the past and be more inclusive, as Epstein has demonstrated, have raised other concerns. This chapter has shown how public and private interests are aligned although their intentions are quite different. This particular aspect of the *CCR5* gene is not one of a neoliberal, laissez-faire government that allows the private sector to call the shot but rather one of a government that insists that the private sector follow its lead in including underrepresented groups of American society. This episode in the story of the *CCR5* gene illustrates how biocapitalism accounts for some but not all of the gene's genealogy. Big pharma and personal genomics firms are two important biocapitalist enterprises. The National Institutes of Health and the Federal Drug Administration, however, are not. They took the lead in setting the agenda for inclusion, not the other way around.

Epilogue: The End of an Error?

If the object of history is to be blasted out of the continuum of historical succession, that is because its monadological structure demands it. This structure first comes to light in the extracted object itself. And it does so in the form of the historical confrontation that makes up the interior (and, as it were, the bowels) of the historical object, and into which enter all the forces and interests of history on a reduced scale.

—Walter Benjamin, *The Arcades Project*, 475.

On a cool, cloudy morning in early February 2010, I journeyed to lower Manhattan, the site of the Southern District Court of New York. The court guards told me that it was an atypically busy day. I stood on line as scores of people went through the security checkpoint and headed for courtroom 18C. By the time I arrived at the courtroom, slightly before 10 a.m., it was packed with reporters, scientists, biotech representatives, and lawyers. I wondered, "What in the world am I, a historian (albeit of science), doing here?" Everyone in the courtroom was waiting for Judge Robert Sweet to open proceedings for *Association for Molecular Pathology et al. v. U.S. Patent and Trademark Office, Myriad Genetics et al.*[1] For the first time, a court of law would determine whether genes (in this case, two breast cancer genes, *BRCA1* and *BRCA2*, which were patented by Myriad Genetics of Utah) should be considered products of nature and therefore fall outside the domain of patentable subject matter.[2] The plaintiffs included women who received false negative reports from Myriad and numerous biomedical researchers who were prohibited from creating additional diagnostic tests for the genes' mutations. These biomedical researchers argued that, in this particular case, patents were stymieing downstream research on diagnostics.

The previous August, Tania Simoncelli, who was working with the American Civil Liberties Union (ACLU) at the time, asked me if I would be interested in writing a deposition in *Association for Molecular Pathology v. USPTO, Myriad Genetics* on behalf of the ACLU. Because I was working on the early stages of this book, I agreed. Tania introduced me to Chris Hansen and Sandra Park, two ACLU attorneys who were assigned to the case. I then began to think about how genes were deemed patentable by the U.S. Patent and Trademark Office, the European Patent Office, and the Japanese Patent Office by studying other historical cases that were relevant to patentable subject matter. At that hearing at the Southern District Court of New York, it struck me that my background (some graduate training in molecular biology and a Ph.D. in history and philosophy of science, specializing in late eighteenth- and early nineteenth-century German physics) might allow me to contribute something relevant to the history of science, medicine, science and technology studies, molecular biology, bioethics, law, and policy studies.

Commercialism was not always a component of genetics. As Robert Kohler demonstrates in *Lords of the Fly: Drosophila Genetics and the Experimental Life*, the Drosophilists of the early twentieth century had a network of credit based on the sharing of mutant flies, techniques, and data. Personal credit and commercialism were deemed antithetical to the collective spirit of scientific research.[3] At that time, geneticists enjoyed the openness of a scientific republic.

Not surprisingly, the U.S. Patent and Trademark Office is loath to encourage Congress to create a new, specialized patent law for biotechnology, claiming that chemical intellectual property should remain the model. John J. Doll, who was the director of biotechnology examinations at the USPTO and went on to become its commissioner of patents and its acting director, uses history to defend his stance, asserting that some forty years earlier, scholars argued that broad utility patents would "devastate the industry" of polymer chemistry.[4] However, "just as the issuing of broad product claims at the early stages of this technology [polymer chemistry] did not deter development of other new vulcanized copolymers, the issuing of relatively broad utility claims in genomic technology should not deter inventions in genomics."[5] Perhaps Doll best summed up the threat that would loom if the patent system made changes:

Without the incentive of patents, there would be less investment in DNA research, and scientists might not disclose their new DNA products to the public. Issuance of patents to such products not only results in the dissemination of technological information to the scientific community for use as a basis for further research but also stimulates investment in the research, development, and commercialization of new biologics. It is only with the patenting of DNA technology that some companies, particularly smaller ones, can raise sufficient venture capital to bring beneficial products to the marketplace or fund further research. A strong U.S. patent system is critical for the continued development and dissemination to the public of information on DNA sequence elements.[6]

The vice president of government relations of the U.S. trade group Biotechnology Industry Organization (BIO), Chuck Ludlam, has similarly predicted disaster for those who wish to tinker with the patent system: "Any move that compromises issuance of patents on genetic tests could have an impact on drug research. They are not separable. If there is an idea around of changing the law of the licensing on diagnostics, I think that is dangerous and misguided."[7]

Patent owners' prognostications of doom and gloom in response to the possible revocation of their gene patents have now become mundane. To them, disallowing product (or composition-of-matter) claims on genes would be financially disastrous and would impede scientific progress. Historians need to analyze that statement rather than simply assume prima facie its accuracy: things that seem intuitive are not always true. In 1900, two countries led the world in the production of pharmaceuticals—Germany and Switzerland, which was a distant second. German law did not permit the patenting of drugs at the time. Only their processes were patentable. Switzerland's chemical industry initially opposed the patent system and then demanded to be kept outside of it. Even chemical processes were not patentable in Switzerland until 1907.[8] Both German and Swiss industries excelled without product patents for pharmaceuticals. French patent law, on the other hand, was so broad in scope that process patents included the resulting product. Likewise, a patented product included all of possible manufacturing methods. Companies enviously guarded their intellectual property to such an extent that monopolies were created that forced competing chemists and dyers from other companies to relocate to other countries. As a result, France's chemical industries suffered.[9] It is therefore not necessarily the case that product patents will either guarantee future income or foster scientific and technological development. And recall that during the early twentieth century, American pharmaceutical companies lobbied against patenting chemical substances because they were facing what they claimed was unfair competition from German companies, which sought such product patents outside of Germany.[10] In short, different patent regimes cater to the interests and abilities of various nations. One size does not fit all.

Some recent studies refute Doll and Ludlam's predictions and suggest that gene patents actually have hampered research on diagnostics and therapeutics. One issue is whether gene patents impede the sharing of scientific knowledge. Some studies suggest that patents do not prohibit the flow information, and others argue the opposite.[11] In a survey of clinical laboratory directors, Stanford University bioethicist Mildred Cho and her colleagues found that 85% of the respondents felt that gene patents have resulted in less knowledge sharing[12] and 67% claimed that patents resulted in a decreased ability to conduct research.[13] Although conflicting evidence addresses the fear of increased secrecy, studies have demonstrated that patents on genetic tests have been deleterious. Patents on genetic tests can stymie downstream research on diagnostics and therapeutics. In fact, 37% of clinical labs either abandoned or ceased developing tests for the human hemochromatosis (HFE) gene after it was patented.[14] Cho reported that 25% of 122 of laboratory directors telephone surveyed claimed that their labs had ceased performing clinical genetic tests as a result of a notification from a patent holder or licensee, and 53% decided not to develop a new clinical genetic test for the same reason. There are a total of twelve genetic tests on which biomedical scientists were prevented from working. Cho and her colleagues concluded "that patents and licenses have had a significant effect on the ability of clinical laboratories to develop and provide genetic tests. Furthermore, our findings suggest that clinical geneticists feel that their research is inhibited by patents."[15] And these findings have been corroborated by a study of the American Society of Human Genetics, which found that 47% of the respondents maintained that patents have delayed or limited their research, and two-thirds of lab directors surveyed asserted that patents inhibit research.[16]

Although many in the biotech sector argue that Myriad Genetics is a unique bête noir, several companies have taken their cue from Myriad's patent-protection practice, and some are even more aggressive. Diagnostic companies Athena Diagnostics and PGxHealth have excluded university laboratories from offering genetic tests for long QT syndrome and Alzheimer's disease.[17] The genes for Alzheimer's disease were patented by Duke University and other academic institutions and licensed exclusively to Athena Diagnostics, which in turn exploited its patents to preclude others from offering the test.[18] GeneDx and university laboratories stopped testing for long QT syndrome after receiving cease-and-desist letters following the gene patent in 2002 even though no commercial test was marketed until 2004.[19] Similarly, companies holding patents for the genetic tests associated with genetic hearing loss, Canavan disease, in which sufferers cannot metabolize aspartic acid, and asthma have used their exclusive rights to prohibit other laboratories from offering genetic testing.[20]

In autumn 2002, the Advisory Committee on Genetics, Health, and Society (SACGHS) was given the charge to advise the Department of Health and Human Services on the ethical, legal, social, and medical issues that are created by technological advances in the field of human genetics. In particular, they were asked to determine the effects of both gene patenting on research and of patents on genetic tests on healthcare. On March 31, 2010, the SACGHS delivered its report to the Department of Health and Human Services.[21] SACGHS based its findings on eight case studies of particular genetic tests for ten clinical conditions conducted by Robert Cook-Deegan and his research team at Duke University's Center for Genome Ethics, Law, and Policy.[22] Their report made a number of critical and informative points, many of which dispelled the myths both of the importance of gene patenting to research and development and of the necessity of patenting for the creation of genetic tests. First, the federal government is the major supporter of basic genetic research in the United States. In 2006, the federal government funded 59% of basic research.[23] The claim that patents might stimulate private investment in genetics research seems to be irrelevant. Scientists have reasons to invent that are independent of patents. For example, biomedical researchers who are racing to find the genes associated with Alzheimer's disease argue that the competition was fueled by "wanting priority of scientific discovery, prestige, scientific credit, and the ability to secure funding for additional research based on scientific achievement."[24] Patenting was not listed as a reason. As the president of PreventionGenetics, a leader in offering tests for genetic ailments, declared:

DNA patents are not needed as motivation for identification of disease genes. Nearly all disease genes are identified not by private industry, but by researchers working at non-profit institutions. These researchers are motivated primarily by competition with their peers for faculty positions at top ranked institutions, for publication space in top journals, and for grants. Profit motive from patents plays only a very minor motivational role at best.[25]

SACGHS concluded that although patents might stimulate private funding to add to the substantially greater amount of money provided by the federal government, private investment rarely is devoted exclusively to diagnostics.[26]

Second, evidence strongly suggests that gene patents discourage subsequent research. Scientists rarely consult patents and patent applications because they disclose significantly less information than a publication. As

K. G. Huang and F. E. Murray have shown, gene patents have a "negative impact on follow-on public research, which results in less public knowledge than would occur if the patented genes were only published and not patented."[27]

Third, there is no evidence to suggest that the possession of exclusive rights was necessary for the development of a genetic test. For example, more than fifty private and public entities offer tests for both cystic fibrosis and Huntington's disease.[28] When exclusive rights are granted, however, there is only one provider of the test, which has proven to be problematic in a number of cases. And exclusive rights do not speed up test development.[29] Moreover, if market forces are allowed to dictate research, tests for rare hereditary disorders will most likely not be developed.[30]

Fourth, not only are patents unnecessary for the creation and development of genetic tests, but they actually threaten the development of new testing technologies. The American College of Medical Genetics is adamant that "genetic tests are typically well-developed and being delivered BEFORE patent holders seek to control the testing. Therefore, it is self-evident that gene patents are not needed to stimulate the development of tests."[31] Such a sentiment was backed by the president of PreventionGenetics and the College of American Pathologists.[32] When gene tests were patented, patent-rights holders can jealously enforce their rights.[33] This is particularly true of multiplex tests, parallel sequencing, and whole-genome sequencing. These techniques involve testing numerous genes, all of which may be patented.[34] Developers of those tests will need to pay royalties or licensing fees for each patented gene. SACGHS found instances where laboratories decided not to report medically significant results relevant to patented genes for fear of infringement liability.[35] SACGHS concluded that "Based on all of the above information, patent-derived exclusive rights are neither necessary nor sufficient conditions for the development of genetic test kits and laboratory-developed tests. In the area of laboratory-developed tests particularly, where development costs are not substantial, patents were not necessary for the development of several genetic tests."[36]

Fifth, when exclusive rights are granted for a genetic test, if the tester does not accept the patient's insurance, then the patient must pay out of pocket.[37] Also, a second opinion is rendered impossible, as was the case with Myriad Genetics' *BRCA1* and *BRCA2* gene tests.[38] Some patents have limited clinical access to genetic tests, particularly when exclusive licenses are granted.[39]

SACGHS made six recommendations to the Secretary of Health and Human Services:

1. The Secretary of Health and Human Services (HHS) should support and work with the Secretary of Commerce to promote the following statutory changes:

A. The creation of an exemption from liability for infringement of patent claims on genes for anyone making, using, ordering, offering for sale, or selling a test developed under the patent for patient-care purposes.

B. The creation of an exemption from patent infringement liability for those who use patent-protected genes in pursuit of research.

...

2. Using relevant authorities and necessary resources, the Secretary should explore, identify, and implement mechanisms that will increase adherence to current guidelines that promote nonexclusive licensing of diagnostic genetic/genomic technologies.

The Secretary should convene stakeholders—for example, representatives from industry and academic institutions, researchers, and patients—to develop a code of conduct that will further broad access to such technologies.

...

3. Using relevant authorities and necessary resources, the Secretary should explore, identify, and implement mechanisms that will make information about the type of license and the field of use for which rights were granted readily available to the public.

...

4. The Secretary should establish an advisory board to provide ongoing advice about the health impact of gene patenting and licensing practices. The advisory board also could provide input on the implementation of any future policy changes, including the other recommendations in this report.

...

5. The Secretary should work with the Secretary of Commerce to ensure that the USPTO is kept apprised of scientific and technological developments related to genetic testing and technology.

...

6. Given that genetic tests will be increasingly incorporated into medical care, the Secretary should ensure that those tests shown to have clinical utility are equitably available and accessible to patients.[40]

Not surprisingly, Europeans are dealing with the same issues. On November 29, 2005, the European Society of Human Genetics (ESHG) Public and Professional Policy Committee and the Patenting and Licensing Committee initiated a meeting on the patenting and licensing of gene testing. A year later, it convened a workshop, and the recommendations agreed on by both groups were endorsed by the board of the ESHG in June 2007.[41] Although the ESHG Working Party on Patenting and Licensing (WPPL) felt that gene and gene-testing patents challenge existing intellectual property law, it did not wish to propose a new model of intellectual property that catered specifically to genetics. Rather, it wanted to work within the existing intellectual property guidelines, seeking different types of licensing models that would enhance access to the patented materials.[42] The WPPL recommended that the European Patent Office not permit broad utility claims on gene patents: "It has been sufficiently illustrated that overly broad claims negatively impact development."[43] As mentioned previously, Germany and France have adopted purpose-bound patent protection that affords protection only to situations in which the nucleic-acid sequence is performing the functions described in the patent.[44] The WPPL also suggested that the European Patent Office prohibit the patenting of individual mutations in known disease genes due to a lack of novelty, adding that a "more important and socially acceptable ruling would be to consider that establishing a link between a disease and a genetic sequence or defect is merely a discovery and therefore not patentable, unless the identification of this link includes a real conceptual innovation."[45]

The Working Party on Patenting and Licensing also was concerned with establishing guidelines for licensing in reasonable terms, which would include the implementation of alternative licensing models. Compulsory licenses help prevent patentees from exerting monopoly rights. Several European countries have tailored models for compulsory licenses applicable to healthcare.[46] Other recommendations included reducing the backlog of examinations, reconsidering the ethical issues involved in gene patenting, promoting access to information on gene patents and patent applications, defining the scope of research exemption more explicitly, requesting stakeholders to develop a code of conduct, and implementing a required course for Ph.D. students on intellectual property.[47]

Although it might be argued that the number of problems with gene patents is dwarfed by the overwhelming number of patents that have not thwarted research and diagnostics, that would be missing the point. Of course, there are numerous examples in which patent holders have permitted access to their patents at a reasonable price. We are only now beginning to see the effects of patenting on research on diagnostic testing. And the future of phenotypic testing based on numerous genes will exacerbate the problem. Myriad Genetics, Athena Diagnostics, and PGxHealth did nothing illegal: they simply guarded and enforced their intellectual property rights. It strikes me that leaving the accessibility of genetic testing to the goodwill of for-profit entities is problematic, if not outright foolish. These small companies that Doll wishes to protect are precisely the problem. As Boston University economist Iain Cockburn argues, "There are a lot of small, hungry companies out there whose only asset is intellectual property. It's less likely that broad cross-licensing agreements can happen. If you have too many people owning small, overlapping slices of the same pie, there could be a breakdown."[48] In addition, absence of evidence does not necessarily mean absence of harm. As summarized below, it took the backing of the ACLU to draw the public's attention to the problems that are inherent with gene patenting. Although, in principle, anyone may challenge a patent, it is difficult to do so without financial and intellectual resources.

There is some light at the end of the tunnel, and it might not be one of an oncoming train. The major patent offices have become more stringent with adjudicating gene patents over the past decade. Although the number of gene patents increased considerably in the United States during the 1990s, that number has decreased significantly during the first decade of the new millennium.[49] The proportion of gene-patent applications granted by the European Patent Office by September 2005 decreased from 45% of those submitted in the 1980s to 8% of those submitted between 1996 and 2000.[50] And some conjecture that a number of patents will be abandoned prematurely as either technical problems prove insurmountable or commercial viability becomes limited. For example, only 70% of the U.S. Patent and Trademark Office DNA patents awarded in the early 1990s were still maintained by 2005.[51] Gene-patent filing at all three major patent offices declined sharply after the Human Genome Project made the human genome sequence public in 2001, thereby rendering it difficult to satisfy the novelty criterion.[52] The number of composition-of-matter claims for DNA and RNA sequences decreased significantly in the United States after 2000, but method claims increased significantly, particularly after 2005. And the percentage of human nucleic-acid-sequence patents declined from 58% of all nucleotide-sequence patents in 2000 to 19% in 2010.[53] Numerous patentees who were interviewed felt that they were now faced with significant challenges, such as more rigorous criteria for demonstrating utility, novelty, nonobviousness, full written description, and unity of invention (the parts of the invention are intrinsically linked). And some argued that the USPTO's Revised Utility Guidelines of 2001 had raised the bar on patent eligibility.[54] That said, data have suggested that U.S.-based biotech firms are still successful in obtaining gene patents from the USPTO, whereas the EPO and JPO grant a far lower percentage.[55]

In short, the publication of the human genome and the stricter requirements placed on gene patent applications have resulted in a decrease in the number of applications and the number of patents awarded during the first decade of the century. Speculative, broad utility claims (such as the ones granted by the USPTO in early 2000 for the *CCR5* gene) are now much more difficult to pass examination. Nevertheless, such changes in policy, Hopkins has argued, will have little effect "on the legacy of specific concerns about the patenting of disease-associated, and other genes for diagnostic purposes (e.g., cancer genes such as *BRCA1*, and the hemochromatosis gene *HFE*). In these cases, it may be necessary to resort to compulsory licensing or other measures to ensure that the benefits of DNA-based diagnostics are not unduly monopolized."[56] Ironically, the CCR5 patent might become emblematic again—this time for the promises (as Fortun calls them) that never materialized after the initial euphoria of the 1990s. After a struggle of several months to acquire Human Genome Sciences, GlaxoSmithKline finally took control of the sequencing company on August 3, 2012, for $3.6 billion on an equity basis, or $3 billion net of cash and debt.

On May 12, 2009, the ACLU and the Public Patent Foundation (PUBPAT) filed a lawsuit against the U.S. Patent and Trademark Office and Myriad Genetics of Utah in the Second Circuit Court of Appeals in Manhattan. Their strategy to torpedo the patents was twofold: they argued that the patents on the genes and their mutations were unconstitutional and that genes are products of nature and therefore not patent eligible. In March 2010, Judge Robert Sweet ruled that U.S. Supreme Court precedents declare that products of nature are not patentable unless "a change [is made] that results in the creation of a fundamentally new product."[57] Because Myriad made no change to the patented sequences, Judge Sweet ruled against the patents. Not surprisingly, Myriad appealed the case to the U.S. Court of Appeals for the Federal Circuit (CAFC).

The acting solicit general, Neal Katyal, intervened on April 4, 2011, which was the first time that the top legal advocate of the executive branch appeared before the U.S. CAFC.[58] He did not support the U.S. Patent and Trademark Office's stance that isolated DNA molecules are patentable; he urged a compromise via the so-called magic microsope test. If an imaginary microscope could focus on a claimed DNA sequence as it exists in the human body, then the DNA is a product of nature and therefore not patentable.[59] *BRCA1* and *BRCA2* genes could, in principle, be seen with this magical telescope; therefore, they should not be patentable. This microscope, however, could not find cDNA sequences in the human genome because cDNA is the product of the human hand and is, in his view, therefore patentable.

The CAFC did not seem to be persuaded by this analogy. By a vote of two to one, the court opined on July 29, 2011, that Myriad's patents on isolated sequences of DNA were patent eligible, thereby reversing Judge Sweet's decision of March 2010.

In December 2011, the ACLU appealed the Court of Appeals for the Federal Circuit's ruling to the U.S. Supreme Court, which granted a writ of certiorari on March 26, 2012. The case was remanded back to the CAFC for further consideration in light of *Mayo Collaborative Services v. Prometheus Laboratories*, 566 U.S. —, 132 S. Ct. 1289 (2012), in which the Supreme Court ruled 9 to 0 that natural laws may not be patented standing alone or in connection with processes that involve "well-understood, routine, conventional activity."[60] This case dealt with Prometheus's method claims for administering a drug to a subject, determining a metabolite concentration in the subject's blood, and inferring the need for a change in dosage based on concentration. The Court ruled that the methods were not patent-eligible subject matter because they contributed nothing inventive to the law of nature that formed the basis of their claimed invention.

On July 20, the CCAF reconsidered the BRCA1 and BRCA2 patent case, and on August 16, the court offered its ruling. The three judges' opinions remained unchanged, confirming their original decision that genes are patent eligible by a vote of two to one.

The ACLU then appealed the Court of Appeals for the Federal Circuit's second decision to the U.S. Supreme Court, which in November 2012 decided that it would hear the case, conceding that the Court would not consider the constitutionality of human gene patents. The issue for the Supreme Court was solely one of patent eligibility. On June 13, 2013, the Supreme Court ruled unanimously that genes that were isolated from the human genome were not patentable.[61] The decision, written by Justice Clarence Thomas, held that a "naturally occurring DNA segment is a product of nature and not patent eligible merely because it has been isolated."[62] Because Myriad genetics neither created nor altered the DNA sequence coding for the *BRCA1* and *BRCA2* genes, there was no invention. The Court felt that the rule against the patenting of natural products was not without limits, however. The key was to strike a balance between creating incentives for discoveries and inventions and hindering the spread of information (which might otherwise create new inventions).[63] In essence, the Court deemed that mere isolation was not sufficient for patent eligibility. In its ruling, the Court drew on two main precedent cases—*Diamond v. Chakrabarty* and *Funk Brothers Seed Co. v. Kalo Inoculant Co.* It underscored that the key to the *Chakrabarty* ruling was that the newly created bacterium possessed "markedly different characteristics from any found in nature."[64] In contrast, Myriad did not create anything novel. Kalo Inoculant's claim in *Funk* was referring to a law of nature; the Court reckoned that Myriad's patents were as well. Like Kalo Inoculant's mixture of six bacterial strains, Myriad's genes were not eligible subject matter for patents.[65]

The decision was somewhat of a compromise. Echoing the opinions of all three Federal Circuit judges and Katyal, the Supreme Court found that cDNA is indeed patent eligible because it is created in the laboratory and differs from the naturally occurring DNA because the introns are excised.[66] Even though the sequence of cDNA is determined by nature,

the lab technician unquestionably creates something new when cDNA is made. cDNA retains the naturally occurring exons of DNA, but it is distinct from the DNA from which it was derived. As a result, cDNA is not a "product of nature" and is patent eligible under §101, except insofar as very short series of DNA may have no intervening introns to remove when creating cDNA. In that situation, a short strand of cDNA may be indistinguishable from natural DNA.[67]

For those suffering from AIDS, perhaps the most exciting chapter of the story of the *CCR5* gene grabbed worldwide headlines in 2010 and still awaits its conclusion. In 2007, a forty-year-old white male, Timothy Ray Brown—who was born in Seattle, resided in San Francisco, and was diagnosed with acute myeloid leukemia—entered the Charité Universitätsmedizin in Berlin, Germany. He had been identified as HIV+ in 1995, and he had been treated daily with HAART (efavirenz, emtricitabine, and tenofir) from 2003 to 2007. In 2007 and 2008 biomedical researchers in Berlin performed two bone-marrow transplantations from a donor who was homozygous for *CCR5-Δ32*. The patient did not experience viral rebound twenty months after the transplantation and discontinuation of HAART.[68] In December 2010, German physicians declared their HIV+ patient "cured."[69] To date, the patient remains HIV–. The donor's marrow was able to generate new CD4 cells that remained uninfected by the virus.[70] Although some saw this as a breakthrough in patient treatment, many warned that bone-marrow transplantations are a treatment of last resort for cancers such as leukemia. As Robert Gallo observed: "It's not practical and it can kill people.... I don't want to throw cold water on an interesting thing, but that's what it is—an interesting thing."[71] The results need to be replicated, and skeptics point out that extremely low levels of virus might be present that have not yet been detected. In addition, because about 1% of northeastern Europeans are homozygous for *CCR5-Δ32*, finding relevant donors will not be easy.

And in the age of biocapitalism, race has also become a commodity. Race has been used strategically as a genetic category to obtain both patent protection and drug approval, as was the case with BiDil. Ironically, the age of personalized genomic medicine tends to create medical diagnoses and medical care based on groups that have diverse genetic and health risks.[72] How we use the tools of molecular biology to examine and characterize genetic differences among humans has critical sociocultural and political consequences. There is nothing inevitable about using race as a major category of classification and differentiation, and we need to understand the economic and political interests that provide the impetus for making those choices as well as appreciate that there are alternatives.

As has been noted in earlier chapters of this book, sociologists and anthropologists of science have expressed concerns over privileging racial categories over others in understanding and explaining human diversity. They fear that other important aspects of healthcare and diversity will be ignored. They have also warned that although the government's effort is a noble one (and that of pharmaceutical and personal genomics companies less so), privileging race as a category of differentiation introduces a myriad of undesired consequences. Some bioethicists and biomedical researchers feel that scientists tend merely to give lip service to the ethical considerations of biotechnology. Racial categories (when properly defined and implemented) might be one (as opposed to the only) appropriate tool for certain studies on human diversity; however, financial interests cannot be the driving force. Big pharma and personal genomics companies tend to feature race when advertising their products. Even though the federal government initiated such a move, private interests are increasingly determining how scientific knowledge is constructed. This cannot remain unchallenged, particularly when it comes to health, identities, histories, and genealogies.

On November 22, 2013, the Food and Drug Administration sent 23andMe a letter demanding that it cease marketing and selling its DNA testing service until the company received FDA approval for medical tests.[73] Less than two weeks later, 23andMe acquiesced and decided that it would continue to test for ancestry and offer customers their "raw genetic" information but would not divulge any "genetic profiles that predispose them to particular illnesses, or predict their responses to prescription drugs."[74]

In conclusion, this book has gestured at the role of history in public policy, much in the spirit of works in the history and sociology of science. It also has told the tale of historical alternatives. Governments and industries of the developed world have been efficient at effacing the past. As a historian, I have attempted to resurrect the past to illustrate the paths not taken and to explain why they were never taken. As Walter Benjamin reminds us, histories that feature only the victors and that forget objects often can be exploited by those in power with sinister results. Too much is at stake to remain silent until all is settled. Surely our calling is, to paraphrase Karl Marx, not simply to interpret the world but to change it.

List of Abbreviations

AAMC	Association of American Medical Colleges
ACMG	American College of Medical Genetics
A-HeFT	African-American Heart Failure Trial
AIDS	Acquired Immunodeficiency Syndrome
AIMs	ancestry-informative markers
ATCC	American Type Culture Collection
AZT	azidothymidine
BIO	Biotechnology Industry Organization
BPAI	Board of Patent Appeals and Interferences
CAFC	Court of Appeals for the Federal Circuit
cART	combination antiretroviral treatment
cDNA	complementary DNA
Chem13	an earlier name for CCR5
DNA	deoxyribonucleic acid
ELSI	Ethical, Legal, and Social Implications (ELSI) Group (associated with the Human Genome Project and the International Haplotype Map)
EPC	European Patent Commission
EPO	European Patent Office
ESHG	European Society of Human Genetics
ESTs	expressed sequence tags
FDA	Food and Drug Administration
gp	glycoprotein
GPCR	G protein-coupled receptor
HAART	highly active antiretroviral therapy
HapMap	International Haplotype Map
HEK cells	human embryonic kidney cells
HGDP	Human Genome Diversity Project
HGP	Human Genome Project

HGS	Human Genome Sciences, Inc.
HIV	Human Immunodeficiency Virus
HRI	Health Research Incorporated
HTA	heteroduplexing tracking assay
HTS	high-throughput screening
JPO	Japanese Patent Office
LTNP	long-term nonprogressors
mAB	monoclonal antibodies
MCP-1	monocyte chemotactic (or chemoattractant) protein-1
MIP	macrophage inflammatory protein
mRNA	messenger RNA
NACHGR	National Advisory Council for Human Genome Research
NARTIs (also NRTIs)	nucleoside analog reserve-transcriptase inhibitors
NCI	National Cancer Institute
NDA	new drug application
NHGRI	National Human Genome Research Institute
NIH	National Institutes of Health
NNRTIs	nonnucleoside reverse-transcriptase inhibitors
NtARTIs (also NtRTIs)	nucleotide analog reverse-transcriptase inhibitors
OD	Opposition Division of the European Patent Office
ORF	open reading frame
PCR	polymerase chain reaction
PD	priority date of a patent
PI	protease inhibitor
PP	patent proprietor
RANTES	regulated on activation, normal T cell expressed and secreted
RNA	ribonucleic acid
SACGHS	Secretary's Advisory Committee on Genetics, Health, and Society
SAR	structure-activity relationship
SNP	single-nucleotide polymorphism
STR	short tandem repeat polymorphism
TAG	Treatment Action Group

TIGR	The Institute for Genomic Research
TRIPS	Agreement on Trade-Related Aspects of Intellectual Property Rights
UPVO	Union International pour la Protection des Obtentions Végétales
USPTO	United States Patent and Trademark Office
WPPL	Working Party on Patenting and Licensing

Notes

Chapter 1

1. James Shreeve, *The Genome War: How Craig Venter Tried to Capture the Code of Life and Save the World* (New York: Knopf, 2004), 85–86. See also Kevin Davies, *Cracking the Genome: Inside the Race to Crack the Human Genome* (Baltimore, MD: Johns Hopkins University Press, 2001), 64–65.

2. As quoted in Davies, *Cracking the Genome*, 64–65. See also Shreeve, *The Genome War*, 85–86.

3. Shreeve, *The Genome War*, 86.

4. Ibid., 86–88.

5. As quoted in ibid., 87.

6. As quoted in ibid., 88. Genetic transduction is the process whereby DNA is transferred from one bacterium to another via a virus. It also can refer to the process by which foreign DNA is introduced into a cell by means of a viral vector.

7. M. D. Adams, Jenny M. Kelley, Jeannine D. Gocayne, et al., "Complementary DNA Sequencing: Expressed Sequence Tags and Human Genome Project," *Science* 252, no. 5013 (1991): 1651–1652.

8. Shreeve, *The Genome War*, 82–84; Robert Cook-Deegan, *The Gene Wars: Science, Politics, and the Human Genome* (New York: Norton, 1994), 309.

9. Shreeve, *The Genome War*, 88.

10. Steven Shapin, *The Scientific Life: A Moral History of a Late Modern Vocation* (Chicago: University of Chicago Press, 2008), 209–268.

11. Ibid., 210 (emphasis in the original).

12. Sheila Jasanoff, *Designs on Nature: Science and Democracy in Europe and the United State* (Princeton, NJ: Princeton University Press, 2005), 42–45.

13. Philip J. Hilts, *Scientific Temperaments: Three Lives in Contemporary Science* (New York: Simon & Schuster, 1982), 176–77, as quoted in Shapin, *The Scientific Life*, 222.

14. Shapin, *The Scientific Life*, 254–255. Although I concur with Shapin that for-profit research is no more corrupt than nonprofit university research, innovations in for-profit companies generally benefit only those who invest in those companies. They are not interested in the public good. For a good account of secrecy at universities, particularly when private interests are at stake, see Sheldon Krimsky, *Science in the Private Interest: Has the Lure of Profits Corrupted Biomedical Research?* (Lanham, MD: Rowman & Littlefield, 2003), 82–86.

15. "Incyte Genomics, Inc. History," available at http://www.fundinguniverse.com/company-histories/incyte-genomics-inc-history/, accessed January 22, 2014, original source International Directory of Company Histories, vol. 52 (Farmington Hills, MI: St. James Press, 2003).

16. Michael Fortun, *Promising Genomics: Iceland and deCODE Genetics in a World of Speculation* (Berkeley: University of California Press, 2009), 51.

17. Stephen A. Merrill and Anne-Marie Mazza, eds., *Reaping the Benefits of Genomic and Proteomic Research* (Washington, DC: National Academies Press, 2006), 48.

18. Michael M. Hopkins, Surya Mahdi, Pari Patel, et al., "DNA Patenting: The End of an Era?," *Nature Biotechnology* 25, no. 2 (2007): 187. See also Antonio Regalado, "The Great Gene Grab," *MIT Technology Review* 103, no. 5 (September–October 2000): 48–55, available at http://www.technologyreview.com/featuredstory/400800/the-great-gene-grab, accessed January 21, 2014. By 2000 the University of California had 253 patents, GlaxoSmithKlein 248, the U.S. Department of Health and Human Services 205, Novo Nordisk 196, Genentech 165, Isis Pharmaceuticals 146, Chiron 135, American Home Products 130, and Novartis 128. By the end of the decade, big pharma dominated the list of leading DNA patent holders—DuPont, Roche, the University of California, Merck, Novartis, GlaxoSmithKline, Pfizer, Isis Pharmaceuticals, Sanofi Aventis, Incyte, Takeda Pharmaceuticals, Life Technologies, Amgen, and Human Genome Sciences. See Robert Cook-Deegan and Christopher Heaney, "Patents in Genomics and Human Genetics," *Annual Review of Genomics and Human Genetics* 11 (2010): 383–425, here 388. See also Gregory D. Graff, Devon Phillips, Zhen Lei, et al., "Not Quite a Myriad of Gene Patents," *Nature Biotechnology* 31, no. 5 (2013): 404–410, here 409; Donna M. Gitter, "International Conflicts over Patenting Human DNA Sequences in the United States and the European Union: An Argument for Compulsory Licensing and a Fair-Use Exemption," *NYU Law Review* 76, no. 6 (2001): 1631; Paul Smaglik, "Could AIDS Treatments Slip through Patents Loophole?," *Nature* 404, no. 6776 (2000): 322.

19. Shreeve, *The Genome War*, 89; Fortun, *Promising Genomics*, 39–40.

20. "Incyte Genomics, Inc. History," available at http://www.fundinguniverse.com/company-histories/incyte-genomics-inc-history/, accessed January 22, 2014, original

source International Directory of Company Histories, vol. 52 (Farmington Hills, MI: St. James Press, 2003).

21. Fortun, *Promising Genomics*, 40–41.

22. As quoted in ibid., 41, original in Joan O. Hamilton, "How SmithKline and Incyte Became Lab Partners," *Signals Magazine*, December 22, 1997.

23. Nicolas Wade, "Assembling of the Genome Is at Hand," *New York Times*, April 7, 2000, A20; Gitter, "International Conflicts," 1631. See also Regalado, *The Great Gene Grab*, 50.

24. Fortun, *Promising Genomics*, 41.

25. Cook-Deegan, *The Gene Wars*, 65.

26. Ibid.

27. For a more complete history of gene sequencing, see Shreeve, *The Genome War*, 57–67.

28. Cook-Deegan, *The Gene Wars*, 70–71.

29. S. F. Altschul, W. Gish, W. Miller, et al., "Basic Local Alignment Search Tool," *Journal of Molecular Biology* 215, no. 3 (1990): 403–410.

30. *CCR5*, when italicized, refers to the gene and its alleles, and CCR5 refers to the protein product, the chemokine receptor that is discussed in further detail in the ensuing chapters. I do not italicize CCR5 when I am speaking of the patent portfolio, as the patent includes the gene and its product as well as other claims.

31. Elliot Marshall, "Patent on HIV Receptor Provokes Outcry," *Science* 287, no. 5457 (2000): 1375–1377. See also U.S. Patent 6,025,154, available at http://www .patents.com/us-6025154.html, accessed January 22, 2014.

32. Marshall, "Patent on HIV Receptor," 1377.

33. Paul Jacobs and Peter G. Gosselin, "'Robber Barons of the Genetic Age': Experts Fret over the Effect of Gene Patents of Research," *Los Angeles Times*, February 28, 2000, available at http://articles.latimes.com/2000/feb/28/news/mn-3512, accessed January 21, 2014.

34. Note that this would represent a low-sequence homology and that the U.S. Patent and Trademark Office requires a much high percentage of sequence homology to grant a patent. See John C. Wooley and Herbert S. Lin, eds., *Catalyzing Inquiry at the Interface of Computing and Biology* (Washington, DC: National Academies Press, 2005), 105.

35. U.S. Patent 6,025,154, available at http://www.patents.com/us-6025154.html, accessed January 22, 2014.

36. Edward A. Berger, Philip M. Murphy, and Joshua M. Farber, "Chemokine Receptors as HIV-1 Coreceptors: Roles in Viral Entry, Tropism, and Disease," *Annual Review of Immunology* 17 (1999): 660; Marco Baggiolini, "Introduction," in *Chemokine Biology: Basic Research and Clinical Application*, ed. Bernhard Moser, Gordon L. Letts, and Kuldeep Neote, 3–15 (Basel: Birkhäuser, 2006), here 4.

37. James M. Fox and James E. Pease, "The Molecular and Cellular Biology of CC Chemokines and Their Receptors," in *Chemokines, Chemokine Receptors, and Disease: Current Topics in Membranes*, ed. Lisa M. Schwiebert, 73–102 (San Diego: Elsevier Academic Press, 2005), here 75. In 2005, there were forty-four known chemokines and eighteen receptors. See also Iain Comerford and Shaun R. McColl, "Mini Review Series: Focus on Chemokines," *Immunology and Cell Biology* 89 (2011): 183.

38. Baggiolini, "Introduction," 7.

39. Krishna Vaddi, Margaret Keller, and Robert C. Newton, *The Chemokine Facts Book* (San Diego, CA: Academic Press, 1997), 10.

40. Baggiolini, "Introduction," 3.

41. Tina M. Caledron and Joan W. Berman, "Overview and History of Chemokines and Their Receptors," in *Chemokines, Chemokine Receptors, and Disease*, ed. Lisa M. Schwiebert (San Diego: Elsevier Academic Press, 2005), 1.

42. U.S. Patent 6,025,154, available at http://www.patents.com/us-6025154.html, accessed January 22, 2014.

43. Richard Horuk, "Chemokine Receptors and HIV-1: The Fusion of Two Major Research Fields," *Immunology Today* 20, no. 2 (1999): 89–94.

44. A word concerning nomenclature is in order. When the abbreviation HIV is used, it generally refers to HIV-1, the virus responsible for most AIDS cases worldwide. HIV-2, another form of the virus, is associated with a slower onset of AIDS and is restricted to certain areas of Africa.

45. Berger, Murphy, and Farber, "Chemokine Receptors," 658.

46. Joseph P. McGowan and Sanjiv Shah, "Understanding HIV Tropism," *Physicians Research Network (PRN) Notebook* 15 (January 2010), available at http://www.prn.org/index.php/management/article/hiv_tropism_1002, accessed January 21, 2014.

47. Berger, Murphy, and Farber, "Chemokine Receptors," 658.

48. McGowan and Shah, "Understanding HIV Tropism."

49. Peter Radetsky, "Immune to a Plague," *Discover*, June 1997, available at http://discovermagazine.com/1997/jun/immunetoaplague1147, accessed January 21, 2014.

50. Ibid.

51. Fiorenza Cocchi, Anthony L. DeVico, Alfredo Garzino-Demo, et al., "Identification of RANTES, MIP-1α, and MIP-1β as the Major HIV-Suppressive Factors Produced by CD8+ T Cells," *Science* 270, no. 5243 (1995): 1811–1815; Jay A. Levy, Carl E. Mackewicz, and Edward Barker, "Controlling HIV Pathogenesis: The Role of the Noncytotoxic Anti-HIV Response of CD8(+) T Cells," *Immunology Today* 17, no. 5 (1996): 217–224; Radetsky, "Immune to a Plague."

52. Yu Feng, Christopher C. Broder, Paul E. Kennedy, et al., "HIV-1 Entry Cofactor: Functional cDNA Cloning of a Seven-Transmembrane, G Protein-Coupled Receptor," *Science* 272, no. 5263 (1996): 872–877; Radetsky, "Immune to a Plague."

53. Berger, Murphy, and Farber, "Chemokine Receptors," 600.

54. Hongkui Deng, Rong Liu, Willfried Ellmeier, et al., "Identification of a Major Co-receptor for Primary Isolates of HIV-1," *Nature* 381, no. 6584 (1996): 661–666; Tatjana Dragic, Virginia Litwin, Graham P. Allaway, et al., "HIV-1 Entry into CD4+ Cells Is Mediated by the Chemokine Receptor CC-CKR-5," *Nature* 381, no. 6584 (1996): 667–673; Ghalib Alkhatib, Christophe Combadiere, Yu Feng, et al., "CC CKR5: A RANTES, MIP-1α, MIP-1β Receptor as a Fusion Cofactor for Macrophage-Tropic HIV-1," *Science* 272, no. 5270 (1996): 1955–1958; Hyeryun Choe, Michael Farzan, Ying Sun, et al., "The β-Chemokine Receptors CCR3 and CCR5 Facilitate Infection by Primary HIV-1 Isolates," *Cell* 85, no. 7 (1996): 1135–1148; B. J. Doranz, J. Rucker, F. R. Jirik, et al., "A Dual-Tropic Primary HIV-1 Isolate That Uses Fusin and the Beta-Chemokine Receptors CKR-5, CKR-3, and CKR-2b as Fusion Cofactors," *Cell* 85, no. 7 (1996): 1149–1158.

55. Interview with Robert Doms, University of Pennsylvania School of Medicine, March 19, 2013.

56. Dragic, Litwin, Allaway, et al., "HIV-1 Entry into CD4+ Cell," 667–673.

57. Doranz, Rucker, Jirik, et al., "A Dual-Tropic Primary HIV-1 Isolate," 1149–1158.

58. Alkhatib, Combadiere, Feng, et al., "CC CKR5," 1955–1958.

59. Choe, Farzan, Sun, et al., "The β-Chemokine Receptors," 1135–1148.

60. As quoted in Radetsky, "Immune to a Plague."

61. As quoted in ibid.

62. Interview with Ned Landau, New York University School of Medicine, February 28, 2013.

63. Michael Dean, Mary Carrington, Cheryl Winkler, et al. "Genetic Restriction of HIV-1 Infection and Progression to AIDS by a Deletion Allele of the *CKR5* [*CCR5*] Structural Gene," *Science* 273, no. 5283 (1996): 1856–1862, here 1858; Michel Samson, Frédérick Libert, Benjamin J. Doranz, et al., "Resistance to HIV-1 Infection in Caucasian Individuals Bearing Mutant Alleles of the CCR-5 Chemokine Receptor

Gene," *Nature* 382, no. 6593 (1996): 722–725; Doranz, Rucker, Jirik, et al., "A Dual-Tropic Primary HIV-1 Isolate," 1149–1158; Rong Liu, William A. Paxton, Sunny Choe, et al., "Homozygous Defect in HIV-1 Coreceptor Accounts for Resistance of Some Multiply-Exposed Individuals to HIV-Infection," *Cell* 86, no. 3 (1996): 367–377. See also William A. Paxton, S. R. Martin, D. Tse, et al., "Relative Resistance to HIV-1 Infection of CD4 Lymphocytes from Persons Who Remain Uninfected Despite Multiple High-Risk Sexual Exposures," *Nature Medicine* 2, no. 4 (1996): 412–417.

64. Interview with Robert Doms, University of Pennsylvania School of Medicine, March 19, 2013.

65. Ibid.

66. Michel Samson, Olivier Labbe, Catherine Mollereau, et al., "Molecular Cloning and Functional Expression of a New Human CC-Chemokine Receptor Gene," *Biochemistry* 35, no. 11 (1996): 3362–3367.

67. U.S. Patent 6,448,375, available at http://www.patents.com/us-6448375.html, accessed January 22, 2014.

68. The eighteen-month rule applied at the time only for those seeking international patents in addition to U.S. patents. By November 2000, that rule applied to all patents submitted to the U.S. Patent and Trademark Office, regardless of whether the patentee sought international patent protection as well. See Human Genome Sciences' international patent filing, WO 96/39437, at Eliot Marshall, "HIV Experts vs. Sequencers in Patent Race," *Science* 275, no. 5304 (1997): 1263. See also http://www.uspto.gov/faq/patents.jsp, accessed January 22, 2014.

69. Carol J. Raport, Jennifa Gosling, Vicki L. Schweickart, et al., "Molecular Cloning and Functional Characterization of a Novel Human CC Chemokine Receptor (CCR5) for RANTES, MIP-1β, and MIP-1α," *Journal of Biological Chemistry* 271, no. 29 (1996): 17,161–17,166.

70. See http://patents.justia.com/examiner/garnette-d-draper?page=4, accessed January 22, 2014.

71. Jean-Paul Gaudillière, "Professional or Industrial Order? Patents, Biological Drugs, and Pharmaceutical Capitalism in Early Twentieth-Century Germany," *History and Technology* 24, no. 2 (2008): 126.

72. Edward Yoxen, "Life as a Productive Force: Capitalizing upon Research in Molecular Biology," in *Science, Technology and the Labour Process*, ed. L. Levidow and R. Young, 66–122 (London: Blackrose Press, 1981); Gaudillière, "Professional or Industrial Order?," 107–133.

73. Peter Drahos with John Braithwaite, *Information Feudalism: Who Owns the Knowledge Economy?* (New York: New Press, 2002), 158.

74. For an outstanding volume dedicated to the history of the natural-versus-artificial distinction, see Bernadette Bensaude-Vincent and William R. Newman, eds., *The Artificial and the Natural: An Evolving Polarity* (Cambridge, MA: MIT Press, 2007). For a detailed account of this distinction in the early modern period, see William R. Newman, *Promethean Ambitions: Alchemy and the Quest to Perfect Nature* (Chicago: University of Chicago Press, 2004).

75. "Secrets of the Dead: Mystery of the Black Death," produced and written by Emma Faure Whitlock, a Tigress Production (New York: WNET New York, Educational Broadcasting Corporation, 2002).

76. O'Brien was the last author of Dean, Carrington, Winkler, et al., "Genetic Restriction of HIV-1 Infection," 1856–1862. See also Stephen J. O'Brien and Michael Dean, "In Search of AIDS-Resistance Genes," *Scientific American* (September 1997), available at http://www.ncoic.com/0997obrien.html, accessed January 21, 2014.

77. J. Claiborne Stephens, David E. Reich, David B. Goldstein, et al. "Dating the Origin of the *CCR5-Δ32* AIDS-Resistance Allele in the Coalescence of Haplotypes." *American Journal of Human Genetics* 62, no. 26 (1998): 1507–1515; Dean, Carrington, Winkler, et al., "Genetic Restriction of HIV-1 Infection," 1856–1862; Samson, Libert, Doranz, et al., "Resistance to HIV-1 Infection," 722–725; Liu, Paxton, Choe, et al., "Homozygous Defect in HIV-1 Coreceptor," 367–377; Peter A. Zimmerman, Alicia Buckler-White, Ghalib Alkhatib, et al.,"Inherited Resistance to HIV-1 Conferred by an Inactivating Mutation in CC Chemokine Receptor 5: Studies in Populations with Contrasting Clinical Phenotypes, Defined Racial Background, and Quantified Risk," *Molecular Medicine* 3, no. 1 (1997): 23–36. On rare occasions, HIV infection has been detected in individuals who are homozygous for the *Δ32* mutation. The viral isolates in all cases were of the T-tropic (or syncytium-inducing, X4) variety, gaining entry into the CD4 cells via the CXCR4 receptor. See Robyn Biti, Rosemary Ffrench, Judy Young, et al., "HIV-1 Infection in an Individual Homozygous for the *CCR5* Deletion Allele," *Nature Medicine* 3, no. 3 (1997): 252–253; Ioannis Theodorou, Laurence Meyer, Magdalena Magierowskia, et al., "HIV-1 Infection in an Individual Homozygous for *CCR5Δ32*: Seroco Study Group," *Lancet* 349, no. 9060 (1997): 1219–1220 and Thomas R. O'Brien, Cheryl Winkler, Michael Dean, et al. "HIV-1 Infection in a Man Homozygous for *CCR5Δ32*." *Lancet* 349, no. 9060 (1997): 1219.

78. Usually *race* refers to the biological characteristics relevant to the physical appearance of a particular group, and *ethnicity* refers to a shared culture, nationality, and ancestry. Biomedical researchers often conflate the two in their analyses.

79. Personal genomics companies specialize in sequencing and analyzing human DNA to determine ancestry and search for alleles that are linked to disease. 23andMe is an example of such a company.

80. Duana Fullwiley, "The Molecularization of Race: Institutionalizing Human Difference in Pharmacogenetics Practice," *Science in Culture* 16, no. 1 (2007): 1–30.

81. Steven Epstein, *Inclusion: The Politics of Difference in Medical Research* (Chicago: University of Chicago Press, 2007), 79–87.

82. Steven Epstein, *Impure Science: AIDS, Activism, and the Politics of Knowledge* (Los Angeles: University of California Press, 1996); Shobita Parthasarathy, *Building Genetic Medicine: Breast Cancer, Technology, and the Comparative Politics of Health Care* (Cambridge, MA: MIT Press, 2007).

83. See, for example, Jasanoff, *Designs on Nature*; Sheila Jasanoff, *The Fifth Branch: Science Advisers as Policymakers* (Cambridge, MA: Harvard University Press, 1990); Sheila Jasanoff, *Science at the Bar: Law, Science, and Technology in America* (Cambridge, MA: Harvard University Press, 1995); Naomi Oreskes and Erik M. Conway, *Merchants of Doubt: How a Handful of Scientists Obscured the Truth on Issues from Tobacco Smoke to Global Warming* (New York: Bloomsbury Press, 2010); D. Winickoff, Sheila Jasanoff, Lawrence Busch, et al., "Adjudicating the GM Food Wars: Science, Risk and Democracy in World Trade Law," *Yale Journal of International Law* 30, no. 1 (2005): 81–123; Brian Wynne, "Public Engagement as a Means of Restoring Public Trust in Science: Hitting the Notes, but Missing the Music?," *Community Genetics* 9, no. 3 (2006): 211–220; Brian Wynne, "Risky Delusions: Misunderstanding Science and Misperforming Publics in the GE Crops Issue," in *Genetically Engineered Crops: Interim Policies, Uncertain Legislation*, ed. I. E. P. Taylor, 258–281 (Vancouver, BC: UBC Haworth Press, 2007); Robert N. Proctor, *Cancer Wars: How Politics Shapes What We Know and Don't Know about Cancer* (New York: Basic Books, 1996).

84. See Bruno Latour, *Science in Action: How to Follow Scientists and Engineers Through Society* (Cambridge, MA: Harvard University Press, 1987), 97. For other classic works on controversies, see, among others, Steven Shapin and Simon Schaffer, *Leviathan and the Air-Pump: Hobbes, Boyle, and the Experimental Life* (Princeton, NJ: Princeton University Press, 1987); Brian Martin and Evelleen Richards, "Scientific Knowledge, Controversy, and Public Decision Making," in *Handbook of Science and Technology Studies*, ed. Sheila Jasanoff, Gerald E. Markle, James C. Petersen, et al., 506–522 (Newbury Park, CA: Sage, 1995).

85. In this sense, this work is closer to Oreskes and Conway, *Merchants of Doubt*, and Proctor, *Cancer Wars*, than it is to the other works.

86. Sheila Jasanoff, "The Idiom of Co-Production," 1–12; see also Sheila Jasanoff, "Introduction," in *Reframing Rights: Bioconstitutionalism in the Genetic Age*, ed. Sheila Jasanoff, 1–28 (Cambridge, MA: MIT Press, 2011).

87. Donald MacKenzie, *Inventing Accuracy: A Historical Sociology of Nuclear Missile Guidance* (Cambridge, MA: MIT Press, 1990).

88. MacKenzie's work belonged to the Edinburgh School's sociology of scientific knowledge (SSK), which argued for the importance of interests and led to their so-called interest theory. Here is where I part company with those of the older SSK tra-

dition. Social interests can be evoked to explain everything and therefore explain nothing.

89. See, for example, Kaushik Sunder Rajan, *Biocapital: The Constitution of Postgenomic Life* (Rayleigh, NC: Duke University Press, 2006).

90. Stefan Helmreich, "Species of Biocapital," *Science as Culture* 17, no. 4 (2008): 463–478, here 463–464.

91. Ibid., 464, 467. See also Yoxen, "Life as a Productive Force," 112.

92. Helmreich, "Species of Biocapital," 464 and 467; Michel Foucault, *The History of Sexuality*, vol. 1 (New York: Vintage, 1978), 143.

93. In this respect, my story is similar to David F. Noble, *America by Design: Science, Technology and the Rise of Corporate Capitalism* (New York: Oxford University Press, 1977). I thank Ken Alder for pointing this out.

94. Hannah Landecker, *Culturing Life: How Cells Became Technologies* (Cambridge, MA: Harvard University Press, 2007), 3.

95. Rebecca Skloot, *The Immortal Life of Henrietta Lacks* (New York: Broadway Paperbacks, 2010).

96. Nikolas Rose, *The Politics of Life Itself: Biomedicine, Power, and Subjectivity in the Twenty-First Century* (Princeton, NJ: Princeton University Press, 2007), 6–7.

97. This part of my story owes much to the scholarship of Lorraine Daston, Ted Porter, Bruno Latour, and particularly Hans-Jörg Rheinberger. See Lorraine Daston, ed., *Biographies of Scientific Objects* (Chicago: University of Chicago Press, 2000); Lorraine Daston, "The Coming into Being of Scientific Objects," in Daston, *Biographies of Scientific Objects*, 1–14; Theodore M. Porter, "Life Insurance, Medical Testing, and the Management of Morality," in Daston, *Biographies of Scientific Objects*, 226–246; Bruno Latour, "On the Partial Existence of Existing and Nonexisting Objects," in Daston, *Biographies of Scientific Objects*, 247–269; Hans-Jörg Rheinberger, "Cytoplasmic Particles," in Daston, *Biographies of Scientific Objects*, 270–294; Hans-Jörg Rheinberger, *Toward a History of Epistemic Things: Synthesizing Proteins in the Test Tube* (Stanford, CA: Stanford University Press, 1994).

98. Porter "Life Insurance," 226.

99. Rheinberger, "Cytoplasmic Particles," 273.

100. Latour, "On the Partial Existence," 252.

101. I agree with Arabatzis's view. In his account of the history of the electron, Arabatzis offers an interesting biography of a theoretical entity. Such a historiography empowers theoretical entities as explanatory resources, and therefore they become tools for the historian. Also, the biographic approach takes seriously the various

problems that scientists face as they attempt to manipulate representations of an unobservable entity. Such biographies also render concepts of unobservable entities as active agents. I share Arabatzis's skepticism about attributing intentionality to objects. Arabatzis is dealing with theoretical entities, while I am dealing with very real, material objects. See Theodore Arabatzis, "Towards a Historical Ontology?," *Studies in the History and Philosophy of Science* 34, no. 2 (2003): 431–442, here 441; see also Theodore Arabatzis, *Representing Electrons: A Biographical Approach to Theoretical Entities* (Chicago: University of Chicago Press, 2006), 36–52.

102. For an outstanding account of the biography of a scientific object, the *TMV* gene, see Angela N. H. Creager, *The Life of a Virus: Tobacco Mosaic Virus as an Experimental Model* (Chicago: University of Chicago Press, 2002). See also, for example, Daston, *Biographies of Scientific Objects*. For biographies of objects in general, see Igor Kopytoff, "The Cultural Biography of Things," in *The Social Life of Things: Commodities in Cultural Perspective*, ed. Arjun Appadurai, 64–91 (New York: Cambridge University Press, 1988); Peter Stallybrass, "Marx's Coat," in *Border Fetishisms: Material Objects in Unstable Spaces*, ed. Patricia Spyer, 183–207 (New York: Routledge, 1998); Pietra Rivoli, *The Travels of a T-Shirt in the Global Economy*, 2nd ed. (Hoboken, NJ: Wiley, 2009); Neil MacGregor, *A History of the World in One Hundred Objects* (New York: Viking Penguin, 2011); Edmund De Waal, *The Hare with Amber Eyes: A Family's Century of Art and Loss* (New York: Farrar, Straus, and Giroux, 2010); Mark Kurlansky, *Salt: A World History* (New York: Penguin, 2002); Chris Gosden and Yvonne Marshall, "The Cultural Biography of Objects," *World Archaeology* 31, no. 2 (1999): 169–178; Bill Brown, "Thing Theory," *Critical Inquiry* 28, no. 1 (2001): 1–22.

103. Friedrich Nietzsche, *Zur Genealogie der Moral* (Leipzig: Naumann, 1887); Michel Foucault, "Nietzsche, la généalogie, l'histoire," in *Hommage à Jean Hyppolite*, 145–172 (Paris: Presses Universitaires de France, 1971).

104. Michel Foucault, *Work of Foucault: Ethics, Subjectivity, and Truth*, ed. Paul Rabinow, vol. 1 (London: Penguin, 1997), 31.

105. Michel Foucault, "Nietzsche, Genealogy, History," in *The Foucault Reader*, ed. Paul Rabinow (New York: Pantheon Books, 1984), 88.

106. Ibid.

107. My account differs from Nietzsche's and Foucault's in important ways. For example, I do not use the genealogical approach "to identify the accidents, the minute deviations—or conversely, the complete reversals—the errors, the false appraisals, and the faulty calculations." Foucault, "Nietzsche, Genealogy, History," 81. And I do not search for discontinuities or raptures, which are important to Foucault's account. See Gary Gutting, "Foucault's Genealogical Method," *Midwest Studies in Philosophy* 15, no. 15 (1990): 327–343, here 333.

108. Foucault, "Nietzsche, Genealogy, History," 83.

Chapter 2

1. For an excellent history of the origins and beginnings of the Human Genome Project, see Daniel J. Kevles, "Out of Eugenics: The Historical Politics of the Human Genome," in *The Code of Codes: Scientific and Social Issues in the Human Genome Project*, ed. Daniel J. Kevles and Leroy Hood, 3–36 (Cambridge, MA: Harvard University Press, 1992); Davies, *Cracking the Genome*.

2. Kevles, "Out of Eugenics," 18.

3. Ibid., 19; Davies, *Cracking the Genome*, 17.

4. The Human Genome Project finished ahead of schedule in 2003 and ended up costing $2.7 billion in fiscal year 1991 dollars. See http://www.genome.gov/11006943, accessed January 22, 2014.

5. Ibid. Collins's National Human Genome Research Initiative started the sequencing component as a pilot project among six institutions—the Massachusetts Institute of Technology, Stanford University, Washington University, the University of Washington, Baylor College of Medicine, and the Institute for Genomic Research. Shreeve, *The Genome War*, 44–45.

6. For a thorough account of the tensions that arise from the public and private aspects of the Human Genome Project, see Shreeve, *The Genome War*, 52–93. See also http://www.hhs.gov/asl/testify/t980617a.html, accessed January 22, 2014.

7. As quoted in Cook-Deegan, *The Gene Wars*, 309.

8. As quoted in ibid., 309.

9. As quoted in ibid., 310.

10. Ibid., 311.

11. Shreeve, *The Genome War*, 83–84.

12. For the National Institutes of Health's attempt to patent 2,750 partial cDNA sequences of unknown function, see Rebecca S. Eisenberg, "Genes, Patents, and Product Developments," *Science* 257, no. 5072 (1992): 903–908; Thomas D. Kiley, "Patent on Random Complementary DNA Fragments?," *Science* 257, no. 5072 (1992): 915–918.

13. Drahos with Braithwaite, *Information Feudalism*, 156–157.

14. Shreeve, *The Genome War*, 83–84.

15. Davies, *Cracking the Genome*, 62, and Cook-Deegan, *The Gene Wars*, 311–312. See also J. Craig Venter, *A Life Decoded: My Genome, My Life* (New York: Viking, 2007), 123, 133, 135–136, 175.

16. Cook-Deegan, *The Gene Wars*, 281–282.

17. Ibid., 282.

18. Reid G. Adler, "Genome Research: Fulfilling the Public's Expectation for Knowledge and Commercialization," *Science* 257, no. 5072 (1992): 908–914.

19. Office of Technology Assessment, U.S. Congress, *Mapping Our Genes: The Genome Projects—How Big, How Fast?* OTA-BA-373 (Washington, DC: U.S. Government Printing Office, 1988), 6; Adler, "Genome Research," 908.

20. Adler, "Genome Research," 908.

21. Bruce Alberts, *Report of the Committee on Mapping and Sequencing the Human Genome of the Board on Basic Biology, Commission on Life Sciences, National Research Council* (Washington, DC: National Academy Press, 1988), 91; Adler, "Genome Research," 908.

22. Marshall, "Patent on HIV Receptor," 1377.

23. Wendy J. Bailey, William B. Vanti, Susan R. George, et al., "Patent Status of Therapeutically Important G Protein-Coupled Receptors," *Expert Opinion on Therapeutic Patents* 11, no. 12 (2001): 1861–1887, here 1861.

24. "But the patent office is swamped. Patent examiners devote on average only 17 hours to checking an inventor's claim to some unique product, process or idea. They are working through a backlog of more than 400,000 patent claims." Jim Landers, "Trouble Impending in Patent Process," *Dallas Morning News*, May 1, 2007, cited in http://www.inventionstatistics.com/Patent_Office.html and http://www.inventionstatistics.com/Patent_Backlog_Patent_Office_Backlog.html, both accessed January 21, 2014. Similarly, Drahos reports the average time spent on the examination of applications by U.S. Patent and Trademark Office examiners is between ten and twenty hours. See Peter Drahos, *The Global Governance of Knowledge: Patent Offices and Their Clients* (New York: Cambridge University Press, 2010), 74.

25. Robert P. Merges, "As Many as Six Impossible Patents before Breakfast: Property Rights for Business Concepts and Patent System Reform," *Berkeley Technology Law Journal* 14 (1999): 577–615, here 601.

26. Drahos, *The Global Governance*, 68–69.

27. Ibid., 153.

28. Ron D. Katznelson, "Bad Science in Search of 'Bad' Patents," *Federal Circuit Bar Journal* 17, no. 1 (2007): 1–30, here 23 and 30. Note that Katznelson argues that some evidence suggests that this increase has resulted not because the USPTO relaxed its standards but because there was a reduction in the scope of the patent claims and an increase in the number of claims per application. Ibid., 22. Drahos disagrees. See Drahos, *The Global Governance*, 74.

29. Drahos, *The Global Governance*, 35.

30. Ibid., 36.

31. Draper served as the primary examiner for 531 patents and as the assistant examiner for 240 patents. See http://patents.com/us-6025154.html and http://patents.justia.com/examiner/garnette-d-draper?page=1, both accessed March 30, 2014. The patents that she reviewed were in the biotech sector. Draper is a coauthor on two biomedical papers: Stephen P. Bruttig, Garnette D. Draper, and Murray P. Hamlet, "Platelet-Endothelial Function in Relation to Environmental Temperature," *Medical Research and Development to Environmental Temperature* 84 (1983): 1–27, and Margaret E. M. Tolbert, Johnston A. Ramalu, and Garnette D. Draper, "Effects of Cadmium, Zinc, Copper, and Manganese on Hepatic Parenchymal Cell Gluconeogenesis," *Journal of Environmental Science and Health* 16, 5 pt. B (1981): 575–585.

32. http://patents.com/us-6025154.html, accessed March 30, 2014. The original patent was listed as a "related patent" in the later application.

33. "Human Genome Sciences Receives Patent on AIDS Virus Entry Point," February 16, 2000, available at http://www.prnewswire.com/news-releases/human-genome-sciences-receives-patent-on-aids-virus-entry-point-72613242.html, accessed on January 24, 2014; Paul Jacobs and Peter G. Gosselin,"'Robber Barons of the Genetic Age': Experts Fret over the Effect of Gene Patents of Research," *Los Angeles Times*, February 28, 2000, available at http://articles.latimes.com/2000/feb/28/news/mn-3512, accessed January 21, 2014.

34. Jacobs and Gosselin, "'Robber Barons of the Genetic Age'". See also Marshall, "Patent on the HIV Receptor," 1375–1377; Sabra Chartrand, "A Human Gene Is Patented as a Potential Tool against AIDS, but Ethical Questions Remain," *New York Times*, March 6, 2000, available at http://www.nytimes.com/2000/03/06/business/patents-human-gene-patented-potential-tool-against-aids-but-ethical-questions.html?pagewanted=all&src=pm, accessed January 20, 2014.

35. Robert Langreth, "Beyond Talk," *Forbes* 172 (2003): 72–75, here 72.

36. As cited in Jacobs and Gosselin "'Robber Barons of the Genetic Age.'"

37. Marshall, "Patent on HIV Receptor," 1375–1377.

38. Ibid.

39. Chartrand, "A Human Gene Is Patented."

40. Ibid.

41. "Euroscreen CCR5 Agonist Program Available for Out-Licensing," available at http://www.euroscreen.com/index.php/Euroscreen-News/Euroscreen-CCR5-Agonist-program-available-for-out-licensing.html, accessed January 22, 2014.

42. Marshall, "HIV Experts," 1263.

43. As cited in Jacobs and Gosselin, "'Robber Barons of the Genetic Age.'"

44. As cited in Marshall, "Patent on HIV Receptor," 1377.

45. Tom Reynolds, "Gene Patent Race Speeds Ahead amid Controversy," *Journal of the National Cancer Institute* 92, no. 8 (2000): 184–186, here 185.

46. As cited in Jacobs and Gosselin, "'Robber Barons of the Genetic Age.'"

47. Telephone interview with Dan Littman of New York University School of Medicine, March 1, 2013.

48. Regalado, "The Great Gene Grab," 51. Human Genome Sciences filed its patent on CCR5 on June 6, 1995, or two days before the statutory changes were made requiring the publication of the patent application eighteen months after the filing date. The point is moot, however. Because HGS filed a patent with the European Patent Office as well, the application was required to be made public eighteen months later in any case.

49. Jacobs and Gosselin, "'Robber Barons of the Genetic Age.'"

50. Smaglik, "Could AIDS Treatment Slip," 322.

51. Jordan J. Cohen, former president of the Association of American Medical Colleges, as quoted in David Dickson, "NIH Opposes Plans for Patenting 'Similar' Gene Sequences," *Nature* 405, no. 6782 (2000): 3. See also Martin Enserink, "Patent Office May Raise Bar on Gene Claims," *Science* 287, no. 5456 (2000): 1196–1197; Gitter, "International Conflicts over Patenting Human DNA," 1627.

52. Nell Boyce and Andy Coghlan, "Your Genes in Their Hands," *New Scientist* 2239 (May 15, 2000): 15; Smagli, "Could AIDS Treatments Slip," 322; Michael Waldholz, "Right to Life: Genes Are Patentable; Less Clear Is If Finder Must Know Their Role," *Wall Street Journal*, March 16, 2000: A1; Gitter, "International Conflicts over Patenting Human DNA," 1627.

53. Marshall, "HIV Experts," 1263.

54. Jacobs and Gosselin, "'Robber Barons of the Genetic Age.'"

55. "HGS Patent on HIV Sequence Found to Contain Sequence Errors," 2000, 602–603, here 602, available at http://online.liebertpub.com/doi/pdf/10.1089/073003100750036717, accessed January 22, 2014. For the work of Broder's lab on the role of CCR5 as a coreceptor for HIV-1, see Feng, Broder, Kennedy, et al., "HIV-1 Entry Cofactor," 872–877; Alkhatib, Combadiere, Feng, et al., "CC CKR5," 1955. See also Marshall, "Patent on HIV Receptor," 1377.

56. Marshall, "Patent on HIV Receptor," 1377.

57. Ibid.

58. Private email correspondence with John P. Moore and Tanya Dragic, November 26, 2007.

59. Paul Jacobs and Peter G. Gosselin, "Profiteering and Shoddy Science: Errors Found in Patent of AIDS Gene, Scientists Say; News Comes amid Concerns That Genomics Race Could Lead to Shoddy Science and Profiteering," *Los Angeles Times*, March 21, 2000, available at http://www.commondreams.org/headlines/032100-02 .htm, accessed January 21, 2014; private email correspondence with John P. Moore and Tanya Dragic, November 26, 2007.

60. Jacobs and Gosselin, "Profiteering and Shoddy Science."

61. As cited in Jacobs and Gosselin, "Profiteering and Shoddy Science." See also "HGS Patent on HIV Sequence Found to Contain Sequence Errors," 2000, 603, available at http://online.liebertpub.com/doi/pdf/10.1089/073003100750036717, accessed January 22, 2014; for two outstanding articles on the relationship between deposits and written descriptions, see Alain Pottage, "Law Machines: Scale Models, Forensic Materiality and the Making of Modern Patent Law," *Social Studies of Science* 41, no. 5 (2011): 621–643; Kendall J. Dood, "Patent Models and the Patent Law: 1790–1880 (pt. 1)" and "Patent Models and the Patent Law: 1790–1880 (pt. 2– conclusion)," *Journal of the Patent Office Society* 65 (1983): 187–216, 234–274.

62. As quoted in Jacobs and Gosselin, "Profiteering and Shoddy Science." See also "HGS Patent on HIV Sequence Found to Contain Sequence Errors," 2000, 603, available at http://online.liebertpub.com/doi/pdf/10.1089/073003100750036717, accessed January 23, 2014.

63. "HGS Patent on HIV Sequence," 603. See also Jacobs and Gosselin, "Profiteering and Shoddy Science."

64. http://www.google.com/patents/us6448375, accessed January 24, 2014.

65. Ibid.

66. http://www.commondreams.org/headlines/032100-02.htm, accessed May 30, 2012. See also http://www.drugdiscoveryonline.com/article.mvc/Euroscreen-Awarded -US-Patent-Covering-Key-Hiv-0001, accessed January 24, 2014.

67. http://www.pharmaceuticalonline.com/doc/euroscreen-awarded-us-patent -covering-key-hiv-0001, accessed January 24, 2014.

68. http://www.google.com/patents/us6265184, http://www.google.com/patents/ us6268477.html, and http://www.google.com/patents/us6797811.html, all accessed January 24, 2014.

69. "Human G-Protein Chemokine Receptor HDGNR10 (CCR5 Receptor)," http:// patents.justia.com/2004/06800729.html, accessed January 24, 2014.

70. It became U.S. Patent 5,932,703. See http://patents.justia.com/examiner/garnette -d-draper?page=4, accessed January 24, 2014.

71. In 2012, that fact became irrelevant. The United States is now in line with Europe because priority is given to the first to submit the application. But at the time, it was relevant.

72. Drahos, *The Global Governance*, 72–73.

73. Ibid., 72.

74. http://www.uspto.gov/ip/boards/bpai/stats/process/fy2011sepb.jsp, accessed January 24, 2014.

75. Euroscreen owns the *CCR5* sequences, antibodies to CCR5, and HIV-1 screening methods in Europe, Australia, Canada, and Japan. Interview with Vincent Lannoy, Euroscreen's intellectual property lawyer responsible for the CCR5 patent portfolio, Gosselies, Belgium, March 12, 2012.

76. Interview with Vincent Lannoy, Euroscreen's intellectual property lawyer responsible for the CCR5 patent portfolio, Gosselies, Belgium, March 12, 2012.

77. Drahos, *The Global Governance*, 10.

78. http://www.prweb.com/releases/2007/10/prweb562529.htm, accessed January 24, 2014. On June 18, 2004, Euroscreen acquired exclusive rights from ICOS Corporation to the antibodies, which bind to CCR5. Euroscreen sublicenses the CCR5 patent portfolio to biotechnology and pharmaceutical partners for commercialization. See "Euroscreen Licenses Patent Rights for CCR5 Antibodies from ICOS," available at http://www.prweb.com/releases/2004/06/prweb133216.htm, accessed January 24, 2014.

79. See http://www.drugdiscoveryonline.com/article.mvc/Euroscreen-Awarded-US -Patent-Covering-Key-Hiv-0001, accessed January 24, 2014.

80. Shreeve, *The Genome War*, 231–233.

81. Bailey, Vanti, George, et al., "Patent Status of Therapeutically Important," 1861.

82. Shreeve, *The Genome War*, 232.

83. Bailey, Vanti, George, et al., "Patent Status of Therapeutically Important," 1872–1873.

84. Ibid., 1862.

Chapter 3

1. http://www.usconstitution.net/xconst_A1Sec8.html, accessed January 24, 2014.

2. See, for example, http://www.patentapplications.net, accessed January 24, 2014. As is stated in 35 U.S.C. section 101: "Whoever invents or discovers any new and useful process, machine, manufacture, or composition of matter, or any new and useful

improvement thereof, may obtain a patent therefore, subject to the conditions and requirements of this title." See http://www.law.cornell.edu/uscode/text/35/101, accessed January 24, 2014. For a helpful introduction to patent law, see Arthur R. Miller and Michael H. Davis, *Intellectual Property: Patents, Trademarks, and Copyrights in a Nutshell*, 2nd ed. (St. Paul, MN: West, 1990), 4–18.

3. William A. Knudson, "An Introduction to Patents, Brands, Trade Secrets, Trademarks, and Intellectual Property Rights Issues," August 2006, 2–3, available at http://productcenter.msu.edu/uploads/files/ippaper%202.pdf, accessed January 21, 2014. In addition, the U.S. Patent and Trademark Office awards reissue patents, which correct errors in the initial patent; defensive publications (DEFs), which proffer limited protection from others patenting an invention, design, or plant; and statutory invention registrations (SIRs), which replaced DEFs in 1986 and offer similar protection. See "Types of Patents," available at http://www.uspto.gov/web/offices/ac/ido/oeip/taf/patdesc.htm, accessed January 24, 2014.

4. That changed in 2012, when the Patent Reform Act of 2011 was passed. Congress changed the law from first to invent to first to file to harmonize with the European Patent Office.

5. For example, "Excluded from such patent protection are laws of nature, natural phenomena, and abstract ideas." See *Parker v. Flook*, 437 U.S. 584 (1978); *Gottschalk v. Benson* 409 U.S. 67 (1972); *Funk Bros. Seed Co. v. Kalo Inoculant Co.*, 333 U.S. 127 (1948), and *Diamond v. Diehr*, 450 U.S. 175 (1981). See also *Le Roy v. Tatham*, 55 U.S. 156 (1852) ("A principle, in the abstract, is a fundamental truth; an original cause, a motive; these cannot be patented"), available at http://supreme.justia.com/cases/federal/us/55/156/case.html, accessed January 23, 2014. Later in the ruling, however, the Court argued that "where a person discovers a principle or property of nature, or where he conceives of a new application of a well-known principle of property of nature, and also, of some mode of carrying it out into practice ... he is entitled to protection." Ibid., 185.

6. http://www.uspto.gov/web/offices/pac/mpep/s2104.html, accessed January 24, 2014.

7. *United States Statutes at Large*, vol. 1, 1st Cong., sess. 2, chap. 7 (April 10, 1790), available at http://en.wikisource.org/wiki/United_States_Statutes_at_Large/Volume_1/1st_Congress/2nd_Session/Chapter_7, accessed on January 20, 2014.

8. Jane Calvert and Pierre-Benoît Joly, "How Did the Gene Become a Chemical Compound? The Ontology of the Gene and the Patenting of DNA," *Social Science Information* 50, no. 2 (2011): 1–21, here 5. See also "Adrenocorticotropin-lipotropin Precursor Gene," which became U.S. Patent 4,322,499, granted March 30, 1982, and "DNA Transfer Vector and Transformed Microorganism Containing Human Proinsulin and Pre-proinsulin Genes," filed September 12, 1979, which became U.S. Patent 4,431,740, granted February 14, 1984. Also in 1984, the gene for human

chorionic somatomammotropin was patented, U.S. Patent 4,447,538. See James DeGiulio, "The Genomic Research and Accessibility Act: More Science Fiction Than Fact," *Northwestern Journal of Technology and Intellectual Property* 8 (2010): 292–306, here 292; Leslie Gladstone Restaino and Theresa Tackeuchi, "Gene Patents and Global Competition Issues: Protection of Biotechnology under Patent Law," *Legal Affairs* 26, no. 1, available at http://www.genengnews.com/articles/chitem .aspx?aid=1163&chid=0. See also http://www.google.com/patents/us4322499 and http://www.google.com/patents/us4431740, all accessed January 24, 2014.

9. Tony West, Beth S. Brinkmann, Scott R. McIntosh, et al., "In the United States Court of Appeals for the Federal Circuit, the Association for Molecular Pathology et al., Plaintiffs-Appellees v. United States Patent and Trademark Office, Defendant, Myriad Genetics, Inc., et al., Defendant-Appellant. Appeal of Case No. 09-CV-4515, Senior Judge Robert W. Sweet, Brief for the United States as Amicus Curiae in Support of Neither Party. No. 2010-1406" (2010), available at http://graphics8.nytimes .com/packages/pdf/business/genepatents-USamicusbrief.pdf, accessed January 21, 2014.

10. See, for example, the patent for the malolactic gene issued September 18, 1984, U.S. Patent 4,472,502 and ibid.

11. West, Brinkmann, McIntosh, et al., "In the United States Court of Appeals"; U.S. Patent 4,680,264, available at http://www.google.it/patents/US4680264, accessed January 24, 2014.

12. "Trilateral Co-operation of the U.S., European and Japanese Patent Offices," *Biotechnology Law Review* 7 (1988): 159–193. See http://www.alrc.gov.au/publications/ 6-patentability-genetic-materials-and-technologies/patentable-subject-matter, accessed January 24, 2014. Also cited in R. Stephen Crespi, "Patenting and Ethics: A Dubious Connection," *Journal of the Patent and Trademark Office Society* 85 (2003): 31–43, here 40; Luigi Palombi, "The Patenting of Biological Materials in the Context of the Agreement on Trade-Related Aspects of Intellectual Property Rights," Ph.D. dissertation, Law School of the University of New South Wales, Australia, 2004, 6.

13. John J. Doll, "Biotechnology: The Patenting of DNA," *Science* 280, no. 5364 (1998): 689–690, here 689.

14. Rebecca S. Eisenberg, "Patenting the Human Genome," *Emory Law Journal* 39, no. 3 (1990): 721–745, as cited in Cook-Deegan, *The Gene Wars*, 310.

15. Cook-Deegan, *The Gene Wars*, 307.

16. Franklin Hoke, "Gene Patenting Is on the Rise, But Scientists Are Unimpressed," *The Scientist* 9 (1995): 1, 6–7, here 6. See also Cook-Deegan and Heaney, "Patents in Genomics," 383–425.

17. Ying Pan, "A Post-*KSR* Consideration of Gene Patenting: The 'Obvious to Try' Standard Limits the Patentability of Genes," *Marquette Law Review* 93, no. 1 (2009):

285–308, here 293. Note that DNA-based patents do not necessarily mean gene patents. Gene patents were first granted in 1982.

18. Cook-Deegan and Heaney, "Patents in Genomics," 384. Calvert and Joly, however, argue that the U.S. Patent and Trademark Office was approaching the 50,000th patent in 2011. See Calvert and Joly, "How Did the Gene," 6. By 2000, over 355,000 sequences were published in patents worldwide, an increase of 5,000% over 1990. See Graham Dutfield, *Intellectual Property Rights and the Life Science Industries: Past, Present and Future*, 2nd ed. (Hackensack, NJ: World Scientific, 2009), 194. See also Hopkins et al., "DNA Patenting," 185; Tom Abate, "Call It the Gene Rush: Patent Stakes Run High," *San Francisco Chronicle*, April 20, 2000, A8.

19. Kyle Jensen and Fiona Murray, "Intellectual Property Enhanced: Intellectual Property Landscape of the Human Genome," *Science* 310, no. 5746 (2005): 239–240.

20. Jeffrey Rosenfeld and Christopher E. Mason, "Pervasive Sequence Patents Cover the Entire Human Genome," *Genome Medicine* 5, no.3 (2013): 27–33.

21. Examples include the two breast cancers genes, *BRCA1* and *2*, *HNCC* and *FAP* linked to colon cancer, *CRTP* linked to cystic fibrosis, *Apo-E* responsible for late onset Alzheimer's disease, and *SMA1*, which gives rise to spinal muscular dystrophy.

22. Restaino and Tackeuchi, "Gene Patents and Global Competition Issues."

23. Dutfield, *Intellectual Property Rights*, 300. Original source: D. C. Mowery and N. Rosenberg, *Paths of Innovation: Technological Change in Twentieth-Century America* (New York: Cambridge University Press, 1988), 96.

24. Hamilton Moses III, E. R. Dorsey, D. H. Matheson, et al., "Financial Anatomy of Biomedical Research," *Journal of the American Medical Association* 294, no. 3 (2005): 1333–1342, here 1336. It should be noted that for basic research in molecular biology, National Institutes of Health funding is far greater than any private source.

25. In terms of percentages, not much changed between 1994 and 2003. For example, in 1994, 40% of applied and basic biomedical research funding was supplied by public dollars, 56% by for-profit firms and foundations, and 4% by charities and other private funds. In 2003, 40% was funded by public dollars, 57% by for-profit firms, and 3% by foundations, charities, and other private funds. Ibid.

26. Sheldon Krimsky, *Science in the Private Interest: Has the Lure of Profits Corrupted Biomedical Research?* (Lanham, MD: Rowman & Littlefield, 2003), 79–80.

27. Bryn Williams-Jones, "History of a Gene Patent: Tracing the Development and Application of Commercial BRCA Testing," *Health Law Journal* 10 (2002): 123–146, available at http://www.academia.edu/634302/History_of_a_Gene_Patent_Tracing _the_Development_and_Application_of_Commercial_BRCA_Testing, accessed January 24, 2014.

28. Ibid.

29. Adler, "Genome Research," 909.

30. Rose, *The Politics of Life*, 35.

31. Ibid., 34.

32. Dutfield, *Intellectual Property Rights*, 170, 296.

33. "Clinton Proclaims Biotech Month, Wants $340 Million to Fight Bioterrorism," *Environmental News Service*, January 20, 2000," available at http://www.ens-newswire.com/ens/jan2000/2000-01-20-02.html, accessed January 24, 2014.

34. David Holtzman, "Gene Patenting Guidelines: 'Magna Carta of Biotechnology,'" *Genetic Engineering News*, February 1, 2001, available at http://www.mindfully.org/GE/Biotech-Magna-Carta.htm, accessed January 20, 2014.

35. Ibid.

36. Ibid.

37. Lewis Hyde, *Common as Air: Revolution, Art, and Ownership* (New York: Farrar, Straus and Giroux, 2010).

38. Daniel J. Kevles, "Inventions, Yes: Nature, No: The Birth of the Products-of-Nature Doctrine in the American Colonies and Courts," forthcoming in *Perspectives on Science* 23, no. 1 (2014).

39. For an excellent article on the topic, see Christopher Beauchamp, "Patenting Nature: A Problem of History," *Stanford Technology Law Review* 16, no. 2 (2013): 257–311.

40. *American Wood Paper v. Fiber Disintegrating*, 90 U.S. 566 (1874), available at http://supreme.justia.com/cases/federal/us/90/566/case.html, accessed January 23, 2014.

41. Ibid., 593–594.

42. Ibid., 594.

43. Beauchamp, "Patenting Nature," 272.

44. *Cochrane v. Badische Anilin & Soda Fabrik*, 111 U.S. 293 (1884), available at http://scholar.google.com/scholar_case?case=18061865851672104499&hl=en&as_sdt=2&as_vis=1&oi=scholarr, accessed January 23, 2014.

45. Beauchamp, "Patenting Nature," 272.

46. 111 U.S. 293, 311 (1884). The Court cited *American Wood-Paper Patent* as the precedent.

47. Beauchamp, "Patenting Nature," 272.

48. *Ex parte Latimer*, 1889 Dec. Comm'r Pat. 123 (1889); Jon M. Harkness, "Dicta on Adrenalin(e): Myriad Problems with Learned Hand's Product-of-Nature Pronounce-

ments in *Parke-Davis v. Mulford*," *Journal of the Patent and Trademark Office Society* 93, no. 4 (2011): 363–399.

49. Beauchamp, "Patenting Nature," 274–275.

50. Ibid., 276.

51. Ibid.

52. 171 F.887, 890 (C.C.N.D. Ill. 1909), as cited in ibid., 278.

53. 189 Fed. Reg. 95 (April 28, 1911).

54. See, for example, Lori B. Andrews, "Genes and Patent Policy: Rethinking Intellectual Property Rights," *Nature Reviews: Genetics* 3, no. 10 (2002): 803–807, here 804; Doll, "Biotechnology," 698–690. For Lourie's view, see "U.S. Court of Appeals for the Federal Circuit, The Association for Molecular Pathology, et al., v. the U.S. Patent and Trademark Office and Myriad Genetics, Inc. et al., decided on 29 July 2011, Opinion for the court filed by Circuit Court Lourie," 38, available at http:// www.genomicslawreport.com/wp-content/uploads/2011/07/Decision-in-USPTO-vs -MYGN.pdf, accessed January 23, 2014.

55. 189 Fed. Reg. 95 (April 28, 1911).

56. Ibid., 103.

57. Littlewood to Takamine, December 7, 1900, Transcript of Record, at 878. *Parke-Davis v. Mulford & Co.*, 196 F. 496 (2d Cir. 1912) (No. 4363). See also Harkness, "Dicta on Adrenalin(e)," 376.

58. Harkness, "Dicta on Adrenalin(e)," 383.

59. Ibid., 387, original quote from *Ex parte Latimer*, 1889 Dec. Comm'r Pat. 123, 124 (1889).

60. Dutfield, *Intellectual Property Rights*, 108.

61. As cited in Gaudillière, "Professional or Industrial Order?," 107.

62. Schering was able to patent hormones in the 1920s and 1930s, thereby establishing the precedents in Germany for subsequent patenting of purified biological substances used as pharmaceuticals. Ibid., 125.

63. Preamble to the German Patent Law of 1877. See ibid., 109.

64. German Patent Law Reform of 1891 conferred to patent holders the limited rights to the products made by the patented processes as well as the processes themselves; however, the patenting of pharmaceuticals was still not permitted. See Joseph Kaiser, *Das Deutsche Patentgesetz vom 7. April 1891* (Leipzig: A. Deichert'sche Verlagsbuchhandlung Nachf. Georg Böhme, 1907), 1–2. See also Arndt Fleischer, *Patentgesetzgebung und chemisch-pharmazeutische Industrie im deutschen Kaiserreich*

(1871–1918). Mit einem Geleitwort von Rudolf Schmitz (Stuttgart: Deutscher Apotheker Verlag, 1984), 165. Two relevant German cases here are the so-called methylene blue case of 1888 and the red congo case of 1889. See Gaudillière, "Professional or Industrial Order?," 109–110.

65. Dutfield, *Intellectual Property Rights*, 75. See also Jeffrey Alan Johnson, *The Kaiser's Chemists: Science and Modernization in Imperial Germany* (Chapel Hill, NC: University of North Carolina Press, 1990); Catherine M. Jackson, "Re-examining the Research School: August Wilhelm Hoffmann and the Re-creation of a Creation of a Liebigian Research School in London," *History of Science* 44 (2006): 281–319; Alan Rocke, *The Quiet Revolution: Hermann Kolbe and the Science of Organic Chemistry* (Berkeley: University of California Press, 1993).

66. Gaudillière "Professional or Industrial Order?," 107.

67. Dutfield, *Intellectual Property Rights*, 75.

68. Ibid., 93. For example, of the 862 U.S. organic colors chemical patents granted between 1900 and 1910, 81.3% were held by Germans, 13.3% by the Swiss, 2.2% by Americans, 1.3% by Britons, and 1.9% by citizens of other countries. See Jonathan Liebenau, "Patents and the Chemical Industry: Tools of Business Strategy," in *The Challenge of New Technology: Innovation in British Business since 1850*, ed. Jonathan Liebenau, 135–150 (Brookfield, VT: Gower, 1988), 139, 143. See also L. E. Sayre, "Patent Laws in Regard to the Protection of Chemical Industry," *Transactions of the Kansas Academy of Science* 30 (1919): 39–44; Floyd L. Vaughan, "Suppression and Non-Working of Patents, with Special Reference to the Dye and Chemical Industries," *American Economic Review* 9, no. 4 (1919): 693–700.

69. Beauchamp, "Patenting Nature," 283.

70. John E. Lesch, *The First Miracle Drugs: How the Sulpha Drugs Transformed Medicine* (New York: Oxford University Press, 2007), 5.

71. Dutfield, *Intellectual Property Rights*, 86.

72. Jonathan Liebenau, "Industrial R&D in Pharmaceutical Firms in the Early Twentieth Century," *Business History* 26 (1984), no. 3: 329–346, here 341. See also Dutfield, *Intellectual Property Rights*, 86; http://history.nih.gov/exhibits/history/docs/page_03.html, accessed January 23, 2014.

73. Liebenau, "Industrial R&D," 341.

74. Dutfield, *Intellectual Property Rights*, 106.

75. Ibid.

76. Basil Achilladelis, "The Dynamics of Technological Innovation: The Sector of Antibacterial Medicines," *Research Policy* 22, no. 4 (1993): 279–308, here 282 and 284.

77. Ibid., 283.

78. Ibid.

79. 189 Fed. Reg. 95, at 103 (April 28, 1911).

80. Dutfield, *Intellectual Property Rights*, 107.

81. Achilladelis, "The Dynamics of Technological Innovation," 282–285. See also Dutfield, *Intellectual Property Rights*, 110–154. Penicillin was never patented, although the processes for its mass production were. Most antibiotics thereafter were patented despite being products of nature. Dutfield, *Intellectual Property Rights*, 141.

82. As quoted in Daniel J. Kevles, "Patents, Protections, and Privileges: The Establishment of Intellectual Property in Animals and Plants," *Isis* 98, no. 2 (2007): 323–331, here 330. See the original, U.S.C. title 35, section 161, available at http://www.law.cornell.edu/uscode/text/35/161, accessed October 6, 2013. See also Glenn E. Bugos and Daniel J. Kevles, "Plants as Intellectual Property: American Practice, Law, and Policy in World Context," *Osiris*, 2nd ser., 7 (1992): 75–104. These two articles provide the historical background for plant patents.

83. U.S.C. title 35, section 161, available at http://www.law.cornell.edu/uscode/text/35/161, accessed October 6, 2013.

84. Bugos and Kevles, "Plants as Intellectual Property," 82.

85. House Committee on Patents, Plant Patents, House Report 1129, 16–17, as quoted in Bugos and Kevles, "Plants as Intellectual Property," 82.

86. Beauchamp, "Patenting Nature," 299–300.

87. 28 F.2d 641, 642 (3d Cir. 1928). See also *United States Industrial Chemical Co. v. Theroz Co.*, 25 F.2d 387 (C.C.A. 4th Circuit, 1928). The U.S. Supreme Court reviewed *General Electric Co. v. De Forest Radio Co.* three years later and ruled against the patent on the grounds of a lack of invention and the existence of prior art. See 283 U.S. 664 (1931), available at http://www.law.cornell.edu/supremecourt/text/283/664, accessed January 23, 2014.

88. *General Electric Co. v. De Forest Radio Co.*, 28 F.2d 641 (3d Cir. 1928), 643.

89. Pasquale J. Federico, "Patents for New Chemical Compounds," *Journal of the Patent Office Society* 21 (1939): 544–549.

90. Ibid., 549.

91. Ibid., 549, n. 10. See also *Kuehmsted v. Farbenfabriken of Elberfeld Co.*, 171 Fed. 887 (1909), and 179 Fed. 701 (1910). The patent for acetylsalicylic acid was upheld.

92. Philip McGarrigle and Vern Norviel, "Laws of Nature and the Business of Biotechnology," *Santa Clara Computer and High Technology Law Journal* 24, no. 2 (2008):

275–334, here 281, available at http://digitalcommons.law.scu.edu/chtlj/vol24/iss2/ ·
2/, accessed January 23, 2014.

93. McGarrigle and Norviel, "Laws of Nature," 282.

94. *Funk Brothers Seed Co. v. Kalo Inoculant Co.*, 333 U.S. 127 (1948), 130–131, available at http://caselaw.lp.findlaw.com/scripts/getcase.pl?court=us&vol=333&invol
=127, last accessed on 23 January 2014.

95. Ibid., 131.

96. Ibid.; Palombi, "The Patenting of Biological Materials," 32.

97. *Merck Co. v. Olin Mathieson Chemical Corp.*, 253 F.2d 156 (4th Cir. 1958), available at http://scholar.google.com/scholar_case?case=9565897413783842026&hl=en
&as_sdt=6&as_vis=1&oi=scholarr, accessed January 23, 2014.

98. Ibid., 159.

99. Ibid., 161–162.

100. Ibid., 161.

101. Ibid., 162–163.

102. Ibid., 163, original at 179 F. 701, 705 (7th Cir. 1910). A similar precedent mentioned by the Court was *Union Carbide Co. v. American Carbide Co.*, 181 F. 104, 106–
107 (2d Cir. 1910).

103. 253 F.2d 156, 162.

104. W. Kingston, "Removing Some Harm from the World Trade Organization,"
Oxford Development Studies 32, no. 2 (2004): 309–320, here 310. See also Dutfield,
Intellectual Property Rights, 142.

105. Dutfield, *Intellectual Property Rights*, 144.

106. Bugos and Kevles, "Plants as Intellectual Property," 89.

107. Ibid., 91–96.

108. Ibid., 95–96.

109. "Application of Malcolm E. Bergy," June 10, 1974, in U.S. Court of Customs
and Patent Appeals, Patent Appeal 76–712, *In re Application of Malcolm E. Bergy et al.*,
Transcript of Record, filed August 16, 1976, 6, as cited in Bugos and Kevles, "Plants
as Intellectual Property," 96.

110. *In the Matter of the Application of Malcolm E. Bergy et al.*, *Federal Reporter*, 2nd
ser., 1977 563: 1037–1038, as cited in Bugos and Kevles, "Plants as Intellectual Property," 97.

111. Bugos and Kevles, "Plants as Intellectual Property," 97.

112. *In re Bergstrom*, 427 F.2d 1394, 166 USPQ 256 (CCPA 1970), and http://www
.uspto.gov/web/offices/pac/mpep/documents/2100_2144_04.htm, accessed January
23, 2014.

113. Palombi, "The Patenting of Biological Materials," 35–36.

114. West, Brinkmann, McIntosh, et al., 30.

115. Rebecca Eisenberg, "Re-Examining the Role of Patents in Appropriating the
Value of DNA Sequences," *Emory Law Journal* 49 (3) (2000): 783-800, here 786. Note
that this quotation is taken from Lori B. Andrews, "Genes and Patent Policy:
Rethinking Intellectual Property Rights." *Nature Reviews: Genetics* 3, no. 10 (2002):
803–807, here 804. Short sequences of DNA, expressed sequence tags (ESTs), can be
used as probes to find other genes. Although they are more difficult to patent now,
that was not the case in the mid-1990s.

116. 409 U.S. 63 (1972).

117. 437 U.S. 584 (1978).

118. Ibid.

119. Merrill and Mazza, *Reaping the Benefits*, 73.

120. 450 U.S. 175 (1981).

121. *Diamond v. Chakrabarty*, 447 U.S. 303 (1980).

122. Daniel J. Kevles, "Ananda M. Chakrabarty Wins a Patent: Biotechnology, Law,
and Society," *Historical Studies in the Physical and Biological Sciences* 25, no. 1 (1994):
111–135, here 113.

123. *Diamond v. Chakrabarty*, 447 U.S. 303, 310 (1980); Palombi, "The Patenting of
Biological Molecules," 33.

124. I thank Rochelle Dreyfuss for pointing this out to me.

125. Palombi, "The Patenting of Biological Molecules," 36.

126. *Diamond v. Chakrabarty*, U.S. 303, 310 (1980); Palombi, "The Patenting of Biological Molecules," 28.

127. Palombi, "The Patenting of Biological Materials," 29–30.

128. Dutfield, *Intellectual Property Rights*, 197.

129. See Calvert and Joly, "How Did the Gene," 5.

130. Ibid. See also John M. Conley and Roberte Makowski, "Back to the Future:
Rethinking the Product of Nature Doctrine as a Barrier to Biotechnology Patents,"
Journal of the Patent and Trademark Office Society 85 (2003): 301–370 (pt. 1) and 371–
398 (pt. 2); L. J. Demaine and A. X. Fellmeth, "Reinventing the Double Helix: A

Novel and Nonobvious Reconceptualization of the Biotechnology Patent," *Stanford Law Review* 55, no. 2 (2002): 303–462.

131. Calvert and Joly, "How Did the Gene," 10–11.

132. See Daniel J. Kevles, "Of Mice and Money: The Story of the World's First Animal Patent," *Daedalus* 131, no. 2 (2002): 78–88.

133. Ibid., 84.

134. Fiona Murray, "Patenting Life: The Oncomouse," in *Making and Unmaking Intellectual Property: Creative Production in Legal and Cultural Perspective*, ed. Mario Biagioli, Peter Jaszi, and Martha Woodmansee, 399–411 (Chicago: University of Chicago Press, 2011).

135. 927 F.2d 1200, *Amgen Inc. v. Chugai Pharmaceutical Co., Ltd., and Genetics Institute, Inc.*, 927 F.2d 1200, para. 45 (Fed. Cir. 1991), available at http://openjurist .org/927/f2d/1200/amgen-inc-v-chugai-pharmaceutical-co-ltd, accessed January 23, 2014. See also Robert M. Schulman, Parker H. Bagley, and Tara Agnew, "The Written Description Requirement: Federal Circuit May Be Recognizing That Biotechnology Is Not Amenable to the Same Rules as Chemistry," *National Law Journal*, May 31, 2004, available at http://www.bakerbotts.com/infocenter/ publications/detail.aspx?id=345304c2-ff97-4fde-a023-909338bd2d57, accessed January 21, 2014.

136. 927 F.2d 1200, 1202, 1204, 1206 (Fed. Cir. 1991).

137. Ibid., 1200, 1206.

138. *Schering Corp. v. Amgen Inc.*, 222 F.3d 1347 (Fed. Cir. 2000); *Schering Corp. v. Amgen Inc.*, 18 F. Supp. 2d 372, 400 (D. Del. 1998). See also Can Cui, "Patentability of Molecules," available at http://jipel.law.nyu.edu/2011/04/patent-eligibility-of -molecules-"product-of-nature"-doctrine-after-myriad/#FN21, accessed January 23, 2014.

139. Beauchamp, "Patenting Nature," 310.

140. Hopkins, Mahdi, Patel, et al., "DNA Patenting," 185.

Chapter 4

1. See Sheila Jasanoff's notion of coproduction in Jasanoff, "The Idiom of Co-Production," 1–12.

2. C. Sheridan, "Curie's Victory over *BRCA1*," *Nature Biotechnology* 22, no. 7 (2004): 797.

3. Alison Abbott, "Europe to Pay Royalties for Cancer Gene: *BRCA1* Patent Decision May Be Ignored in Clinics," *Nature* 456, no. 456 (2008): 556.

4. "In accordance with an aspect of the present invention, there is provided an iso-lated nucleic acid (polynucleotide) which encodes for the mature polypeptide having the deduced amino acid sequence of FIGS. 1A-1B (SEQ ID NO: 2) or for the mature polypeptide encoded by the cDNA of the clone deposited as ATCC Deposit No. 97183 on Jun.1, 1995 at the American Type Culture Collection, Patent Deposi-tory, 10801 University Boulevard, Manassas, Va. 20110-2209," available at http://www.patents.com/us-6025154.html, accessed January 23, 2014.

5. "Examiner Reissue/Reexam Amendment Training for 'Changes to Patent Practice and Procedure' Final Rule Package," available at http://www.uspto.gov/web/offices/pac/dapp/opla/frule/rerex.pdf, accessed January 23, 2014. This rule has a long history. The Patent Act of 1836 permitted changes in the patent specification after a patent had been awarded provided that the mistakes arose "by inadvertency, accident, or mistake, and without any fraudulent intention" and no new matter was added. See Dood, "Patent Models and the Patent Law," 252.

6. U.S. Patent 6,025,154, available at http://www.patents.com/us-6025154.html, accessed January 23, 2014.

7. Burton A. Amernick, *Patent Law for the Nonlawyer: A Guide for the Engineer, Tech-nologist, and Manager*, 2nd ed. (New York: Van Nostrand Reinhold, 1991), 59–60.

8. "Searching Patent Data for Biological Sequences," available at http://www.patentlens.net/daisy/ipsearch/ipsearch/1706/1739/1744.html, accessed January 23, 2014; U.S. Patent 6,025,154, available at http://www.patents.com/us-6025154.html, accessed January 23, 2014.

9. http://www.uspto.gov/web/offices/pac/mpep/s2161.html, accessed January 23, 2014.

10. Sasha Blaug, Michael Shuster, and Henry Su, "*Enzo Biochem v. Gen-Probe*: Com-plying with the Written Description Requirement under U.S. Patent Law," *Nature Biotechnology* 21, no. 1 (2003): 97–99.

11. Kenneth J. Burchfiel, *Biotechnology and the Federal Circuit* (Washington DC: Bureau of National Affairs, 1995/2001), 147.

12. 54 F.2d 400 (1931).

13. Burchfiel, *Biotechnology*, 158.

14. Ibid.

15. 434 F.2d at 1393 (9th Cir. 1972); Burchfiel, *Biotechnology*, 159.

16. Burchfiel, *Biotechnology*, 159.

17. *Brunswick Corp. v. United States*, 34 Fed. Cl. 532, 584 (1995).

18. 427 F.2d 833 (1970).

19. Burchfiel, *Biotechnology*, 149.

20. The U.S. Court of Customs and Patent Appeals was abolished in 1982 by the Federal Courts Improvement Act, which created the U.S. Court of Appeals for the Federal Circuit, merging the CCPA with the appellate division of the U.S. Court of Claims.

21. Burchfiel, *Biotechnology*, 150.

22. Ibid.

23. "'Possession' of a chemical or biotechnology compound, and a written description of it, do not require knowledge or description of its particular chemical structure." Ibid., 151.

24. Ibid., 155.

25. Ibid., 154–156.

26. *Ex parte Maizel*, 27 USPQ2d at 1665 (Bd. Pat. App. & Inter. 1992).

27. Burchfiel, *Biotechnology*, 154, original at 27 USPQ2d at 1665.

28. 984 F.2d 1164 at 1171 (1993), as quoted in Burchfiel, *Biotechnology*, 150.

29. 984 F.2d 1164 at 1174, and Burchfiel, *Biotechnology*, 151.

30. Burchfiel, *Biotechnology*, 151.

31. I would like to thank Rochelle Dreyfuss for pointing that out to me.

32. Kenneth J. Burchfiel, *Biotechnology and the Federal Circuit: 2005 Cumulative Supplement* (Washington, DC: Bureau of National Affairs, 2005), 92.

33. 119 F.3d 1559 (Fed. Cir. 1997).

34. Ibid. See Burchfiel, *Cumulative Supplement*, 92.

35. The redundancy or degeneracy of the genetic code refers to the fact that more than one codon (or a group of three nucleotides) can code for the same amino acid.

36. 119 F.3d at 1566–1567. The judges were citing *Fiers v. Revel*, 984 F.2d 1164, 1171 and 117 (Fed. Cir. 1993). See Burchfiel, *Cumulative Supplement*, 93.

37. 984 F.2d 1164, 1170 (Fed. Cir. 1993); Burchfiel, *Cumulative Supplement*, 93.

38. 119 F.3d at 1569, as cited in Burchfiel, *Cumulative Supplement*, 94.

39. Burchfiel, *Cumulative Supplement*, 95.

40. Q. Todd Dickinson, "Guidelines for Examination of Patent Applications under 35 U.S.C. 112, paragraph 1, 'Written Description' Requirement, USPTO," 66 *Federal Register* 1099–1111 (January 5, 2001), Notices, here 1100.

41. Ibid., 1101. The Guidelines cite *Eli Lilly* as the precedent here. 119 F.3d at 1566.

42. Dickinson, "Guidelines," 1101 (italics in the USPTO Guidelines, not in the original court case).

43. *Enzo Biochem v. Gen-Probe Incorporated, Chugai Pharma U.S.A., Chugai Pharmaceutical Co., BioMérieux, and Becton Dickinson and Company, Defendants-Appellees, and BioMérieux SA, Defendant.*, No. 01–1230, U.S. Court of Appeals (henceforth *Enzo I*), 285 F.3d 1013 (Fed. Cir. April 2, 2002), available at http://openjurist.org/285/f3d/1013/enzo-biochem-inc-v-gen-probe-incorporated-usa-sa, accessed on January 24, 2014.

44. Ibid.

45. Ibid., 1016. See also William C. Mull, "Note: Using the Written Description Requirement to Limit Broad Patent Scope, Allow Competition, and Encourage Innovation in Biotechnology," *Health Matrix* 14 (2004): 393–435, here 410.

46. *Enzo I*, 285 F.3d at 1022; Mull, "Note," 411.

47. Blaug, Shuster, and Su, "*Enzo Biochem*," 97–99.

48. *Enzo I*, 285 F.3d at 1027 (J. Dyk, dissenting); Mull, "Note," 411.

49. 323 F.3d 956; *Enzo Biochem v. Gen-Probe Incorporated, Chugai Pharma U.S.A., Chugai Pharmaceutical Co., BioMérieux, and Becton Dickinson and Company, Defendants-Appellees, and BioMérieux SA, Defendant.*, No. 01–1230, U.S. Court of Appeals, Federal Circuit, decided July 15, 2002, here paragraph 30, (henceforth *Enzo II*), available at https://law.resource.org/pub/us/case/reporter/F3/323/323.F3d.956.01-1230 .html, accessed on January 24, 2014. See also Blaug, Shuster, and Su, "*Enzo Biochem*"; Mull, "Note," 424.

50. I would like to thank Rochelle Dreyfuss for pointing that out to me.

51. *Enzo II*, 323 F.3d 956; Mull, "Note," 424. See also Blaug, Shuster, and Su, "*Enzo Biochem*." Contrary to what Durack has argued, this decision has more to do with reduction to practice than with notions of tacit knowledge. See Katherine T. Durack, "Tacit Knowledge in Patent Applications: Observations on the Value of Models to Early U.S. Patent Office Practice and Potential Implications for the Twenty-first Century," *World Patent Information* 26, no. 2 (2004): 131–136.

52. Robert P. Merges, Peter S. Menell, and Mark A. Lemley, *Intellectual Property in the New Technological Age*, 4th ed. (New York: Aspen, 2004), 181.

53. This point was raised by a letter from W. Robinson H. Clark, Jeremy McKorm, and Sean Wooden of Dorsey & Whitney, LLP., to Stephen Walsh and Linda Therkorn of the USPTO, in Public Comments on the United States Patent and Trademark Office, "Revised Interim Guidelines for Examination of Patent Applications under the 35 U.S.C. § 112, ¶1 'Written Description' Requirement," 64 *Federal Register*

71,427 (December 21, 1999), comment 8, available at http://www.uspto.gov/web/offices/com/sol/comments/utilitywd/wrhc.pdf, accessed January 23, 2014.

54. Harold C. Wegner, "The Disclosure Requirements of the 1952 Patent Act: Looking Back and a New Statute for the Next Fifty Years," *Akron Law Review* 37 (2004): 243–261, here 248.

55. Blaug, Shuster, and Su, "*Enzo Biochem*," 97–99.

56. Ibid.

57. Robert C. Scheinfeld, "Enzo Biochem: What Direction Is Written Description Taking?," Baker Botts Publications, September 25, 2002, available at http://www.bakerbotts.com/infocenter/publications/detail.aspx?id=345304c2-ff97-4fde-a023-909338bd2d57, accessed January 21, 2014.

58. Blaug, Shuster, and Su, "*Enzo Biochem*," 2003, 97–99.

59. I would like to thank Rochelle Dreyfuss for pointing that out to me.

60. *Ariad Pharmaceuticals v. Eli Lilly & Co.*, 560 F.3d 1366 (Fed. Cir. 2009), available at https://www.casetext.com/case/ariad-pharmaceuticals-inc-v-eli-lilly-and-co/, accessed January 23, 2014.

61. *Festo Corp. v. Shoketsu Kinzoku Kogyo Kabushiki Co.*, 535 U.S. 722, 736 (2002). See also *Ariad Pharmaceuticals v. Eli Lilly & Co.*, 560 F.3d 1366, 1380–1381 (Fed. Cir. 2009).

62. Julia Carbone, E. Richard, Bhaven Sampat, et al., "DNA Patents and Diagnostics: Not a Pretty Picture," *Nature Biotechnology* 28, no. 8 (2010): 784–791.

63. *Ariad Pharmaceuticals v. Eli Lilly & Co.*, 560 F.3d 1366 (Fed. Cir. 2009), available at https://www.casetext.com/case/ariad-pharmaceuticals-inc-v-eli-lilly-and-co/, accessed January 23, 2014.

64. "Utility Examination Guidelines," 66 *Federal Register* 1093 (January 5, 2001): 1093, available at http://www.uspto.gov/web/offices/com/sol/notices/utilexmguide.pdf, accessed August 29, 2013.

65. Ibid.

66. http://blast.ncbi.nlm.nih.gov/Blast.cgi, accessed January 23, 2014.

67. Linda L. McCabe and Edward R. B. McCabe, *DNA: Promise and Peril* (Berkeley: University of California Press, 2008), 165.

68. "Revised Interim Utility Guidelines Training Materials," available at http://www.uspto.gov/web/offices/pac/utility/utilityguide.pdf, 53–55, accessed January 23, 2014.

69. Ibid., 54.

70. Ibid., 54–55.

71. Jack Spiegel, Public Comments on the United States Patent and Trademark Office, "Revised Interim Guidelines for Examination of Patent Applications under the 35 U.S.C. § 112, ¶1 'Written Description' Requirement," 64 *Federal Register* 71,427 (December 21, 1999), comment 64 on the Interim Utility Guidelines 10–11, March 22, 2000, available at http://www.uspto.gov/web/offices/com/sol/comments/ utilitywd/nihjs.pdf, esp. 151, accessed January 23, 2014 (henceforth cited as Spiegel, Public Comments). The document can also be found with different page numbers as comment 44 at http://www.uspto.gov/web/offices/com/sol/comments/utilguide/ nih2.pdf. See also David Dickson, "NIH Opposes Plans for Patenting 'Similar' Gene Sequences," *Nature* 405, no. 6782 (2000): 3.

72. Spiegel, Public Comments, 152–153.

73. 383 U.S. 519 (1966). Warren A. Kaplan and Sheldon Krimsky, "Patentability of Biotechnology Inventions and the PTO Utility Guidelines: Still Uncertain after All These Years?" (2001), available at http://www.tufts.edu/~skrimsky/PDF/patentability .PDF, accessed January 21, 2014.

74. 383 U.S. 519 (1966), available at http://supreme.justia.com/cases/federal/us/ 383/519/case.html, accessed January 23, 2014.

75. Spiegel, Public Comments.

76. Ibid., 153.

77. As quoted in ibid., 153.

78. Gitter, "International Conflicts," 1664.

79. 145 USPQ 390, 393 (CCPA 1965).

80. 34 USPQ2d 1436.1441 (Fed. Cir. 1995).

81. Spiegel, Public Comments, 154.

82. Ibid.

83. Ibid.

84. Ibid., 155.

85. Ibid., 156.

86. Ibid.

87. Ibid.

88. *In re Wilder*, 563 F.2d 457 (CCPA 1977); *In re May*, 574 F.2d 1082, 197 (CCPA 1978), available at http://www.uspto.gov/web/offices/pac/mpep/documents/2100 _2144_09.htm, accessed January 23, 2014.

89. Spiegel, Public Comments, 153.

90. It should be noted, however, that the Federal Circuit recognizes the degeneracy of the genetic code: "A prior art disclosure of the amino acid sequence of a protein does not necessarily render particular DNA molecules encoding the protein obvious because the redundancy of the genetic code permits one to hypothesize an enormous number of DNA sequences coding for the protein." *In re Deuel*, 51 F.3d 1552, 1558–1559 (Fed. Cir. 1995). See http://www.uspto.gov/web/offices/pac/ mpep/documents/2100_2144_09.htm, accessed January 23, 2014. See also Ying Pan, "A Post-*KSR* Consideration of Gene Patenting: The 'Obvious to Try' Standard Limits the Patentability of Genes," *Marquette Law Review* 93, no. 1 (2009): 285–308, here 292.

91. Spiegel, Public Comments, 156.

92. George Corey, Letter to the USPTO, March 22, 2000, in Public Comments on the United States Patent and Trademark Office, "Revised Interim Guidelines for Examination of Patent Applications under the 35 U.S.C. § 112, ¶1 'Written Description' Requirement," 64 *Federal Register* 71,427 (December 21, 1999), comment 12, available at http://www.uspto.gov/web/offices/com/sol/comments/utilitywd/gcorey .pdf, accessed January 23, 2014.

93. Ibid.

94. Spiegel, Public Comments, 156–157.

95. Ibid., 157.

96. Ibid., 158.

97. Dickson, "NIH Opposes," 3. See also Ronald Worton of the American Society of Human Genetics, Public Comments on the United States Patent and Trademark Office, "Revised Interim Guidelines for Examination of Patent Applications under the 35 U.S.C. § 112, ¶1 'Written Description' Requirement," 64 *Federal Register* 71,427 (December 21, 1999), comment 52, available at http://www.uspto.gov/web/ offices/com/sol/comments/utilitywd/ashg.pdf, accessed January 23, 2014.

98. R. Rodney Howell, Public Comments on the United States Patent and Trademark Office, "Revised Interim Guidelines for Examination of Patent Applications under the 35 U.S.C. § 112, ¶1 'Written Description' Requirement," 64 *Federal Register* 71,427 (December 21, 1999), comment 50, available at http://www.uspto.gov/web/ offices/com/sol/comments/utilitywd/acmg.pdf, accessed January 23, 2014. See also Julie Grisham, "New Rules for Gene Patents," *Nature Biotechnology* 18, no. 9 (2000): 921.

99. Jordan J. Cohen, Public Comments on the United States Patent and Trademark Office, "Revised Interim Guidelines for Examination of Patent Applications under the 35 U.S.C. § 112, ¶1 'Written Description' Requirement," 64 *Federal Register* 71,427 (December 21, 1999), comment 53, available at http://www.uspto.gov/web/

offices/com/sol/comments/utilitywd/aamc.pdf, accessed August 28, 2013; Dickson, "NIH Opposes," 3.

100. Dickson, "NIH Opposes," 3.

101. Charles E. Ludlam, Public Comments on the United States Patent and Trademark Office, "Revised Interim Guidelines for Examination of Patent Applications under the 35 U.S.C. § 112, ¶1 'Written Description' Requirement," 64 *Federal Register* 71,427 (December 21, 1999), comment 55, http://www.uspto.gov/web/offices/com/sol/comments/utilitywd/bio.pdf, accessed January 23, 2014.

102. Sean A. Johnston, Public Comments on the United States Patent and Trademark Office, "Revised Interim Guidelines for Examination of Patent Applications under the 35 U.S.C. § 112, ¶1 'Written Description' Requirement," Letter to Mark Nagumo, Steven Walsh, and Linda Therkorn, March 22, 2000, 64 *Federal Register* 71,427 (December 21, 1999), comment 59, http://www.uspto.gov/web/offices/com/sol/comments/utilitywd/genentech.pdf, accessed January 24, 2014.

103. Grisham, "New Rule," 921.

104. Dickson, "NIH Opposes," 3.

105. This point was raised in *PharmaStem Therapeutics v. Viacell,* 491 F.3d 1342, 1364–65 (Fed. Cir. 2007). The court ruled that a gene whose utility was ascertained solely by sequence analogy was unpatented as its utility was obvious. See also Pan, "A Post-*KSR* Consideration," 304. In 2008, the British Royal Courts of Justice revoked a genome patent owned by Human Genome Sciences, Inc. because its utility was based on sequence homology. The British Court ruled that the claims lacked industrial applicability (or utility in the language of U.S. patent law), insufficiency (enablement), and obviousness. See Chris Holman, "Holman's Biotech IP Blog, Genomics-Based Patents: Are Prophetic Assertions of Utility Enough?," December 1, 2008, available at http://holmansbiotechipblog.blogspot.com/2008/12/genomics-based-patents-are-prophetic.html, accessed January 20, 2014.

106. Drahos with Braithwaite, *Information Feudalism*, 43.

107. Cook-Deegan, *The Gene Wars*, 311.

108. Palombi, "The Patenting of Biological Materials," 11–25.

109. Reid G. Adler, "Biotechnology as an Intellectual Property," *Science* 224, no. 4647 (1984): 357–363, here 361. See also *Westinghouse v. Boyden Power Brake Co.*, 170 U.S. 537 (1898), available at http://supreme.justia.com/us/170/537/, access January 23, 2014.

110. As quoted in Drahos with Braithwaite, *Information Feudalism*, 158.

111. Michael A. Kock, "Purpose-Bound Protection for DNA Sequences: In through the Back Door?," *Journal of Intellectual Property Law and Practice* 5, no. 7 (2010): 495–513, here 502.

112. "A gene is a chemical, albeit a complex one." *Genetics Institute v. Amgen*, 502 U.S. 856 (1991). See also *Amgen v. Chugai Pharmaceutical Co.*, 927 F.2d 1200, 1206 (Fed. Cir.).

113. Steven Teutsch and the Secretary's Advisory Committee on Genetics, Health, and Society, "Gene Patents and Licensing Practices and Their Impact on Patient Access to Genetic Tests: Report of the Secretary's Advisory Committee on Genetics, Health, and Society," March 2010, available at http://osp.od.nih.gov/sites/default/files/SACGHS_patents_report_2010.pdf, accessed January 21, 2014, 14.

114. Marshall, "HIV Experts," 1263.

115. As quoted in Jacobs and Gosselin, "'Robber Barons of the Genetic Age.'" At the time, Goldstein was with the Washington, DC, firm of Sterne, Kessler, Goldstein & Fox.

116. John H. Barton, "Patents, Genomics, Research and Diagnostics," *Academic Medicine* 77 no. 12 (1997): 1339–1347, here 1340.

117. Doll, "Biotechnology," 690.

118. Rebecca S. Eisenberg and Robert P. Merges, "Opinion Letter as to the Patentability of Certain Inventions Associated with the Identification of Partial cDNA Sequences," *AIPLA Quarterly Journal* 23, no. 1 (1995): 1–52.

119. Ibid., 9–10.

120. Ibid., 7.

121. Ibid., 9–10. See also PTO Utility Examination Guideline, 60 *Federal Register* 36, 263 (1995). Eisenberg and Merges cite other examples to illustrate the relaxing of the utility requirements during the early 1990s, including *Ex parte Sudilovsky*, 21 USPQ2d (BNA) 1702 (Bd. Pat. App. & Interf. 1992); *Ex parte Aggrawal*, 23 USPQ2d (BNA) 1334 (Bd. Pat. App. & Interf. 1991); *Ex parte Balzarini* 21 USPQ2d 1892 (Bd. Pat. App. & Interf. 1991); *In re Brana* 51 F.3d 1560, 34 USPQ2d (BNA) 1436 (Fed. Cir. 1995).

122. Eisenberg and Merge, "Opinion Letter," 12.

123. National Advisory Council for Human Genome Research NIH/Burke, comment 42, available at http://www.uspto.gov/web/offices/com/sol/comments/utilguide/nih.pdf, accessed January 23, 2014.

124. Ibid.

125. N. Thumm, "Patents for Genetic Inventions: A Tool to Promote Technological Advance or a Limitation for Upstream Inventions?," *Technovation* 25, no. 12 (2005): 1410–1417; Mildred K. Cho, Samantha Illangasekare, Meredith A. Weaver, et al., "Effects of Patents and Licenses on the Provision of Clinical Genetic Testing Ser-

vices," *Journal of Molecular Diagnostics* 5, no. 1 (2003): 3–8; M. Heller and R. Eisenberg, "Can Patents Deter Innovation? The Anti-Commons in Biomedical Research," *Science* 280, no. 5364 (1998): 698–701.

126. Organisation for Economic Co-operation and Development, *Genetic Inventions, Intellectual Property Rights and Licensing Practices: Evidence and Policies* (Paris: Organization for Economic Co-operation and Development, 2002), 77.

127. Thumm, "Patents for Genetic Inventions," 1410–1417; Cho, Illangasekare, Weaver, et al., "Effects on Patents," 3–8; Heller and Eisenberg, "Can Patents Deter Innovation?," 698–701.

128. Merrill and Mazza, *Reaping the Benefits*, 25.

129. Ibid., 63–64.

130. Ibid., 53. See also Grisham, "New Rules," 921.

131. Grisham, "New Rules," 921.

132. "The Fate of Gene Patents under the New Utility Guidelines," *Duke Law and Technology Review* 8 (February 28, 2001), available at http://www.law.duke.edu/journals/dltr/articles/2001dltr0008.html, accessed January 20, 2014.

133. 66 *Federal Register* 1094 (January 5, 2001), Notices, available at http://www.uspto.gov/web/offices/com/sol/notices/utilexmguide.pdf, accessed January 23, 2014.

134. Ibid.

135. Ibid.

136. Ibid., 1095.

137. Ibid.

138. Bruce Alberts and Aaron Klug, "The Human Genome Itself Must Be Freely Available to All Humankind," *Nature* 404, no. 325 (2000): 325. See also Merrill and Mazza, *Reaping the Benefits*, 51–52.

139. Merrill and Mazza, *Reaping the Benefits*, 26.

140. John Sulston, "Heritage of Humanity," *Le Monde diplomatique*, December 2002, available at http://mondediplo.com/2002/12/15genome, accessed January 21, 2014.

141. Ibid.

142. "Utility Examination Guidelines," 66 *Federal Register* 1095 (January 5, 2001), Notices, available at http://www.uspto.gov/web/offices/com/sol/notices/utilexmguide.pdf, accessed January 23, 2014.

143. Ibid. See also 35 USC section 103(a) and *In re Deuel*, 51 F.3d 1552, 1559 (Fed. Cir. 1995): "[T]he existence of a general method of isolating cDNA or DNA

molecules is essentially irrelevant to the question of whether the specific molecules themselves would have been obvious." See also *In re Bell*, 991 F.2d 781 (Fed. Cir. 1993).

144. "Utility Examination Guidelines," 66 *Federal Register* 1094 (January 5, 2001), Notices.

145. Ibid.

146. Ibid., 1096.

147. Ibid.

148. "[T]he USPTO acknowledges the use of homology (similarity due to common descent) as a valid criterion for inferring function. Homology claims cannot be rejected outright because it has not been shown that homology-based assertions of utility are inherently unbelievable or involve implausible scientific evidence." See Bailey, Vanti, George, et al., "Patent Status," 1864.

149. Byran C. Diner and David S. Forman, "Emerging New Biotechnologies and the Patent Attorneys' Struggle to Best Protect Them," *Trends in Biotechnology* (January 2001), available at http://www.finnegan.com/resources/articles/articlesdetail .aspx?news=7a7fdfb3-ce6a-4656-813d-9754f3a5d3af, accessed January 20, 2014.

150. Trilateral Project B3b: "Mutual Understanding in Search and Examination: Nucleic Acid Molecule-Related Inventions Whose Functions Are Inferred Based on Sequence Homology Search," available at http://www.trilateral.net/projects/ biotechnology/mutual.pdf, accessed January 23, 2014.

151. Ibid.

152. Ibid.

153. Ibid.

154. Ibid.

155. Ibid.

156. Bailey, Vanti, George, et al., "Patent Status," 1870.

157. Yvonne Bonnie Eyler, "Proteomics and 'Orphan' Receptors," 2001, available at http://www.powershow.com/view/1add2-NGE1Z/Proteomics_and_Orphan _Receptors_flash_ppt_presentation, accessed January 23, 2014. Eyler recalled that the presentation dates back to 2001 as stated in her email to me on December 29, 2010. See also Dave Nguyen, "101 Sequence Homology," 2007, available at www .cabic.com/bcp/120407/DNguyen_101SH.ppt, accessed October 6, 2013, presented at the Biotechnology and Chemical Pharmaceutical Customer Partnership Meeting, December 4, 2007, U.S. Patent and Trademark Office, 600 Dulany Street, Alexandria, VA and Revised Utility Guidelines Training Materials, especially examples 10 and

12, available at http://www.uspto.gov/web/menu/utility.pdf, accessed August 29, 2013.

158. Sharon Begley, "As Top Court Invalidates Some Gene Patents, Biotech Has Moved On," Reuters, June 13, 2013, available at http://www.reuters.com/article/2013/06/13/us-usa-court-genes-industry-idUSBRE95C1GD20130613, accessed January 20, 2014.

Chapter 5

1. "Decision to Grant a European Patent," 16.09.2004, https://register.epo.org/espacenet/application?number=EP97904948&lng=&tab=main, and https://register .epo.org/espacenet/application?number=EP97904948&lng=en&tab=doclist, accessed January 23, 2014. The examiners were W. K. H. Meyer, H. M. Domingues, and K. H. L. Heckl. For the second patent, see http://google.com/patents/EP1482042A1, accessed January 23, 2014.

2. S. Aymé, G. Matthijs, and S. Soini, "Patenting and Licensing in Genetic Testing: Recommendations of the European Society of Human Genetics," *European Journal of Human Genetics* 16, no. 8 (2008): 405–411, here 406.

3. Ibid., 408.

4. Ibid. Hopkins agrees: "the more stringent approach of European and Japanese patent examiners may in large part allay concerns over DNA patenting in these regions." Hopkins, Mahdi, Patel, et al., "DNA Patenting," 185.

5. http://www.wto.org/english/thewto_e/whatis_e/tif_e/agrm7_e.htm, accessed January 23, 2014.

6. The ensuing paragraph is based on Arnoud Engelfriet, "Differences between U.S. and European Patents," *Ius Mentis: Law and Technology Explained*, October 1, 2005, available at http://www.iusmentis.com/patents/uspto-epodiff/, accessed January 20, 2014.

7. Sullivan & Cromwell LLP, "Congress Passes Historic Patent Reform Legislation," September 8, 2011, http://www.sullcrom.com/files/Publication/b1472d3f-a49c-4e1f -929f-fb85794ae7dc/Presentation/PublicationAttachment/e6112730-4db5-45b9 -b5b2-fb97e38fbc6a/SC_Publication_Congress_Passes_Historic_Patent_Reform _Legislation.pdf, accessed January 23, 2014.

8. Ibid.; Dennis Crouch, "Patent Reform Act of 2011: An Overview," available at http://www.patentlyo.com/patent/2011/02/patent-reform-act-of-2011-an-overview .html, accessed January 23, 2014.

9. "What Are the Differences between the U.S. Patent System and the European Patent System?," May 10, 2004, available at http://www.isarpatent.com/wcm/doc _arch/sommer2002_en.pdf, accessed January 23, 2014.

10. Article 105(1) European Patent Commission, available at http://www.epo.org/law-practice/legal-texts/html/epc/2010/e/ar105.html, accessed January 23, 2014.

11. Engelfriet, "Differences." See also Courtenay C. Brinckerhoff, "Protecting Invention in the U.S. and Europe: Inventors Need to Be Cognizant of Patent Laws on Both Sides of the Atlantic," *Genetic Engineering Biotechnology News* 28 (2008), available at http://www.genengnews.com/gen-articles/protecting-inventions-in-the-u-s-and-europe/2385/, accessed January 20, 2014.

12. See, for example, Brinckerhoff, "Protecting Invention."

13. Ibid.

14. Sheila Jasanoff, *Designs on Nature: Science and Democracy in Europe and the United States* (Princeton, NJ: Princeton University Press, 2005), 217–218.

15. Ibid., 218.

16. As quoted in ibid., 221.

17. Ibid.

18. E. Richard Gold and Alain Gallochat, "The European Biotech Directive: Past as Prologue," *European Law Journal* 7, no. 3 (2001): 331–366, here 351.

19. Ibid.

20. In France, purpose-bound protection is extended to inventions made from isolated material from the human body, and in Germany, it is extended to human/primate gene sequences. See "Report from the Commission to the Council and the European Parliament: Development and Implications of Patent Law in the Field of Biotechnology and Genetic Engineering. SEC (2005) 943," 2005, available at http://eurlex.europa.eu/smartapi/cgi/sga_doc?smartapi!celexplus!prod!DocNumber&type_doc=COMfinal&an_doc=2005&nu_doc=312&lg=en, accessed January 23, 2014.

21. Hopkins, Mahdi, Patel, et al., "DNA Patenting," 185.

22. Ibid., 187.

23. http://www.strawman.info/offer.htm, accessed January 23, 2014.

24. European Patent Registry, Filing of a New Opposition, June 14, 2004, "Opposition to EP-B-0883687 in the Name of Euroscreen S.A. of Route de Lennik 1070 Brussels. Opposition by Strawman Limited of 34 Lovedon Lane, Winchester, Hampshire, SO23 7NU," 4, available at https://register.epo.org/espacenet/application?number=EP97904948&lng=en&tab=doclist, accessed January 20, 2014, underlining in the original.

25. Ibid., 1–2.

26. Ibid., 15–17.

27. Ibid., 18–38.

28. Ibid., 7; Charles A. Janeway, Jr., Paul Travers, Mark Walport, et al., *Immunobiology* (New York: Garland, 1994).

29. European Patent Register, Filing of a New Opposition, June 13, 2004, "Opposition to EP-B-0883687 in the Name of Euroscreen S.A. of Route de Lennik 1070 Brussels. Opposition by Strawman Limited of 34 Lovedon Lane, Winchester, Hampshire, SO23 7NU, 2, available at https://register.epo.org/espacenet/application?number =EP97904948&lng=en&tab=doclist, accessed January 23, 2014.

30. Ibid., 9.

31. Ibid., 13, underlining in the original.

32. Ibid., 14.

33. "Opposition to EP-B-883687 by F. Hoffmann-La Roche AG, Filing of a New Opposition, 26.7.2005," European Patent Register, Filing of a New Opposition, available at https://register.epo.org/espacenet/application?number=EP97904948&lng=en &tab=doclist, accessed January 23, 2014, 2–3.

34. Christophe Combadiere, Sunil K. Ahuja, H. L. Tiffany, et al., "Cloning and Functional Expression of CC-CKR5, a Human Monocyte CC-Chemokine Receptor-Selective for MIP-1-α, MIP-1-β, and RANTES," *Journal of Leukocyte Biology* 60, no. 1 (1996): 147–152; Heidi Heath, S. Qin, P. Rao, et al., "Chemokine Receptor Usage by Human Eosinophils: The Importance of CCR3 Demonstrated Using an Antagonistic Monoclonal Antibody," *Journal of Clinical Investigation* 99, no. 2 (1997): 178–184; Jianglin He, Youzhi Chen, Michael Farzan, et al., "CCR3 and CCR5 Are Co-receptors for HIV-1 Infection of Microglia," *Nature* 385, no. 6617 (1997): 645–649. See European Patent Register, Filing of a New Opposition, 26.7.2005, 1–3, available at https:// register.epo.org/espacenet/application?number=EP97904948&lng=en&tab=doclist, accessed January 23, 2014. For a more detailed attack against the patent's priority, see 19–22, and for novelty, see 22–26.

35. "Opposition to EP-B-883687 by Hoffmann-La Roche," 3.

36. Ibid., 1–3. Here the lawyers cite a classic biochemistry textbook, Lubert Stryer, *Biochemistry*, 3rd ed. (New York: Freeman, 1988), 984–988. They also cite Toru Nakano, Ken-ichi Higashino, Norihisa Kikuchi, et al., "Vascular Smooth Muscle Cell-Derived, Gla-Containing Growth-Potentiating Factor for Ca (2+)-Mobilizing Growth Factors," *Journal of Biological Chemistry* 270, no. 11 (1995): 5702–5705; Israel F. Charo, Scott J. Myers, Ann Herman, et al., "Molecular Cloning and Functional Expression of Two Monocyte Chemoattractant Protein 1 Receptors Reveals Alternative Splicing of the Carboxyl-Terminal Tails," *Proceedings of the National Academy of Sciences (PNAS)-USA* 91, no. 7 (1994): 2752–2756 (note that the patent opposition mistyped the page numbers); S. Yamagami, Y. Tokuda, K. Ishii, et al., "cDNA Cloning and Functional Expression of a Human Monocyte Chemoattractant Protein 1

Receptor," *Biochemical Biophysical Research Communications* 202, no. 2 (1994): 1156–1162; Cocchi, DeVico, Garzino-Demo et al., "Identification," 1811–1815; Christine A. Power, Alexandra Meyer, Karin Nemeth, et al., "Molecular Cloning and Functional Expression of a Novel CC Chemokine Receptor cDNA from a Human Basophilic Cell Line," *Journal of Biological Chemistry* 270, no. 33 (1995): 19495–19500; Christophe Combadiere, Sunil K. Ahuja, and Philip M. Murphy, "Cloning and Functional Expression of a Human Eosinophil CC Chemokine Receptor," *Journal of Biological Chemistry* 270, no. 27 (1995): 16491–16494; Feng, Broder, Kennedy, et al., "HIV-1 Entry Cofactor," 872–877; Samson, Labbe, Mollereau, et al., "Molecular Cloning," 3362–3367; Deng, Liu, Ellmeier, et al., "Identification," 661–666; Dragic, Litwin, Allaway, et al., "HIV-1 Entry," 667–673; Alkhatib, Combadiere, Feng, et al., "CC CKR5," 1955–1958; Choe, Farzan, Sun, et al., "The β-Chemokine Receptors," 1135–1148; Doranz, Rucker, Jirik, et al., "A Dual-Tropic Primary," 1149–1158; and Rucker, Samson, Doranz, et al., "Regions in β-Chemokine," 437–446.

37. "Opposition to EP-B-883687 by Hoffmann-La Roche," 3, underlining in the original, available at https://register.epo.org/espacenet/application?number=EP9790 4948&lng=en&tab=, accessed January 23, 2014.

38. As quoted in ibid., 16.

39. Ibid., 14.

40. Ibid., 16.

41. Ibid., 11–14.

42. Ibid., 21.

43. Ibid., 25.

44. European Patent Office, "Opposition by Progenics Pharmaceuticals, Inc. against European Patent EP 0 883 687 B1 Granted in the Name of Euroscreen S.A.," 27.7.2005, available at https://register.epo.org/espacenet/application?number=EP97 904948&lng=en&tab=doclist, accessed January 23, 2014.

45. Ibid., 2.

46. Claim 25 of EP '687 as cited in ibid., 5.

47. Ibid., 5.

48. Ibid., 6.

49. Ibid., 6–10.

50. Ibid.

51. Ibid., 22.

52. Ibid., 25.

53. European Patent Register, "Notice of Opposition," letter from DeClercq, Brants & Partners (now called De Clercq & Partners), 06.01.2006, available at https://register.epo.org/espacenet/application?number=EP97904948&lng=en&tab=doclist, accessed January 23, 2014.

54. Ibid., 1–2.

55. Ibid., 25, or 1 of "Main Request."

56. Ibid., 25–27, or 1–3 of "Main Request."

57. Claim 9, ibid., 27, or 3 of "Main Request."

58. Claims 16–17, ibid., 27–28, or 3–4 of "Main Request."

59. Claims 26–28, ibid., 29, or 5 of "Main Request."

60. Ibid., 9–11.

61. Ibid., 6.

62. Ibid., 3.

63. Ibid., 15.

64. Ibid., 16.

65. Ibid., 16–21.

66. Ibid., 21–24.

67. Chemokine receptor 88C is CCR5. European Patent Office, "Annex of 26 May 2008, European Patent Register," available at https://register.epo.org/espacenet/application?number=EP97904948&lng=en&tab=doclist, accessed January 23, 2013.

68. Ibid.

69. "Annex to the Communication—Opposition," available at http://www.euroscreen.com/index.php/Euroscreen-News/Euroscreen-wins-the-opposition-related-to-its-CCR5-patent-claims.html, accessed January 23, 2014.

70. https://register.epo.org/espacenet/application?number=EP97904948&lng=en&tab=doclist, 05.08.2011, accessed January 23, 2014.

71. Ibid., 05.08.2011, "Summons to Attend Oral Proceedings," accessed February 3, 2014.

72. As quoted in https://register.epo.org/espacenet/application?number=EP97904948&lng=en&tab=doclist05.08.2011, "Annex to the Communication—Opposition," accessed Janaury 23, 2014, 3.

73. European Patent Register, "Notice of Opposition," letter from DeClercq, Brants & Partners (now called De Clercq & Partners), 06.01.2006, 26–27, 2–3 of

"Main Argument," available at https://register.epo.org/espacenet/application?number =EP97904948&lng=en&tab=doclist, accessed January 23, 2014.

74. https://register.epo.org/espacenet/application?number=EP97904948&lng =en&tab=doclist, 05.08.2011, "Annex to the Communication—Opposition," 3, accessed January 23, 2014.

75. Ibid., 4. See also "Notice of Opposition," 06.01.2006, 10–11, available at https:// register.epo.org/espacenet/application?number=EP97904948&lng=en&tab=doclist, accessed January 23, 2014.

76. "Annex to the Communication—Opposition," 05.08.2011, 4, available at https://register.epo.org/espacenet/application?number=EP97904948&lng=en&tab =doclist, accessed January 23, 2014; https://register.epo.org/espacenet/application? number=EP97904948&lng=en&tab=doclis, 06.01.2008, "Notice of Opposition," 11, accessed January 23, 2014. An antisense oligonucleotide is a sequence of DNA, which is complementary to a gene's mRNA sequence, thereby binding to it and blocking its translation into a protein.

77. "Annex to the Communication—Opposition," 05.08.2011, 5, available at https://register.epo.org/espacenet/application?number=EP97904948&lng=en&tab =doclist, accessed January 23, 2014.

78. Ibid., 6.

79. Ibid. ChemR13 receptor is an earlier name for CCR5.

80. Power, Meyer, Nemeth, et al., "Molecular Cloning," 19495–19500; Combadiere, Ahuja, and Murphy, "Cloning and Functional Expression," 16491–16494. Note that the Opposition Division has its publication date as June 20, 1996, which is a typo: it should be 1995.

81. "The European Patent Convention," available at http://www.epo.org/law -practice/legal-texts/html/epc/2013/e/ar54.html, accessed January 23, 2014.

82. Ibid.

83. "Annex to the Communication—Opposition," 05.08.2011, 6, available at https://register.epo.org/espacenet/application?number=EP97904948&lng=en&tab =doclist, accessed January 23, 2014.

84. Ibid., 4, 6–7.

85. Ibid., 7. See also Power, Meyer, Nemeth, et al., "Molecular Cloning," 19495– 19500; Combadiere, Ahuja, and Murphy, "Cloning and Functional Expression," 16491–16494.

86. "Annex to the Communication—Opposition," 05.08.2011, 7, available at https://register.epo.org/espacenet/application?number=EP97904948&lng=en&tab =doclist, accessed January 23, 2014.

87. Ibid.

88. "Guidelines for Examination, European Patent Office," available at http://www
.epo.org/law-practice/legal-texts/html/guidelines/e/g_vii_5_2.htm, accessed January
23, 2014.

89. "Annex to the Communication—Opposition," 05.08.2011, 8, available at
https://register.epo.org/espacenet/application?number=EP97904948&lng=en&tab
=doclist, accessed January 23, 2014.

90. https://register.epo.org/espacenet/application?number=EP97904948&lng=en&
tab=doclist, accessed January 23, 2014, 16.12.2011, "Request for Revocation of
Patent," accessed January 23, 2013.

91. https://register.epo.org/espacenet/application?number=EP97904948&lng=en
&tab=doclist, accessed January 23, 2014, 20.12.2011, According to the "Letter
Regarding the Opposition Procedure (No Time Limit)," the parties were officially
informed on December 28, 2011. See "Decision Revoking the European Patent,"
28.12.2011, accessed on January 23, 2013.

92. http://www.patentlens.net/patentlens/patents.html?patnums=EP_0811063
_B1&language=& and http://www.patentlens.net/patentlens/patents.html?patnums
=EP_1870465_B1&language=en&, both accessed January 23, 2014.

93. Interview with Vincent Lannoy, Euroscreen, Gosselies, Belgium, March 12, 2012.

Chapter 6

1. http://www.avert.org/india-hiv-aids-statistics.htm, accessed January 24, 2014.

2. For an outstanding account of the history of the controversy of the codiscovery
and the history of the AIDS epidemic in general, see Steven Epstein, *Impure Science:
AIDS, Activism, and the Politics of Knowledge* (Los Angeles: University of California
Press, 1996), 66–75.

3. See, for example, "The Groups of Antiretroviral Drugs," available at http://www
.avert.org/treatment.htm, accessed January 24, 2014; Gary H. Wynn, Michael J.
Zapor, Benjamin H. Smith, et al., "Antiretrovirals: Part I, Overview, History, and
Focus on Protease Inhibitors," *Psychosomatics* 45, no. 3 (2004): 262–270. See also
Samuel Broder, "The Development of Antiretroviral Therapy and Its Impact on the
HIV-1/AIDS Pandemic," *Antiretroviral Research* 85, no. 1 (2010): 1–38, here 5.

4. Broder, "The Development," 2; Erik De Clercq, "The History of Antiretrovirals:
Key Discoveries over the Past Twenty-five Years," *Reviews in Medical Virology* 19, no.
5 (2009): 287–299, here 288.

5. Charles Flexner, "HIV-Protease Inhibitors," *New England Journal of Medicine* 338,
no. 18 (1998): 1281–1292, here 1281. The idea was to replace the peptide linkage of

HIV-1 [-NH-CO-] with an hydroxyethylene group [-CH_2-CH(OH)-] of the drug. On this point, see De Clercq, "The History," 292. See also N. E. Kohl, E. A. Emini, W. A. Schleif, et al., "Active Human Immunodeficiency Virus Protease Is Required for Viral Infectivity," *Proceedings of the National Academy of Sciences (PNAS) USA* 85, no. 13 (1988): 4686–4690; Annemarie M. J. Wensing, Noortje M. van Maarseveen, and Monique Nijhuis, "Fifteen Years of HIV Protease Inhibitors: Raising the Barrier to Resistance," *Antiviral Research* 85, no. 1 (2010): 59–74, here 60; Thomas J. Hope and Didier Trono, "Structure, Expression, and Regulation of the HIV Genome," *UCSF HIVInSite*, November 2000, available at http://hivinsite.ucsf.edu/InSite?page=kb-02-01-02, accessed January 20, 2014; Wynn, Zapor, Smith, et al., "Antiretrovirals," 2004.

6. De Clercq, "The History," 292.

7. http://www.rxlist.com/invirase-drug.htm, accessed January 24, 2014.

8. John C. Tilton and Robert W. Doms, "Entry Inhibitors in the Treatment of HIV-1 Infection," *Antiviral Research* 85, no. 1 (2010): 91–100, here 91–92.

9. Ibid., 92.

10. Ibid., 93.

11. A fifth class of HIV/AIDS drugs was approved by the Food and Drug Administration in 2007—integrase inhibitors, which interfere with the HIV integrase enzyme. This enzyme enables the virus to integrate its genome into the host cell. The first intergrase inhibitor approved was raltegravir (Isentress). See De Clercq, "The History," 294–295.

12. Tilton and Dom, "Entry Inhibitors," 95.

13. Ibid. See also Bryan M. O'Hara and William C. Olson, "HIV Entry Inhibitors in Clinical Development," *Current Opinion in Pharmacology* 2, no. 5 (2002): 523–528, here 525; Kirsten A. Nagashima, "Human Immunodeficiency Virus Type 1 Entry Inhibitors PRO 542 and T-20 Are Potently Synergistic in Blocking Virus-Cell and Cell-Cell Fusion," *Journal of Infectious Diseases* 183, no. 7 (2001): 1121–1125.

14. J. P. Lalezari, J. J. Eron, M. Carlson, et al., "A Phase II Clinical Study of the Long-Term Safety and Antiviral Activity of Enfuvirtide-Based Antiretroviral Therapy," *AIDS* 17, no. 5 (2003): 691–698.

15. Ibid.

16. Ibid. It was later determined that the reason that the viral load was not decreased was that most people suffered from R5 tropism of the virus, which entered the cells via CCR5.

17. Ibid. ADM3100, for example, was discontinued due to reports of cardiac abnormalities with the participants.

18. Recent evidence suggests, however, that they are more likely to become infected with West Nile virus than those who are homozygous for the wild-type *CCR5* gene.

19. For video examples of recent HTS in action, see http://www.youtube.com/watch?v=IgrNF7Gdj4c and http://www.youtube.com/watch?v=xakRli5vxd4, both accessed January 24, 2014. For a history of HTS, see John L. LaMattina, *Drug Truths: Dispelling the Myths about Pharma R&D* (Hoboken, NJ: Wiley, 2009), 64. See also Dennis A. Pereira and John A. Williams, "Origin and Evolution of High Throughput Screening," *British Journal of Pharmacology* 152, no. 1 (2007): 53–61.

20. Ramon Carbó-Droca, Xavier Gironés, and Paul G. Mezey, eds., *Fundamentals of Molecular Similarity* (New York: Kluwer Academic/Plenum, 2001); G. A. Patani and E. J. LaVoie, "Bioisosterism: A Rational Approach in Drug Design," *Chemical Reviews* 96, no. 8 (1996): 3147–3176. See also Jeff C. Watkins, P. Krogsgaard-Larsen, and T. Honoré, "Structure-Activity Relationships in the Development of Excitatory Amino Acid Receptor Agonists and Competitive Antagonists," *Trends in Pharmacological Sciences* 11, no. 1 (1990): 25–33.

21. "Introduction to (Quantitative) Structure Activity Relationships," 2012, available at http://www.oecd.org/document/29/0,3746,en_2649_34379_42675741_1_1_1_1,00.html, accessed January 24, 2014.

22. Carbó-Droca, Gironés, and Mezey, eds., *Fundamentals*; Patani and LaVoie, "Bioisosterism."

23. "The Story of Selzentry: Manos Perros, Anthony Wood, and Elna van der Ryst," 2010, available at http://www.innovation.org/index.cfm/StoriesofInnovation/InnovatorStories/The_Story_of_Selzentry, accessed January 24, 2014.

24. As quoted in ibid.

25. Anthony Wood and Duncan Armour, "The Discovery of the CCR5 Receptor Antagonist, UK-427,857: A New Agent for the Treatment of HIV Infection and AIDS," *Progress in Medicinal Chemistry* 43 (2005): 239–271, here 242. Merck was testing molecules based on inhibition to MIP-1α. Research to that point suggested that the binding sites of HIV-gp120 and MIP-1α were distinct and separate, although MIP-1α could act as an allosteric antagonist to gp120. Ibid.

26. Christopher A. Lipinski's rule of five is used to determine the possibility that a chemical will become an orally active drug that generally has no more than one violation of the following four rules—no more than five hydrogen-bond donors, no more than ten hydrogen-bond acceptors, a mass of less than 500 daltons, and an octanol-water partition coefficient log P < or = 5. All numbers are multiples of five, hence the name.

27. Wood and Armour, "The Discovery," 242.

28. Ricardo Macarron, Martyn N. Banks, Dejan Bojanic, et al., "Impact of High-Throughput Screening in Biomedical Research," *Nature Reviews: Drug Discovery* 10, no. 3 (2011): 188–195, here 191; Tilton and Doms, "Entry Inhibitors," 95.

29. Wood and Armour, "The Discovery," 244.

30. Patrick Dorr, Mike Westby, S. Dobbs, et al., "Maraviroc (UK-427,857): A Potent, Orally Bioavailable, and Selective Small-Molecule Inhibitor of Chemokine Receptor CCR5 with Broad-Spectrum Anti-Human Immunodeficiency Virus Type 1 Activity," *Antimicrobial Agents and Chemotherapy* 49, no. 11 (2005): 4721–4732, here 4724; Macarron, Banks, Bojanic, et al., "Impact of High-Throughput Screening," 191. See also Manos Perros, "CCR5 Antagonists for the Treatment of HIV Infection and AIDS," in *Advances in Antiviral Drug Design*, ed. Erik De Clercq, vol. 5, 185–213, here 197 (Oxford: Elsevier, 2007); Wood and Armour, "The Discovery," 244–261.

31. Wood and Armour, "The Discovery," 268.

32. Dorr, Westby, Dobbs, et al., "Maraviroc," 191.

33. Macarron, Banks, Bojanic, et al., "Impact of High-Throughput Screening," 190; Dorr, Westby, Dobbs, et al., "Maraviroc," 4724. Xenobiotics are drugs such as antibiotics, which are not part of an organism's normal diet.

34. Dorr, Westby, Dobbs, et al., "Maraviroc," 4724.

35. John Spencer, "Case Study on Maraviroc," in *An Introduction to Medicinal Chemistry*, ed. Graham L. Patrick (New York: Oxford University Press, 2009), available at http://fdslive.oup.com/www.oup.com/orc/resources/chemistry/patrick4e/01student/updates/sep09maraviroc.pdf, accessed January 21, 2014. See also Wood and Armour "The Discovery," 244–266.

36. John L. LaMattina, *Drug Truths*, 65; Dorr, Westby, Dobbs, et al., "Maraviroc," 4724.

37. Dorr, Westby, Dobbs, et al., "Maraviroc," 4724.

38. Ibid., 4724–4727.

39. http://www.viivhealthcare.com/about-us/who-we-are.aspx, accessed January 24, 2014.

40. Other examples of success include thrombopoietin (THO) receptor agonists and hepatitis C virus NS5A inhibitors. Macarron, Banks, Bojanic, et al., "Impact of High-Throughput Screening," 190.

41. Ibid., 188–189. See also Roger Lahana, "Who Wants to Be Irrational?," *Drug Discovery Today* 8, no. 15 (2003): 655–656; Landers, "Trouble Impending," A1; Ted T. Ashburn and Karl B. Thor, "Drug Repositioning: Identifying and Developing New Uses for Existing Drugs," *Nature Reviews: Drug Discovery* 3 (2004): 673–683; J.-B. Garnier, "Rebuilding the R&D Engine in Big Pharma," *Harvard Business Review* 86, no. 5

(2008): 68–76; Rick Mullin, "As High-Throughput Screening Draws Fire, Researchers Leverage Science to Put Automation into Perspective," *Chemical Engineering News* 82, no. 30 (2004): 23–32.

42. Macarron, Banks, Bojanic, et al., "Impact of High-Throughput Screening," 194.

43. See, for example, M. Shiraishi, Y. Aramaki, M. Seto, et al., "Discovery of Novel, Potent, and Selective Small-Molecule CCR5 Antagonists as Anti-HIV-1 Agents: Synthesis and Biological Evaluation of Anilide Derivatives with a Quaternary Ammonium Moiety," *Journal of Medicinal Chemistry* 43, no. 10 (2000): 2049–2063; Fadi F. Hamdan, Martin Audet, Philippe Garneau, et al., "High-Throughput Screening of G Protein-Coupled Receptor Antagonists Using a Bioluminescence Resonance Energy Transfer 1-Based ß-Arrestin2 Recruitment Assay," *Journal of Biomolecular Screening* 10, no. 5 (2005): 463–475; Robert G. Wei, Damian O. Arnaiz, You-Ling Chou, et al., "CCR5 Receptor Antagonists: Discovery and SAR Study of Guanylhydrazone Derivatives," *Bioorganic and Medicinal Chemistry Letters* 17, no. 1 (2007): 231–234.

44. Perros, "CCR5 Antagonists," 190.

45. Ibid.

46. Ibid.

47. Duncan Armour, "The Discovery of CCR5 Receptor Antagonists for the Treatment of HIV Infection: Hit-to-Lead Studies," *ChemMedChem* 1, no. 7 (2006): 706–709, here 709; J. G. Cumming, A. E. Cooper, K. Grime, et al., "Modulators of the Human CCR5 Receptor: Part 2, SAR of Substituted 1-(3,3-Diphenylpropyl)-Piperidinyl Phenylacetamides," *Bioorganic and Medicinal Chemistry Letters* 15, no. 22 (2005): 5012–5015; Gebhard Thoma, François Nuninger, Marc Schaefer, et al., "Orally Bioavailable Competitive CCR5 Antagonists," *Journal of Medicinal* Chemistry 47, no. 8 (2004): 1939–1955; Conrad P. Dorn, Paul E. Finke, Bryan Oates, et al., "Antagonists of the Human CCR5 Receptor as Anti-HIV-1 Agents: Part 1, Discovery and Initial Structure-Activity Relationships for 1-Amino-2-Phenyl-4-(Piperidin-1-yl)Butanes," *Bioorganic and Medicinal Chemistry Letters* 11, no. 2 (2001): 259–264; Shon R. Pulley, "CCR5 Antagonists: From Discovery to Clinical Efficacy," in *Chemokine Biology: Basic Research and Clinical Application*, ed. Kuldeep Neote et al., 2 vols. (2006–07), vol. 2 (2007): 145–163, here 146; Perros, "CCR5 Antagonists," 190.

48. Masanori Baba, Osamu Nishimura, Naoyuki Kanzaki, et al., "A Small-Molecule Nonpeptide CCR5 Antagonist with Highly Potent and Selective Anti-HIV-1 Activity," *Proceedings of the National Academy of Sciences (PNAS) USA* 96, no. 10 (1999): 5698–5703; Shiraishi, Aramaki, Seto, et al., "Discovery of Novel," 2049–2063.

49. Masanori Baba, Katsunori Takashima, Hiroshi Miyake, et al., "TAK-652 Inhibits CCR5-Mediated Human Immunodeficiency Virus Type 1 Infection in Vitro and Has Favorable Pharmacokinetics in Humans," *Antimicrobial Agents Chemotherapy* 49, no. 11 (2005): 107–116. See also Perro, "CCR5 Antagonists," 192–193.

50. Dorn, Finke, Oates, et al., "Antagonists of the Human CCR5," 259–264; Dong-Ming Shen, Min Shu, Sander G. Mills, et al., "Antagonists of Human CCR5 Receptor Containing 4-(Pyrazolyl)Piperdine Side Chains: Part 1, Discovery and SAR Study of 4-Pyrazolylpiperdine Side Chains," *Bioorganic and Medicinal Chemistry Letters* 14, no. 4 (2004): 935–939; Dong-Ming Shen, Min Shu, Christopher A. Willoughby, et al., "Antagonists of Human CCR5 Receptor Containing 4-(Pyrazolyl)Piperdine Side Chains: Part 2, Discovery of Potent, Selective, and Orally Bioavailable Compounds," *Bioorganic and Medicinal Chemistry Letters* 14, no. 4 (2004): 941–945; M. Shu, J. L. Loebach, K. A. Parker, et al., "Antagonists of Human CCR5 Receptor Containing 4-(Pyrazolyl)Piperdine Side Chains: Part 3, SAR Studies on the Benzylpyrazole Segment," *Bioorganic and Medicinal Chemistry Letters* 14, no. 4 (2004): 947–952.

51. Perros, "CCR5 Antagonists," 193–194.

52. Anandan Palani, Sherry Shapiro, John W. Clader, et al., "Discovery of 4-[(Z)-(4-Bromophenyl)- (Ethoxyimino)Methyl]-1′-[(2,4-Dimethyl-3- Pyridinyl)Carbonyl]-4′-Methyl-1,4′- Bipiperidine N-Oxide (SCH 351125): An Orally Bioavailable Human CCR5 Antagonist for the Treatment of HIV Infection," *Journal of Medicinal Chemistry* 44, no. 21 (2001): 3339–3342; David Price, "Maraviroc (Selzentry): The First-in-Class CCR5 Antagonist for the Treatment of HIV," in *Modern Drug Synthesis*, ed. Jie Jack Li and Douglas S. Johnson, 17–27, here 18 (New York: Wiley, 2010). See also Pulley, "CCR5 Antagonists," vol. 2 (2007), 152.

53. Jayaram R. Tagat, Stuart W. McCombie, Dennis Nazareno, et al., "Piperazine-Based CCR5 Antagonists as HIV-1 Inhibitors: IV, Discovery of 1-[(4,6-Dimethyl-5-Pyrimidinyl)Carbonyl]- 4-[4-[2-Methoxy-1(R)-4-(Trifluoromethyl)Phenyl]Ethyl-3(S) -Methyl-1-Piperazinyl]- 4-Methylpiperidine (Sch-417690/Sch-D), a Potent, Highly Selective, and Orally Bioavailable CCR5 Antagonist," *Journal of Medicinal Chemistry* 47, no. 10 (2004): 2405–2408; Julie M. Strizki, Cecile Tremblay, Serena Xu, et al., "Discovery and Characterization of Vicriviroc (SCH 417690), a CCR5 Antagonist with Potent Activity against Human Immunodeficiency Virus Type 1," *Antimicrobial Agents and Chemotherapy* 49, no. 12 (2005): 4911–4919; Price, "Maraviroc (Selzentry)," 19. See also O'Hara and Olson, "HIV Entry Inhibitors," 524–525; Perros, "CCR5 Antagonists," 194–195.

54. Vincent Idemyor, "Human Immunodeficiency Virus (HIV) Entry Inhibitors (CCR5 Specific Blockers) in Development: Are They the Next Novel Therapies?," *HIV Clinical Trials* 6, no. 5 (2005): 272–277; Rama Kondru, Jun Zhang, Changhua Ji, et al., "Molecular Interactions of CCR5 with Major Classes of Small-Molecule Anti-HIV CCR5 Antagonists," *Molecular Pharmacology* 73, no. 3 (2008): 789–800.

55. There are four phases of FDA drug testing. Phase 1 studies the efficacy and side effects of the drug on 20 to 80 people; phase 2 studies the drug on 100 to 300 individuals; and phase 3 studies the drug on 1,000 to 3,000, compares the drug with other treatments, and gathers information on its safe use. After drugs pass phase 3,

they normally can be prescribed by physicians. The process can be shortened through accelerated approval. Phase 4 tracks the drug's risks, benefits, and optimal use after approval for prescription.

56. Ronald Baker, "HIVandHepatitis.com," posted November 12, 2007, available at http://web.archive.org/web/20071112031341/http://www.hivandhepatitis.com/recent/2007/091807_a.html, accessed January 20, 2014. See also Tilton and Doms, "Entry Inhibitors," 95; Joel E. Gallant, "VICTOR-E3 and VICTOR-E4: Vicriviroc Plus PI-Based Optimized Background Regimen in Treatment-Experienced Patients," in "The CCO Independent Conference Coverage of the 2010 Conference on Retroviruses and Opportunistic Infections, San Francisco, California, 2010," available at http://www.clinicaloptions.com/login.aspx?item=%2fhiv%2fconference+coverage%2fretroviruses+2010%2fpodium%2fpodium%2fpages%2fpage+11&user=extranet%5cAnonymous&site=website&qs=, accessed January 20, 2014. See also "VICTOR-E3 and VICTOR-E4: Use of Vicriviroc Does Not Improve Virologic Efficacy in CCR5-Tropic HIV-Infected Patients Receiving a PI-Based Optimized Background Regime," February 18, 2010, in "The CCO Independent Conference Coverage of the 2010 Conference on Retrovirus and Opportunistic Infections, San Francisco, CA, February 16–19, 2010," available at http://www.clinicaloptions.com/login.aspx?item=%2fhiv%2fconference+coverage%2fretroviruses+2010%2fpodium%2fcapsules%2f54lb&user=extranet%5cAnonymous&site=website&qs=, accessed January 20, 2014.

57. Liz Highleyman, "Vicriviroc Fails to Beat Stiff Competition, Merck Will Not File for Treatment-Experienced Approval," paper presented at the Seventeenth Conference on Retroviruses and Opportunistic Infections (CROI 2010), February 16–19, 2010, San Francisco, California, February 19, 2010, available at http://www.hivandhepatitis.com/2010_conference/croi/docs/0219_2010_f.html, accessed January 20, 2014.

58. Price, "Maraviroc (Selzentry)," 19; Tilton and Dom, "Entry Inhibitors," 94. See also http://www.gsk-clinicalstudyregister.com/quick-search-list.jsp;jsessionid=4AA8 4A8B295509E21725009075B98E31?item=aplaviroc&type=Compound&letterrange =A-F, accessed January 24, 2014. Symptoms included gastrointestinal side effects such as nausea and vomiting and abdominal pain. See Perros, "CCR5 Antagonists," 197.

59. Price, "Maraviroc (Selzentry)," 19. See also Armour, "The Discovery of CCR5 Receptor," 706–709. 1,4,4-Trisubstituted-Piperazines have a history of activity against a range of GPCRs. Hence, they were chemically optimized. See Perros, "CCR5 Antagonists," 196.

60. Chu-Biao Xue, Lihua Chen, Ganfeng Cao, et al., "Discovery of INCB9471, a Potent, Selective, and Orally Bioavailable CCR5 Antagonist with Potent Anti-HIV-1 Activity," *ACS Medicinal Chemistry Letters* 1, no. 9 (2010): 483–487, here 483. See also Niu Shin, Kim Solomon, Naiming Zhou, et al., "Identification and Characterization of INCB9471, an Allosteric Noncompetitive Small-Molecule Antagonist of C-C

Chemokine Receptor 5 with Potent Inhibitory Activity against Monocyte Migration and HIV-1 Infection," *Journal of Pharmacology and Experimental Therapeutics* 338, no. 1 (2011): 228–239.

61. Liz Highleyman, "Monoclonal Antibody PRO 140 Suppresses HIV Viral Load with Once-Weekly Dosing," May 7, 2010, available at http://www.hivandhepatitis .com/recent/2010/0507_2010_b.html, accessed January 20, 2014; Jeffrey M. Jacobson, Melanie A. Thompson, Jacob P. Lalezari, et al., "Anti-HIV-1 Activity of Weekly or Biweekly Treatment with Subcutaneous PRO 140, a CCR5 Monoclonal Antibody," *Journal of Infectious Diseases* 201, no. 10 (2010): 1481–1487; Tilton and Doms, "Entry Inhibitors," 95.

62. "Phase 2 Clinical Trials Started on PRO 140," *AIDS Patient Care STDs* 22, no. 2 (2008): 159–160.

63. "PRO 140," available at http://www.aidsmeds.com/archive/pro_140_2086.shtml, accessed January 24, 2014.

64. Dragic, the lead author on one of the papers announcing CCR5 as an HIV-1 coreceptor, worked for Progenics.

65. See the previous chapter for their challenge of one of Euroscreen's European patents on CCR5.

66. http://www.prnewswire.com/news-releases/human-genome-sciences-reports -on-progress-toward-commercialization-54521382.html, accessed January 24, 2014.

67. J. P. Lalezari, G. K. Yadavalli, M. Para, et al., "Safety, Pharmacokinetics, and Antiviral Activity of HGS004, a Novel Fully Human IgG4 Monoclonal Antibody against CCR5, in HIV-1-Infected Patients," *Journal of Infectious Diseases* 197, no. 5 (2008): 721–727.

68. Jennifer C. Pai, Jamie N. Sutherland, and Jennifer Maynard, "Progress towards Recombinant Anti-Infective Antibodies," *Recent Patents on Anti-Infective Drug Discovery* 4, no. 1 (2007): 1–17, 3. See also Olga Latinovic, Marvin Reitz, Nhut M. Le, et al., "CCR5 Antibodies HGS004 and HGS101 Preferentially Inhibit Drug-Bound CCR5 Infection and Restore Drug Sensitivity of Maraviroc-Resistant HIV-1 in Primary Cells," *Virology* 411, no. 1 (2011): 32–40.

69. Perros, "CCR5 Antagonists," 202.

70. "Euroscreen Announces CCR5 Licensed to Pfizer," available at http://www .thefreelibrary.com/Euroscreen+announces+CCR5+licensed+to+Pfizer.-a087090688, accessed January 24, 2014. See also "Euroscreen CCR5 Agonist Program Available for Out-Licensing," available at http://www.euroscreen.com/index.php/Euroscreen -News/Euroscreen-CCR5-Agonist-program-available-for-out-licensing.html, accessed January 24, 2014.

71. Jules Vernon, "Motivate 1 Study: Efficacy and Safety of Maraviroc Plus Optimized Background Therapy in Viremic, ART-Experienced Patients Infected with

CCR5-Tropic HIV-1: Twenty-four-Week Results of Phase 2b/3 Studies," paper presented February 27, 2007, at the Fourteenth Conference on Retroviruses and Opportunistic Infections (CROI), Los Angeles, California, February 25–28, 2007, available at http://www.natap.org/2007/CROI/croi_39.htm, accessed January 21, 2014.

72. Roy M. Gulick, Jacob Lalezari, James Goodrich, et al., "Maraviroc for Previously Treated Patients with R5 HIV-1 Infection," *New England Journal of Medicine* 359, no. 14 (2008): 1429–1441, here 1429. "[T]hese results demonstrate that, in treatment-experienced patients with R5 virus, maraviroc combined with OBT provides sustained antiretroviral efficacy and tolerability through 48 weeks," in Jules Levin, "Efficacy and Safety of Maraviroc Plus Optimized Background Therapy in Treatment-Experienced Patients Infected with CCR5-Tropic HIV-1: Forty-eight-week Combined Analysis of the MOTIVATE Studies- Pooled Analysis of MOTIVATE 1 & 2," paper presented at the Fifteenth Annual Meeting of CROI, February 3–6, 2008, Boston, Massachusetts, available at http://www.natap.org/2008/CROI/croi_43.htm, accessed January 21, 2014. See also W. David Hardy, Roy M. Gulick, Howard Mayer, et al., "Two-Year Safety and Virologic Efficacy of Maraviroc in Treatment-Experienced Patients with CCR5-Tropic HIV-1 Infection: Ninety-six-Week Combined Analysis of MOTIVATE 1 and 2," *Journal of Acquired Immune Deficiency Syndromes* 55, no. 5 (2010): 558–564.

73. "AIDSinfo—HIV/AIDS Drug Information—Maraviroc," available at http://www .aidsinfo.nih.gov/DrugsNew/DrugDetailNT.aspx?int_id=408, accessed on January 24, 2014. See also Timothy J. Wilkin, Zhaohui Su, Daniel R. Kuritzkes, et al., "HIV Type 1 Chemokine Coreceptor Use among Antiretroviral-Experienced Patients Screened for a Clinical Trial of a CCR5 Inhibitor: AIDS Clinical Trial Group A5211," *Clinical Infectious Diseases* 44, no. 4 (2007): 591–595; Tim Horn, "Encouraging Data from Two Maraviroc Studies," *AIDSMEDS*, February 28, 2007, available at http://www.aidsmeds.com/articles/1961_11404.shtml, accessed January 20, 2014; Gerd Fätkenheuer, Mark Nelson, Adriano Lazzarin, et al., "Subgroup Analyses of Maraviroc in Previously Treated R5 HIV-1 Infection," *New England Journal of Medicine* 359, no. 14 (2008): 1442–1455.

74. Miranda Hitti, "Selzentry Is First in a New Class of HIV Drugs Made to Slow HIV's Advance, Says FDA," August 7, 2007, available at http://www.webmd.com/ hiv-aids/news/20070807/fda-oks-new-hiv-drug-selzentry, accessed January 20, 2014.

75. http://hivinsite.ucsf.edu/insite?page=ar-06-01, accessed January 24, 2014. See also "FDA Advisory Committee Recommends Approval of Pfizer's Selzentry for Use in Patients Starting HIV Therapy for the First Time," October 8, 2009, available at http://www.businesswire.com/news/home/20091008006176/en/FDA-Advisory -Committee-Recommends-Approval-Pfizer's-Selzentry, accessed January 24, 2014; "Ninety-six-Week MERIT ES [Extra Sensitive] Analysis Shows Efficacy of Pfizer's HIV/ AIDS Treatment Celsentri/Selzentry (Maraviroc) in Treatment-Naïve HIV Patients; Results Consistent with Forty-eight-Week Analysis," June 21, 2009, available at http://www.drugs.com/clinical_trials/96-week-merit-es-analysis-shows-efficacy

-pfizer-s-hiv-aids-celsentri-selzentry-maraviroc-na-ve-hiv-7772.html, accessed January 24, 2014.

76. It should be noted that a subsequent study (MERIT ES, a retrospective analysis of the MERIT with a more sensitive Trofile assay) found that Maraviroc was just as effective as Sustiva. See Liz Highleyman, "MERIT Reanalysis with More Sensitive Trofile Test Shows Maraviroc (Selzentry) Works as Well as Efaviren (Sustiva) in Patients New to Therapy," paper presented at the Fifty-eighth Annual ICAAC and Forty-sixth Annual IDSA Meeting, October 25–28, 2008, Washington, DC, October 28, 2008, available at http://www.hivandhepatitis.com/2008icr/icaac_idsa/docs/102808_c.html, accessed January 20, 2014; Michael Saag, J. Heera, J. Goodrich, et al., "Reanalysis of the MERIT Study with the Enhanced Trofile™ Assay (MERIT ES)," October 28, 2008, paper presented at the 2008 ICAAC/IDSA Annual Meeting, Washington, DC, available at http://www.natap.org/2008/ICAAC/ICAAC_19.htm, accessed January 24, 2014.

77. "Pfizer's Selezentry Poised to Be Most Expensive First-Line AIDS Drug," October 8, 2009, available at http://www.businesswire.com/news/home/20091008006257/en/Pfizer's-Selzentry-Poised-Expensive-First-Line-AIDS-Drug, accessed January 24, 2014.

78. Ibid.

79. Ibid.

80. Daniel Kuritzkes, Santwana Kar, and Peter Kirkpatrick, "Maraviroc," *Nature Reviews: Drug Discovery* 7, no. 1 (2008): 15–16.

81. "Pfizer News: Selzentry Named 'Best Pharmaceutical Agent' at Prix Galien USA 2008 Awards," September 25, 2008, available at http://www.natap.org/2008/newsUpdates/092708_01.htm, accessed January 24, 2014.

82. Alex Shimmings, "2008 Scrip Awards Celebrate Industry's Achievement," December 11, 2008, available at http://www.scripintelligence.com/home/2008-Scrip-Awards-celebrate-industrys-achievements-22020, accessed January 21, 2014.

83. "The Story of Selzentry," 2010, available at http://www.innovation.org/index.cfm/Storiesofinnovation/InnovatorStories/The_Story_of_Selzentry, accessed January 24, 2014.

84. "FDA Panel OKs Pfizer's Selzentry for Broader Us [sic] in HIV Naive Patients but Drug Criticized for Cost," 2010, available at http://www.thepharmaletter.com/article/fda-panel-oks-pfizer-s-selzentry-for-broader-us-in-hiv-naive-patients-but-drug-criticized-for-its-cost. See also http://www.datamonitor.com/store/News/icaac_2010_dominance_of_cross_class_combinations_intensifies_challenges_for_standalone_drugs_in_hiv?productid=B0C029C5-9382-45BF-AD0A-D5B07BD43C7E, both accessed January 24, 2014.

85. See http://www.gsk.com/investors/quarterly-results.html, accessed January 24, 2014.

86. http://www.selzentry.com/patient-assistance.html, accessed January 24, 2014.

87. For a good summary of HIV-1 tropism, see McGowan and Shah, "Understanding HIV Tropism."

88. Ibid.

89. Berger, Murphy, Farber, et al., "Chemokine Receptors," 658; McGowan and Shah, "Understanding HIV Tropism."

90. Edward A. Berger, Robert W. Doms, E.-M. Fenyö, et al., "A New Classification for HIV-1," *Nature* 391 no. 6664 (1998): 240; Gabriella Scarlatti, Eleonora Tresoldi, Asa Björndal, et al., "In Vivo Evolution of HIV-1 Co-receptor Usage and Sensitivity to Chemokine-Mediated Suppression," *Nature Medicine* 3, no. 11 (1997): 1259–1265; Raj Shankarappa, Joseph B. Margolick, Stephen J. Gange, et al., "Consistent Viral Evolutionary Changes Associated with the Progression of Human Immunodeficiency Virus Type 1 Infection," *Journal of Virology* 73, no. 12 (1999): 10489–10502; Svetlana Glushakova, Yanjie Yi, Jean-Charles Grivel, et al., "Preferential Coreceptor Utilization and Cytopathicity by Dual-Tropic HIV-1 in Human Lymphoid Tissue ex Vivo," *Journal of Clinical Investigations* 104, no. 5 (1999): R7-R11; Ruth I. Connor, Kristine E. Sheridan, Daniel Ceradini, et al., "Change in Coreceptor Use Correlates with Disease Progression in HIV-1–Infected Individuals," *Journal of Experimental Medicine* 185, no. 4 (1997): 621–628; McGowan and Shah, "Understanding HIV Tropism."

91. Bonnie Goldman, "A New Way to Fight HIV: CCR5 Inhibitors. An Interview with David Hardy, M.D.," in *The Body: The Complete HIV/AIDS Resource*, April 30, 2008, available at http://www.thebody.com/content/art46473.html, accessed January 20, 2014. See also Hetty Blaak, Angélique B. van't Wout, Margreet Brouwer, et al., "*In vivo* HIV-1 infection of CD45RA+ CD4+ T cells Is Established Primarily by Syncytium-Inducing Variants and Correlates with the Rate of CD4+ T Cell Decline," *Proceedings of the National Academy of Sciences (PNAS) USA* 97, no. 3 (2000): 1269–1274; José A. Esté, Cecilia Cabrera, Julià Blanco, et al., "Shift of Clinical Human Immunodeficiency Virus Type 1 Isolates from X4 to R5 and Prevention of Emergence of the Syncytium-Inducing Phenotype by Blockade of CXCR4," *Journal of Virology* 73, no. 7 (1999): 5577–5585; A. Giovannetti, F. Ensoli, F. Mazzetti, et al., "CCR5 and CXCR4 Chemokine Receptor Expression and β-Chemokine Production during Early T Cell Repopulation Induced by Highly Active Anti-retroviral Therapy," *Clinical Experimental Immunology* 118, no. 1 (1999): 87–94.

92. McGowan and Shah, "Understanding HIV Tropism." This was confirmed during my telephone interview with Don Littmann of New York University School of Medicine, March 1, 2013.

93. McGowan and Shah, "Understanding HIV Tropism." See also Glushakova, "Preferential Coreceptor Utilization," R7-R11; Shankarappa, Margolick, Gange, et al., "Consistent Viral Evolutionary," 10489–10502.

94. Sean Philpott, Barbara Weiser, Kathryn Anastos, et al., "Preferential Suppression of CXCR4-Specific Strains of HIV-1 by Antiviral Therapy," *Journal of Clinical Investigations* 107, no. 4 (2001): 431–437; Ozlem Equils, Eileen Garratty, Lian S. Wei, et al., "Recovery of Replication-Competent Virus from CD4 T Cell Reservoirs and Change in Coreceptor Use in Human Immunodeficiency Virus Type 1-Infected Children Responding to Highly Active Antiretroviral Therapy," *Journal of Infectious Diseases* 182, no. 3 (2000): 751–757; Katharina Skrabal, Virginie Trouplin, Béatrice Labrosse, et al., "Impact of Antiretroviral Treatment on the Tropism of HIV-1 Plasma Virus Populations," *AIDS* 17, no. 6 (2003): 809–814.

95. Harold Burger and Donald Hoover, "HIV-1 Tropism, Disease Progression, and Clinical Management," *Journal of Infectious Diseases* 198, no. 8 (2008): 1095–1097.

96. McGowan and Shah, "Understanding HIV Tropism."

97. Nina H. Lin and Daniel R. Kuritzkes, "Tropism Testing in the Clinical Management of HIV-1 Infection," *Current Opinions in HIV and AIDS* 4, no. 6 (2009): 481–487.

98. Jeannette M. Whitcomb, Wei Huang, Signe Fransen, et al., "Development and Characterization of a Novel Single-Cycle Recombinant-Virus Assay to Determine Human Immunodeficiency Virus Receptor Tropism," *Antimicrobial Agents Chemotherapy* 51, no. 2 (2007): 566–575.

99. "Euroscreen CCR5 Agonist Program Available for Out-Licensing," available at http://www.euroscreen.com/index.php/Euroscreen-News/Euroscreen-CCR5-Agonist -program-available-for-out-licensing.html, accessed January 24, 2014.

100. http://www.healthresearch.org/about-us, accessed 24 January 24, 2014.

101. Eric L. Delwart, Eugene G. Shpaer, Joost Louwagie, et al., "Genetic Relationships Determined by a DNA Heteroduplex Mobility Assay: Analysis of HIV-1 *env* Genes," *Science* 262, no. 5137 (1993): 1257–1261; Eric L. Delwart, Haynes W. Sheppard, Bruce D. Walker, et al., "Human Immunodeficiency Virus Type 1 in Vivo Tracked by DNA Heteroduplex Mobility Assays," *Journal of Virology* 68, no. 10 (1994): 6672–6683.

102. Lin and Kuritzkes, "Tropism Testing," 481–487.

103. Sean Philpott, Barbara Weiser, Harold Burger, et al., "Analysis of HIV-1 Coreceptor Use in the Clinical Care of HIV-1-Infected Patients," U.S. Patent 7,943,297, awarded May 17, 2011, available at http://patents.com/us-7943297.html, accessed January 21, 2014; Sean Philpott, Barbara Weiser, and Harold Burger, "Heteroduplex Tracking Assay," U.S. Patent 7,344,830, awarded March 18, 2008, available at http:// www.google.com/patents/us7344830, accessed January 21, 2014; Sean Philpott,

Barbara Weiser, Harold Burger, et al., "Heteroduplex Tracking Assay Description/ Claims," USPTO Patent Application 20100323341, 2010, available at http://www .freshpatents.com/-dt20101223ptan20100323341.php, accessed January 21, 2014. See also Barbara Weiser, "HIV-1 Receptor Usage and CXCR4-Specific Viral Load Predict Clinical Disease Progression during Combination Antiretroviral Therapy," in *AIDS* 22, no. 4 (2008): 469–479.

104. http://www.thefreelibrary.com/Pathway+Diagnostics+Announces+Patent+Issu ance+for+the+Diagnostic...-a0171417265, accessed January 24, 2014.

105. http://ir.questdiagnostics.com/phoenix.zhtml?c=82068&p=irol-newsArticle &ID=1068390&highlight=, accessed January 24, 2014.

106. Lin and Kuritzke, "Tropism Testing," 481–487.

107. "The Age of AIDS," 2006. See http://www.pbs.org/wgbh/pages/frontline/aids/, accessed January 24, 2014; Matt Mason, *The Pirate's Dilemma: How Youth Is Reinventing Capitalism* (New York: Free Press, 2009), 61–67; http://www.avert.org/generic.htm, accessed January 24, 2014.

108. "Pfizer Gets Patent for New HIV/AIDS Drug in India, Report Says," in *The Body: The Complete HIV/AIDS Resource*, December 11, 2007, available at http://www .thebody.com/content//art44331.html?ts=pf, accessed January 24, 2014.

109. Ibid.

110. "Indian Drugmaker Seeks to Make, Sell Generic Version of Pfizer's Drug," *The Body: The Complete HIV/AIDS Resource*, January 5, 2011, available at http://www .thebody.com/content/art60077.html/ts=pf, accessed January 24, 2014.

111. "ViiV Healthcare Questions Natco's Ability to Make and Sell Selzentry in India; Stays Silent on Voluntary License Issue," in *Pharmasia News*, June 2, 2011, available at http://www.elsevierbi.com/publications/pharmasia-news/2011/6/2/viiv -healthcare-questions-natcos-ability-to-make-and-sell-selzentry-in-india-stays-silent -on-voluntary, accessed January 24, 2014.

112. Khoma Singh, "Natco Seeks Pfizer Nod for Drug Clone," *Economic Times*, January 5, 2011, available at http://articles.economictimes.indiatimes.com/2011-01-05/ news/28426847_1_natco-pharma-pfizer-hiv-patients, accessed January 21, 2014.

113. Rumman Ahmed, "Update: Natco Pharma Seeks 'Compulsory License' for Copy of Pfizer Drug," January 5, 2011, available at http://in.advfn.com/news_UPDATE -Natco-Pharma-Seeks-Compulsory-License-For-Copy-Of-Pfizer-Drug_45882508.html http://online.wsj.com/article/BT-CO-20110105-703261.htmlUPDATE, accessed January 20, 2014.

114. Singh, "Natco Seeks Pfizer."

115. Ibid.

116. Ibid.

117. Eric Palmer, "Natco May Attack Pfizer, Roche Drugs with Compulsory License," *Fierce Pharma*, July 20, 2012, available at http://www.fiercepharma.com/story/natco -may-next-attack-pfizer-roche-drugs-compulsory-license/2012-07-20, accessed January 21, 2014.

118. Editorial Board of the New York Times, April 4, 2013, available at http://www .nytimes.com/2013/04/05/opinion/the-supreme-court-in-india-clarifies-law-in -novartis-decision.html?_r=0, accessed January 24, 2014.

119. Marcia Angell, *The Truth about Drug Companies: How They Deceive Us and What to Do about It* (New York: Random House, 2005).

Chapter 7

1. An allele is one of two or more alternate forms of a gene that are located at the same site on a chromosome. Genes can have many different alleles. A mutation is a change in the DNA sequence of an allele, which may or may not change the protein sequence for which it codes. Scientists refer to *Δ32* as both a mutation and an allele.

2. Yunzhen Cao, Limo Qin, Linqi Zhang, et al., "Virologic and Immunologic Characterization of Long-Term Survivors of Human Immunodeficiency Virus Type 1 Infection," *New England Journal of Medicine* 332, no. 4 (1995): 201–208; Giuseppe Pantaleo, Stefano Menzo, Mauro Vaccarezza, et al., "Studies in Subjects with Long-Term Nonprogressive Human Immunodeficiency Virus Infection," *New England Journal of Medicine* 332, no. 4 (1995): 209–216. Earlier studies detailed very high-risk male subjects who were seronegative despite exposure to HIV-1. See, for example, David T. Imagawa, Moon H. Lee, Steven M. Wolinsky, et al., "Human Immunodeficiency Virus Type 1 in Homosexual Men Who Remain Seronegative for Prolonged Periods," *New England Journal of Medicine* 320, no. 22 (1989): 1458–1462 and 321, no. 24 (1989): 1681; David T. Imagawa and R. Detels, "HIV-1 in Seronegative Homosexual Men," *New England Journal of Medicine* 325, no. 17 (1991): 1250–1251; S. Rowland-Jones, J. Sutton, K. Ariyoshi, et al., "HIV-Specific Cytotoxic T-Cells in HIV-Exposed but Infected Gambian Women," *Nature Medicine* 9, no. 1 (1995): 59–64; P. Langlade-Demoyen, N. Ngo-Giang-Huong, F. Ferchal, et al., "Human Immunodeficiency Virus (HIV) Nef-Specific Cytotoxic T Lymphocytes in Noninfected Heterosexual Contact of HIV-Infected Patients," *Journal of Clinical Investigations* 93, no. 3 (1994): 1293–1297; Mario Clerici, J. V. Giorgi, C. C. Chou, et al., "Cell-Mediated Immune Response to Human Immunodeficiency Virus (HIV) Type 1 in Seronegative Homosexual Men with Recent Sexual Exposure to HIV-1," *Journal of Infectious Diseases* 165, no. 6 (1992): 1012–1019.

3. Pantaleo, Menzo, Vaccarezza, et al., "Studies in Subjects," 213–214; Cao, Qin, Zhang, et al., "Virologic and Immunologic Characterization," 201.

4. William A. Paxton, Scott R. Martin, Doris Tse, et al., "Relative Resistance to HIV-1 Infection of CD4 Lymphocytes from Persons Who Remain Uninfected Despite Multiple High-Risk Sexual Exposures," *Nature Medicine* 2, no. 4 (1996): 412–417.

5. Pantaleo, Menzo, Vaccarezza, et al., "Studies in Subjects," 209.

6. Stephen J. O'Brien and Michael Dean, "In Search of AIDS-Resistance Genes," *Scientific American* (September 1997), available at http://www.ncoic.com/0997obrien.html, accessed January 21, 2014.

7. Ibid.

8. See Richard A. Kaslow, "The Multicenter AIDS Cohort Study: Rationale, Organization, and Selected Characteristics of the Participants," *American Journal of Epidemiology* 126, no. 2 (1986): 310–318. Although only men were initially studied, women were subsequently included.

9. O'Brien and Dean, "In Search of AIDS-Resistance Genes."

10. Radetsky, "Immune to a Plague."

11. Alkhatib, Combadiere, Feng, et al., "CC CKR5," 1955–1958; Choe, Farzan, Sun, et al., "The β-Chemokine Receptors," 1135–1148; Feng, Broder, Kennedy, et al., "HIV-1 Entry Cofactor," 872–877; Dragic, Litwin, Allaway, et al., "HIV-1 Entry," 667-673; Doranz, Rucker, Jirik, et al., "A Dual-Tropic," 1149–1158.

12. Paxton was the second author, Koup the ninth author, and Landau the tenth and final author of Liu, Paxton, Choe, et al., "Homozygous Defect," 367–377.

13. Ibid, 370–371.

14. Ibid., 368–369. Liu referred to CCR5 as CKR-5.

15. Ibid., 372.

16. Ibid.

17. Ibid., 372.

18. Samson, Libert, Doranz, et al., "Resistance to HIV-1 Infection," 722–725.

19. Ibid., 722.

20. O'Brien and Dean, "In Search of AIDS-Resistance Genes."

21. Ibid.

22. They included the Hemophilia Growth and Development Study, Multicenter Hemophilia Cohort Study, D.C. Gay Cohort Study, Multicenter AIDS Cohort Study, San Francisco City Clinic Cohort, and the AIDS Link to the Intravenous Experience.

23. Dean, Carrington, Winkler, et al., "Genetic Restriction," 1858.

24. Ibid., 1859.

25. Ibid., 1861.

26. Yaoxing Huang, William A. Paxton, Steven M. Wolinsky, et al., "The Role of Mutant *CCR5* Allele in HIV-1 Transmission and Disease Progression," *Nature Medicine* 2, no. 11 (1996): 1240–1243, here 1241.

27. Ibid.

28. P. A. Zimmerman, A. Buckler-White, G. Alkhatib, et al., "Inherited Resistance to HIV-1 Conferred by an Inactivating Mutation in CC Chemokine Receptor 5: Studies in Populations with Contrasting Clinical Phenotypes, Defined Racial Background, and Quantified Risk," *Molecular Medicine* 3, no. 1 (1997): 23–36, here 25.

29. Ibid., 25.

30. Ibid., 31.

31. Jeremy J. Martinson, Nicola H. Chapman, David C. Rees, et al., "Global Distribution of the *CCR5* Gene 32-Basepair Deletion," *Nature Genetics* 16, no. 1 (1997): 100–103, here 100. See also Liu, Paxton, Choe, et al., "Homozygous Defect," 367–377; Samson, Liebert, Doranz, et al., "Resistance to HIV-1 Infection," 722–725; and Dean, Carrington, Winkler, et al., "Genetic Restriction of HIV-1 Infection," 1856–1862.

32. Martinson, Chapman, Rees, et al., "Global Distribution of the *CCR5* Gene," 100.

33. For example, see Christina Christodoulou, Marios Poullikas, Avidan U. Neumann, et al., "Low Frequency of *CCR5Δ32* Allele among Greeks in Cyprus," *AIDS Research and Human Retroviruses* 13, no. 16 (1997): 1373–1374; G. Nasioulas, M. Dean, E. Koumbarelis, et al., "Allele Frequency of the CCR5 Mutant Chemokine Receptor in Greek Caucasians," *Journal of Acquired Immune Deficiency Syndromes and Human Retrovirology* 17, no. 2 (1998): 181–182; C. Li, Y. P. Yan, B. Shieh, et al., "Frequency of the *CCR5 Delta 32* Mutant Allele in HIV-1-Positive Patients, Female Sex Workers, and a Normal Population in Taiwan," *Journal of the Formosa Medical Association* 96, no. 12 (1997): 979–984; Martinson, Chapman, Rees, et al., "Global Distribution of the *CCR5* Gene," 100–103; Magda Magierowska, Virginia Lepage, Ludmila Boubnova, et al., "Distribution of the *CCR5* Gene 32 Base Pair Deletion and *SDF1-3'A* Variant in Healthy Individuals from Different Populations," *Immunogenetics* 48, no. 6 (1998): 417–419; Gérard Lucotte and Géraldine Mercier, "Distribution of the *CCR5* Gene 32-bp Deletion in Europe," *Journal of Acquired Immune Deficiency Syndromes and Human Retrovirology* 19 (1998): 174–177; Gérard Lucotte and Géraldine Mercier, "*Δ32* Mutation Frequencies of the CCR5 Coreceptor in Different French Regions," *Comptes rendus de l'Academie des Sciences, Series III, Sciences de la Vie* 321, no. 5 (1998): 409–413; Rita Zamarchi, Stefano Indraccolo, Sonia Minuzzo, et al., "Frequency of a Mutated CCR-5 Allele (*Δ32*) among Italian Healthy Donors and Individuals at Risk of Parenteral HIV Infection," *AIDS Research and Human Retroviruses* 15, no. 4 (1999): 337–344; R. Kantor and J. M. Gershoni, "Distribution of the

CCR5 Gene 32-Base Pair Deletion in Israeli Ethnic Groups," *Journal of Acquired Immune Deficiency Syndromes and Human Retrovirology* 20, no. 1 (1999): 81–84; Frank Struyf, "Prevalence of CCR5 and CCR2 HIV-Coreceptor Gene Polymorphisms in Belgium," *Human Heredity* 50, no. 5 (2000): 304–307; Elmir Elharti, R. Elaouad, M. J. Simons, et al., "Letter to the Editor: Frequency of the CCR5Δ32 Allele in the Moroccan Population," *AIDS Research and Human Retroviruses* 16, no. 1 (2000): 87–89; Carolyn Williamson, S. A. Loubser, B. Brice, et al., "Allelic Frequencies of Host Genetic Variants Influencing Susceptibility to HIV-1 Infection and Disease in South African Populations," *AIDS* 14, no. 4 (2000): 449–451; I. Kalev, A.-V. Mikelsaar, L. Beckman, et al., "High Frequency of the HIV-1 Protective CCR5Δ32 Deletion in Native Estonians," *European Journal of Epidemiology* 16 (2000): 1107–1109; William Klitz, Chaim Brautbar, Anna M. Schito, et al., "Evolution of the CCR5 Δ32 Mutation Based on Haplotype Variation in Jewish and Northern European Population Samples," *Human Immunology* 62, no. 5 (2001): 530–538; F. Wang and D. Liu, "Polymorphism of Human Alleles Associated with Genetic Resistance Against HIV-1 Infection and Its Implications," *Zhonghua Yi Xue Yi Chuan Xue Za Zhi* 17, no. 4 (2000): 285–287; Claude Desgranges, Patricia Carvajal, Alejandro Afani, et al., "Frequency of CCR5 Gene 32-Basepair Deletion in Chilean HIV-1 Infected and Non-infected Individuals," *Immunology Letters* 76, no. 2 (2001): 115–117; Gérard Lucotte, "Frequencies of 32 Base Pair Deletion of the (Δ32) Allele of the CCR5 HIV-1 Co-receptor Gene in Caucasians: A Comparative Analysis," *Infection, Genetics and Evolution* 1, no. 3 (2002): 201–205; G. Lucotte and P. Smets, "CCR5-Δ32 Allele Frequencies in Ashkenazi Jews," *Genetic Testing* 7, no. 4 (2003): 333–337; John Novembre, Alison P. Galvani, and Montgomery Slatkin, "The Geographic Spread of the CCR5 Δ32 HIV-Resistance Allele," *PLoS Biology* 3, no. 11 (2005): 1954–1562; S. M. Muxel, S. D. Borelli, M. K. Amarante, et al., "Association Study of CCR5 Δ32 Polymorphism among the HLA-DRB1 Caucasian Population in Northern Paraná, Brazil," *Journal of Clinical Laboratory Analysis* 22, no. 4 (2008): 229–233; H. Liu, E. E. Nakayama, I. Theodorou, et al., "Polymorphisms in CCR5 Chemokine Receptor Gene in Japan," *International Journal of Immunogenetics* 34, no. 5 (2007): 325–335; Tamira Freitas, António Brehm, and Teresa Fernandes, "Frequency of the CCR5-Δ32 Mutation in the Atlantic Island Populations of Madeira, the Azores, Cabo Verde, and Sao Tomé e Príncipe," *Human Biology* 78, no. 6 (2006): 697–703; A. E. Vargas, A. R. Marrero, F. M. Salzano, et al., "Frequency of CCR5Δ32 in Brazilian Populations," *Brazilian Journal of Medical and Biological Research* 39, no. 3 (2006): 321–325; S. A. Apriatin, E. R. Rakhmanaliev, I. A. Nikolaeva, et al., "Comparison [of] CCR5del32 Mutation[s] in the CCR5 Gene Frequencies in Russians, Tuvinians, and in Different Groups of HIV-Infected Individuals," *Genetika* 41 (2005): 1559–1562; Liying Ma, Michael Marmor, Ping Zhong, et al., "Distribution of CCR2-64I and SDF1-3'A Alleles and HIV Status in Seven Ethnic Populations of Cameroon," *Journal of Acquired Immune Deficiency Syndromes and Human Retrovirology* 40, no. 1 (2005): 89–95; C. Li, S. C. Lu, P. S. Hsieh, et al., "Distribution of Human Chemokine (C-X3-C) Receptor 1 (CX3CR1) Gene Polymorphisms and Haplotypes of the CC Chemokine Receptor 5 (CCR5) Promoter in

Chinese People, and the Effects of CCR5 Haplotypes on CCR5 Expression," *International Journal of Immunogenetics* 32, no. 2 (2005): 99–106; Fernanda Andreza de Pinho Lott Carvalhaes, Greice Lemos Cardoso, Igor Guerreiro Hamoy, et al., "Distribution of *CCR5-Δ32, CCR2-64I*, and *SDF1-3'A* Mutations in Populations from the Brazilian Amazon Region," *Human Biology* 76, no. 4 (2004): 643–646; Tao Feng, Anping Ni, Guocui Yang, et al., "Distribution of the *CCR5* Gene 32-Base Pair Deletion and CCR5 Expression in Chinese Minorities," *JAIDS: Journal of Acquired Immune Deficiency Syndromes* 32, no. 2 (2003): 131–134; A. Mangano, G. Theiler, L. Sala, et al., "Distribution of *CCR5-Δ32* and *CCR2-64I* Alleles in an Argentine Amerindian Population," *Tissue Antigen* 58, no. 2 (2001): 99–102; A. P. M. Leboute, M. W. P. de Carvalho, and A. L. Simoes, "Absence of the *Δccr5* Mutation in Indigenous Populations of the Brazilian Amazon," *Human Genetics* 105, no. 5 (1999): 442–443; Jian-Dong Jiang, Yue Wang, Z.-Z. Wang, et al., "Low Frequency of the *CCR5Δ32* HIV-resistance Allele in Mainland China: Identification of the First Case of *CCR5Δ32* Mutation in the Chinese Population," *Scandinavian Journal of Infectious Disease* 31, no. 4 (1999): 345–348; C. Szalai, A. Czinner, A. Császár, et al., "Frequency of the HIV-1 Resistance *CCR5* Deletion Allele in Hungarian Newborns," *European Journal of Pediatrics* 157, no. 9 (1999): 782; G. Nasioulas, M. Dean, E. Koumbarelis, et al., "Allele Frequency of the CCR5 Mutant Chemokine Receptor in Greek Caucasians," *Journal of Acquired Immune Deficiency Syndromes and Human Retrovirology* 17, no. 2 (1998): 181–182; Sergi Veloso, Montserrat Olona, Felipe García, et al., "Effect of *TNF-α* Genetic Variants and *CCR5Δ32* on the Vulnerability to HIV-1 Infection and Disease Progression in Caucasian Spaniards," *BMC Medical Genetics* 11 (2010): 63–73; A. Sidoti, R. D'Angelo, C. Rinaldi, et al., "Distribution of the Mutated Delta 32 Allele of the *CCR5* Gene in a Sicilian Population," *International Journal of Immunogenetics* 32, no. 3 (2005): 193–198; N. Degerli, E. Yilmaz, F. Bardakci, et al., "The *Δ32* Allele Distribution of the *CCR5* Gene and Its Relationship with Certain Cancers in a Turkish Population," *Clinical Biochemistry* 28 (2005): 248–252; Abdel-Halim Salem and Mark A. Batzer, "Distribution of the HIV Resistance *CCR5-Δ32* Allele among Egyptians and Syrians," *Mutation Research/Fundamental and Molecular Mechanisms of Mutagenesis* 616, nos. 1–2 (2007): 175–180.

34. Frédérick Libert, Pascale Cochaux, Gunhild Beckman, et al., "The *Δccr5* Mutation Conferring Protection against HIV-1 in Caucasian Populations Has a Single and Recent Origin in Northeastern Europe," *Human Molecular Genetics* 7, no. 3 (1998): 399–406.

35. Jeremy J. Martinson, Lily Hong, Rose Karanicolas, et al., "Global Distribution of the *CCR2-64I/CCR5-59653T* HIV-1 Disease-Protective Haplotype," *AIDS* 14, no. 5 (2000): 483–489.

36. Stephens, Reich, Goldstein, et al., "Dating the Origin," 1507–1515.

37. See, for example, M. A. Ansari-Lari, X. M. Liu, M. L. Metzker, et al., "The Extent of Genetic Variation in the *CCR5* Gene," *Nature Genetics* 16, no. 3 (1997): 221–222.

38. Ibid., 221.

39. Ibid., 222.

40. Mary Carrington, Terri Kissner, Bernard Gerrard, et al., "Novel Alleles of the Chemokine-Receptor Gene *CCR5*," *American Journal of Human Genetics* 61, no. 6 (1997): 1261–1267.

41. Ibid., 1262. They noted that one novel mutation was found in a Hispanic but did not state how many Hispanic subjects were studied. See 1262 and 1264.

42. Ibid., 1262.

43. Enrique Gonzalez, Michael Bamshad, Naoko Sato, et al., "Race-Specific HIV-1 Disease-Modifying Effects Associated with *CCR5* Haplotypes," *Proceedings of the National Academy of Sciences (PNAS) USA* 96, no. 21 (1999): 12004–12009.

44. Enrique Gonzalez, Rahul Dhanda, Mike Bamshad, et al., "Global Survey of Genetic Variation in *CCR5*, *RANTES*, and *MIP-1α*: Impact on the Epidemiology of the HIV-1 Pandemic," *Proceedings of the National Academy of Sciences (PNAS) USA* 98, no. 9 (2001): 5199–5204, here 5202.

45. Jianming Tang, Brent Sheldon, Nina J. Makhatadze, et al., "Distribution of Chemokine Receptor *CCR2* and *CCR5* Genotypes and Their Relative Contribution to Human Immunodeficiency Virus Type 1 (HIV-1) Seroconversion, Early HIV-1 RNA Concentration in Plasma, and Later Disease Progression," *Journal of Virology* 76, no. 2 (2002): 662–672, here 662. See also Srinivas Mummidi, Mike Bamshad, Seema S. Ahuja, et al., "Evolution of Human and Non-human Primate CC Chemokine Receptor 5 Gene and mRNA: Potential Roles for Haplotype and mRNA Diversity, Differential Haplotype-Specific Transcriptional Activity, and Altered Transcription Factor Binding to Polymorphic Nucleotides in the Pathogenesis of HIV-1 and Simian Immunodeficiency Virus," *Journal of Biological Chemistry* 275, no. 25 (2000): 18,946–18,961.

46. Gonzalez, Bamshad, Sato, et al., "Race-Specific HIV-1," 12008. On *CCR2* and *CCR5* variants and disease progressions, see Michael W. Smith, Michael Dean, Mary Carrington, et al., "Contrasting Genetic Influence of *CCR2* and *CCR5* Variants on HIV-1 Infection and Disease Progression," *Science* 277, no. 5328 (1997): 959–965.

47. Gonzalez, Bamshad, Sato, et al., "Race-Specific HIV-1," 12,005.

48. See, for example, Gonzalez, Dhanda, Bamshad, et al., "Global Survey," 5199 –5204.

49. Williamson, Loubser, Brice, et al., "Allelic Frequencies of Host Genetic Variants Influencing Susceptibility to HIV-1 Infection," 450. They reported the frequency for Caucasians to be 9.8% on 449, but that is a typo: 1 homozygote + 25 heterozygotes out of 144 = $(1 \times 2 + 25 \times 1)/(144 \times 2) = 9.4\%$.

50. Ibid., 450. Again, there is a typo on 449. In the results, they argue that the allele frequency is 19.8% among Caucasians, whereas they later show it to be 20.3%: 2 homozygotes and 55 heterozygotes = $(2 \times 2 + 55 \times 1)/(145 \times 2) = 20.3\%$.

51. Cecile Masquelier, Jean-Yves Servais, Emmanuel Rusanganwa, et al., "A Novel 24-Base Pair Deletion in the Coding Region of *CCR5* in African Population," *AIDS* 21, no. 1 (2007): 111–113.

52. Desiree C. Petersen, Maritha J. Kotze, Michele D. Zeier, et al., "Novel Mutations Identified Using a Comprehensive *CCR5*-Denaturing Gradient Gel Electrophoresis Assay," *AIDS* 15, no. 2 (2001): 171–177, here 175. "Coloured" was defined as individuals of mixed ancestral descent (including Khoi, San, African Negro, Madagascan, Javanese, and European origin); "South African Africans" referred to South Africans of central African descent; and "South African Caucasians" referred to South Africans of European descent (mainly of Dutch, French, German, and British origin) (172).

53. Ibid., 176. The biomedical researchers stressed that only the nine original subjects of the study plus an additional twenty-eight Caucasians were tested (174).

54. Anabela C. P. Picton, Maria Paximadis, and Caroline T. Tiemessen, "Genetic Variation within the Gene Encoding the HIV-1 CCR5 Coreceptor in Two South African Populations," *Infection, Genetics and Evolution* 10, no. 4 (2010): 487–494, here 489; Petersen, Kotze, Zeier, et al., "Novel Mutations," 174; Fernando Arenzana-Seisdedos and Marc Parmentier, "Genetics of Resistance to HIV Infection: Role of Co-receptors and Co-receptor Ligands," *Seminars in Immunology* 18, no. 6 (2006): 387–403, here 391.

55. Picton, Paximadis, and Tiemeseen, "Genetic Variation within the Gene," 489.

56. Biehuoy, Shieh, Yao-Pei Yan, Nai-Ling Ko, et al., "Detection of Elevated Serum ß-Chemokine Levels in Seronegative Chinese Individuals Exposed to Human Immunodeficiency Virus Type 1," *Clinical Infectious Diseases* 33, no. 3 (2001): 273–279, here 273.

57. Jiang, Wang, Wang, et al., "Low Frequency of the *CCR5Δ32*," 345. Some still argued in 2004 that the mutation had not been found among Han Chinese. Cheryl Winkler, Ping An, and Stephen J. O'Brien, "Patterns of Ethnic Diversity among the Genes That Influence AIDS," *Human Molecular Genetics* 13, supp. 1 (2004): R9–R19, here R13.

58. F. Wang, L. Jin, Z. Lei, et al., "Genotypes and Polymorphisms of Mutant *CCR5-Delta 32, CCR2-64I*, and *SDF1-3'A* HIV-1 Resistance Alleles in Indigenous Han Chinese," *Chinese Medical Journal* 114, no. 11 (2001): 1162–1166.

59. Tao Feng, Anping Ni, Guocui Yang, et al., "Distribution of the *CCR5* Gene 32-Base Pair Deletion and CCR5 Expression in Chinese Minorities," *Journal of Acquired Immune Deficiency Syndromes* 32, no. 2 (2003): 131–134.

60. Srinivas Mummidi, Seema S. Ahuja, Enrique Gonzalez, et al., "Genealogy of the *CCR5* Locus and Chemokine System Gene Variants Associated with Altered Rates of HIV-1 Disease Progression," *Nature Medicine* 4, no. 7 (1998): 786–793. See also M. V. Downer, T. Dodge, D. K. Smith, et al. "Regional Variation in the *CCR5-Δ32* Distribution among Women from the US HIV Epidemiology Research (HERS)," *Genes and Immunology* 3, no. 5 (2002): 295–298.

61. Maureen P. Martin, Michael Dean, Michael W. Smith, et al. "Genetic Acceleration of AIDS Progression by a Promoter Variant of *CCR5*," *Science* 282, no. 5395 (1998): 1907–1911; An Ping, Maureen P. Martin, Mary Carrington, et al. "Influence of *CCR5* Promoter Haplotypes on AIDS Progression in African-Americans," *AIDS* 14, no. 14 (2000): 2117–2122; Winkler, An, O'Brien, et al., "Patterns of Ethnic Diversity," R15.

62. Ping, Nelson, Carrington, et al., "Influence of *CCR5* Promoter,": 2117.

63. Li, Lu, Hsieh, et al., "Distribution of Human Chemokine," 105. Zhao's group found the *CCR5-Δ32* allele in the Chinese subjects that were studied but with a frequency of less than 0.1%. Xiu-Ying Zhao, Shui-Shan Lee, Ka-Hing Wong, et al., "Functional Analysis of Naturally Occurring Mutations in the Open Reading Frame of *CCR5* in HIV-Infected Chinese Patients and Healthy Controls," *Journal of Acquired Immune Deficiency Syndromes* 38, no. 5 (2005): 509–517, 511. See also Lidan Xu, Yuandong Qiao, Xuelong Zhang, et al., "A Haplotype in the *CCR5* Gene Promoter Was Associated with the Susceptibility to HIV-1 Infection in a Northern Chinese Population," *Molecular Biology Reports* 38 no. 1 (2011): 327–332.

64. Zhao, Lee, Wong, et al., "Functional Analysis," 509.

65. Xu, Qiao, Zhang, et al., "A Haplotype," 327.

66. Ibid.; Tatsuo Shioda, Emi E. Nakayama, Yuetsu Takana, et al., "Naturally Occurring Deletional Mutation in the C-terminal Cytoplasmic Tail of CCR5 Affects Surface Trafficking of CCR5," *Journal of Virology* 75, no. 7 (2001): 3462–3468, here 3462.

67. Kalev, Mikelsaar, Beckman, et al., "High Frequency," 1107.

68. Arenzana-Seisdedos and Parmentier, "Genetics of Resistance," 391.

69. Ibid. See also Martinson, Hong, Karanicolas, et al., "Global Distribution of the *CCR2-64I/CCR5-59653T*," 484. Martinson's figures are based on a subject population of 3,923 individuals worldwide. See 486. See also Kalev, Mikelsaar, Beckman, et al., "High Frequency," 1107. See also Pardis C. Sabeti, Emily Walsh, Steve F. Schaffner, et al., "The Case for Selection at *CCR5-Δ32*," *PLoS Biology* 3, no. 11 (2005): 1963–1969, here 1964.

70. James V. Neel, "Diabetes Mellitus: A 'Thrifty' Genotype Rendered Detrimental by 'Progress'?," *American Journal of Human Genetics* 14, no. 4 (1962): 353–362. For

other examples of positive selection of human genes, see Benjamin Voight, Sridhar Kudaravalli, Xiaoquan Wen, et al., "A Map of Recent Positive Selection in the Human Genome," *PLoS Biology* 4, no. 3 (2006): 446–458; Martin Kreitman and Anna Di Rienzo, "Balancing Claims for Balancing Selection," *Trends in Genetics* 20, no. 7 (2004): 300–304.

71. Eric de Silva and Michael P. H. Stumpf, "HIV and the *CCR5-Δ32* Resistance Allele," *FEMS Microbiology Letters* 241, no. 1 (2004): 1–12, here 2.

72. Goldstein and O'Brien used a Markov chain Monte Carlo framework expansion, a group of algorithms that is used in sampling probability distributions. A Markov chain is a mathematical system that randomly transitions between two finite states. It is used in statistical modeling. Stephens, Reich, Goldstein, et al., "Dating the Origin," 1508. Libert and his colleagues genotyped over 2,500 individuals from eighteen European populations confirming that the highest percentage of the *Δ32* allele is found in northeastern Europe. In addition, based on highly polymorphic microsatellites (or short tandem repeats of DNA that are often used as genetic markers) located on either side of the *CCR5* gene locus, the group concluded, unlike most at the time, that the *CCR5-Δ32* allele originated from a single mutation event that most likely occurred "a few thousand years ago in Northeastern Europe," most likely among "the Finno-Ugrian tribes of Russia." For the dating techniques, they used both the crossover recombination rates and the haplotype of two linked, highly polymorphic, microsatellites both upstream and downstream from *CCR5*. In both cases, they employed a Luria-Delbrück (or fluctuation) test. In 1943, Luria and Delbrück had shown that bacterial resistance to phage infection occurs spontaneously and is not induced by virus-bacterium interactions. Darwinian natural selection acting on random mutations could be applied to bacterial genetics. See http://vcp .med.harvard.edu/timeline/luria-delbruck.html, accessed January 25, 2014. Using crossover recombination rates, Libert's group calculated an age of about 3,500 years. Using the mutations of two microsatellites, they came up with 1,400 years and 2,250 years with a plausible range of 375 to 4,800 years. Libert, Cochaux, Beckman, et al., "The *Δccr5* Mutation," 399, 404. Martinson's group, however, in 1997 reckoned (unlike most) that the gene frequency found in Europe was consistent with the effects of genetic drift on a neutral polymorphism conferring neither an advantage nor disadvantage to the host. Martinson, Chapman, Rees, et al., "Global Distribution of the *CCR5* Gene 32-Basepair," 102.

73. Stephens, Reich, Goldstein, et al., "Dating the Origin," 1513.

74. Klitz, Brautbar, Schito, et al., "Evolution of the *CCR5 Δ32*," 530–538, here 535–536; S. Maayan, L. Zhang, E. Shinar, et al., "Evidence for Recent Selection of the *CCR5-Δ32* Deletion from Differences in Its Frequency between Ashkenazi and Sephardic Jews," *Genes and Immunity* 1 no. 6 (2000) 358–361.

75. Klitz, Brautbar, Schito, et al., "Evolution of the *CCR5 Δ32*," 532; Martinson, Hong, Karanicolas, et al., "Global Distribution of the *CCR2-64I/CCR5-59653T*," 485.

Earlier studies had the allele frequency among Ashkenazi Jews as high as 20.9%. See, for example, Martinson, Chapman, Rees, et al., "Global Distribution of the *CCR5* Gene," 100.

76. Klitz, Brautbar, Schito, et al., "Evolution of the *CCR5 Δ32* Mutation," 536.

77. Alshad S. Lalani, Jennefer Masters, Wei Zeng, et al. "Use of Chemokine Receptors by Poxviruses," *Science* 286, no. 5446 (1999): 1968–1971.

78. De Silva and Stumpf, "HIV and the *CCR5-Δ32*," 7. See also Andrea Carfí, Craig A. Smith, Pamela J. Smolak, et al., "Structure of a Soluble Secreted Chemokine Inhibitor vCCI (p35) from Cowpox Virus," *Proceedings of the National Academy of Sciences (PNAS) USA* 96, no. 22 (1999): 12,379–12,383.

79. Lucotte, "Frequencies of 32 Base Pair Deletion," 201–205.

80. Lucotte and Mercier, "Distribution of the *CCR5* Gene," 176–177.

81. Lucotte, "Frequencies of 32 Base Pair Deletion," 204.

82. Ibid.

83. Ibid., 204–205.

84. Gérard Lucotte and Florent Dieterlen, "More about the Viking Hypothesis of Origin of the *Δ32* Mutation in the *CCR5* Gene Conferring Resistance to HIV-1 Infection," *Infection, Genetics, and Evolution* 3, no. 4 (2003): 293–295, here 294.

85. Alison P. Galvani and Montgomery Slatkin, "Evaluating Plague and Smallpox as Historical Selective Pressures for the *CCR5-Δ32* HIV-Resistance Allele," *Proceedings of the National Academy of Sciences (PNAS) USA* 100, no. 25 (2003): 15,276–15,279.

86. Ibid., 15,276. The authors claimed that 15% to 20% of the European population, rather than London's population, had been killed. Also, estimates of Black Death mortality in Europe are usually 30% to 60%, and the plague was present in Marseilles from 1720 to 1721, not 1722.

87. Ibid.

88. Ibid.

89. Ibid., 15,277.

90. Ibid., 15,278.

91. Ibid.

92. Joan Mecsas, Greg Franklin, William A. Kuziel, et al., "Evolutionary Genetics: CCR5 Mutation and Plague Protection," *Nature* 427, no. 6975 (2004): 606. See also S. J. Elvin, E. D. Williamson, J. C. Scott, et al., "Evolutionary Genetics: Ambiguous Role of CCR5 in *Y. pestis* Infection," *Nature* 430, no. 6998 (2004): 417.

93. Mecsas, Franklin, Kuziel, et al., "Evolutionary Genetics," 606.

94. Stumpf and Wilkinson-Herbots, "Allelic Histories," 168.

95. Scott R. Duncan, S. Scott, and C. J. Duncan, "Reappraisal of the Historical Selective Pressures for the *CCR5-Δ32* Mutation," *Journal of Medical Genetics* 42, no. 3 (2005): 205–208.

96. S. R. Scott and C. J. Duncan, *Biology of Plagues: Evidence from Historical Populations* (Cambridge: Cambridge University Press, 2005).

97. Duncan, Scott, and Duncan, "Reappraisal," 205.

98. Ibid., 207.

99. Ibid.

100. Ibid., 205.

101. Ibid.

102. Ibid., 207. See S. Hummel, D. Schmidt, B. Kremeyer, et al., "Detection of the *CCR5-Δ32* HIV Resistance Gene in Bronze Age Skeletons," *Genes and Immunity* 6 (2005): 371–374.

103. Hummel, Schmidt, Kremeyer, et al., "Detection," 371–372.

104. Ibid., 373.

105. Ibid., 374.

106. Przemysław Zawicki and Henryk W. Witas, "HIV-1 Protecting *CCR5–Δ32* Allele in Medieval Poland," *Infection, Genetics, and Evolution* 8, no. 2 (2008): 146–151.

107. Novembre, Galvani, and Slatkin, "The Geographic Spread," 1554–1562.

108. Sabeti, Walsh, Schnaffer, et al., "The Case for Selection," 1963–1969.

109. Ibid, 1963.

110. Ibid., 1964, emphasis in the original.

111. Ibid.

112. Ibid.

113. Ibid., 1966.

114. "First Edition of the HapMap Released, a Catalogue of Human Genetic Variation," October 26, 2005, available at http://www.broadinstitute.org/news/258, accessed January 25, 2014.

115. Eric Faure and Manuela Royer-Carenzi, "Is the European Spatial Distribution of the HIV-1 Resistant *CCR5-Δ32* Allele Formed by a Breakdown of the Pathocenosis

Due to the Historical Roman Expansion?," *Infection, Genetics and Evolution* 8 (2008): 864–874.

116. Francis Alonzo III, Lina Kozhaya, Stephen A. Rawlings, et al., "CCR5 Is a Receptor for *Staphylococcus aureus* Leukotoxin ED," *Nature* 493, no. 7430 (2013): 51–55.

117. S. K. Cohn Jr. and L. T. Weaver, "The Black Death and AIDS: *CCR5–Δ32* in Genetics and History," *Quarterly Journal of Medicine* 99, no. 8 (2006): 497–503, here 501–502.

118. Faure and Royer-Carenzi, "Is the European," 871.

119. Philip W. Hedrick and Brian C. Verrelli, "'Ground Truth' for Selection on *CCR5-Δ32*," *Trends in Genetics* 22, no. 6 (2006): 293–296, here 294.

Chapter 8

1. Niall O'Dowd, "Harvard Professor Gates Is Half-Irish, Related to Cop Who Arrested Him," *ABC News*, July 28, 2009, available at http://abcnews.go.com/Politics/story?id=8195564#.T0AXL1F9m-8, accessed January 21, 2014. The charges were subsequently dropped.

2. https://www.23andme.com/reasons/3/, accessed January 25, 2014.

3. https://www.23andme.com/reasons/2/, accessed January 25, 2014.

4. https://www.23andme.com/ancestry/origins/, accessed January 25, 2014.

5. Ibid.

6. For the commercialization of genetic ancestral testing, see Henry T. Greely, "Genetic Genealogy: Genetics Meets the Marketplace," in *Revisiting Race in a Genomic Age*, ed. Barbara A. Koenig, Sandra Soo-Jin Lee, and Sarah S. Richardson, 215–234. New Brunswick, NJ: Rutgers University Press, 2008.

7. Rose, *The Politics of Life*, 185.

8. T. Grodzicker, J. Williams, P. Sharp, et al., "Physical Mapping of Temperature Sensitive Mutations," *Cold Spring Harbor Symposium Quarterly Biology* 39, no. 1 (1975): 439–446.

9. A. J. Jeffrey, "DNA Sequence Variants in the $^G\gamma$-, $^A\gamma$-, δ- and β-Globin Genes of Man," *Cell* 18, no. 1 (1979): 1–10.

10. D. Botstein, R. L. White, M. Skolnick, et al., "Construction of a Genetic Linkage Map in Man Using Restriction Fragment Length Polymorphisms," *American Journal of Human Genetics* 32 (1980): 314–331.

11. STPs are a type of microsatellite polymorphism consisting of two to six nucleotides that are repeated numerous times.

12. *Alu* insertion polymorphisms are a family of DNA repeats that are scattered throughout the genome that are mobilized by a few so-called master genes. See M. A. Batzer, "African Origin of Human-Specific Polymorphic *Alu* Insertions," *Proceedings of the National Academy of Sciences (PNAS) USA* 91, no. 25 (1994): 12,288–12,292; N. T. Perna, M. A. Batzer, P. L. Deininger, et al., "*Alu* Insertion Polymorphism: A New Type of Marker for Human Population Studies," *Human Biology* 64, no. 5 (1992): 641–648.

13. D. G. Wang, J. B. Fan, C. J. Siao, et al., "Large-Scale Identification, Mapping and Genotyping of Single-Nucleotide Polymorphisms in the Human Genome," *Science* 280, no. 5366 (1998): 1077–1082; Leonid Kruglyak, "The Use of a Genetic Map of Biallelic Markers in Linkage Studies," *Nature Genetics* 17, no. 1 (1997): 21–24; Kruglyak, "The Road," 316.

14. Gary H. Gibbons, Choong Chin Liew, Mark O. Goodarzi, et al., "Markers of Malign across the Cardiovascular Continuum: Interpretation and Application," *Circulation* 109 (2004): IV-47–IV-58.

15. Ibid., IV-47.

16. Ibid., IV-51.

17. J. L. Weber and P. E. May, "Abundant Class of Human DNA Polymorphisms Which Can Be Typed Using the Polymerase Chain Reaction," *American Journal of Human Genetics* 44, no. 3 (1989): 388–396; J. Weissenbach, G. Gyapay, A. Vignil, et al., "A Second-Generation Linkage Map of the Human Genome Project," *Nature* 359, no. 6398 (1992): 794–801; Kruglyak, "The Road," 316.

18. Ainsley Weston, James Ensey, Kathleen Kreiss, et al., "Racial Differences in Prevalence of a Supratypic HLA-Genetic Marker Immaterial to Pre-Employment Testing for Susceptibility to Chronic Beryllium Disease," *American Journal of Industrial Medicine* 41, no. 6 (2002): 457–465.

19. Duana Fullwiley, "The Biologistical Construction of Race: 'Admixture Technology' and the New Genetic Medicine," *Social Studies of Science* 38, no. 5 (2008): 695–735, here 714–715. For the original research, see Esteban González Burchard, E. K. Silverman, L. R. Rosenwasser, et al., "Association between a Sequence Variant in the IL-4 Gene Promoter and FEV_1 in Asthma," *American Journal of Respiratory and Critical Care Medicine* 160, no. 3 (1999): 919–922.

20. James F. Wilson, Michael E. Weale, Alice C. Smith, et al., "Population Genetic Structure of Variable Drug Response," *Nature Genetics* 29, no. 3 (2001): 265–269.

21. Michael Montoya, *Making the Mexican Diabetic: Race, Science, and the Genetics of Inequality* (Berkeley: University of California Press, 2011), 40–68.

22. Early in the millennium, most gene-testing companies used lineage-based tests, which focused on mitochrondrial DNA and the nonrecombining Y chromosome, to

search for SNPs and AIMs. More recently, genetic-testing companies (such as 23andMe and decODEme) rely more on autosomal marker-based tests. See Mark D. Shriver and Rick A. Kittles, "Genetic Ancestry and the Search for Personalized Genetic Histories," in *Revisiting Race in a Genomic Age*, ed. Barbara Koenig, Sandra Soo-Jin Lee, and Sarah S. Richardson, 201–214, here 202 (New Brunswick, NJ: Rutgers University Press, 2008). See also Greely, "Genetic Genealogy," 216–223; "Genotyping Technology of 23andMe.com," available at https://www.23andme.com/more/genotyping/, accessed January 25, 2014.

23. Steven Epstein, *Inclusion: The Politics of Difference in Medical Research* (Chicago: University of Chicago Press, 2007).

24. For a summary, see Joan H. Fujimura, Troy Duster, and Ramya Rajagopalan, "Race, Human Genomics, and Biomedicine," *Social Studies of Science* 38, no. 5 (2008): 643–656, here 643–644.

25. Biomedical researchers are not blind to these questions. See, for example, Michael J. Bamshad, Stephen Wooding, Benjamin A. Salisbury, et al., "Deconstructing the Relationship between Genetics and Race," *Nature Review-Genetics* 5, no. 8 (2004): 598–609. See also Fujimura, Duster, and Rajagopalan, "Race," 644.

26. Samuel Levy, Granger Sutton, Pauline C. Ng, et al., "The Diploid Genome Sequence of an Individual Human," *PLoS Biology* 5 no. 10 (2007): 2113–2144. In 2001, scientists had thought that the percentage was closer to 99.9%. See Morris W. Foster, "Integrating Ethics and Science in the International HapMap Project," *Nature Reviews: Genetics* 5, no. 6 (2004): 467–475.

27. Foster, "Integrating Ethics and Science," 467.

28. David R. Bentley and The International HapMap Consortium, "The International HapMap Project," *Nature* 426, no. 6968 (2003): 789–796, here 790.

29. Foster, "Integrating Ethics and Science," 467. See also David Secko, "Phase I of HapMap Complete," *News from The Scientist* 6 (October 26, 2005): 1026.

30. Although some archeologists claim that the migration occurred as long as 125,000 years ago, most archeologists and geneticists argue that the first successful migration out of Africa occurred about 60,000 years ago.

31. Genetic bottlenecking occurs when there is a substantial decrease in the size of a population due to a cataclysmic environmental mishap, such as an earthquake or volcanic eruption. This results in decreased variation in the population's gene pool.

32. The term *founder effects* refers to the lack of genetic variation that occurs when a new population is created by a number of individuals from another, larger population.

33. Foster, "Integrating Ethics and Science," 474.

34. "Developing a Haplotype Map of the Human Genome for Finding Genes Related to Health and Disease," July 18–19, 2001, available at http://www.genome.gov/10001665, accessed January 25, 2014.

35. David A. Altshuler and The International HapMap Consortium, "A Haplotype Map of the Human Genome," *Nature* 437, no. 7063 (2005): 1299–1320, here 1300. See also International HapMap Project, "What Is the HapMap?," available at http://hapmap.ncbi.nlm.nih.gov/whatishapmap.html.en, accessed January 25, 2014.

36. Bentley and The International HapMap Consortium, "The International HapMap Project," 789.

37. Ibid., 792.

38. Altshuler and The International HapMap Consortium, "A Haplotype Map," 1315.

39. Fuijumura, Duster, and Rajagopalan, "Race," 646.

40. Ibid., 646–647.

41. Bentley and the International HapMap Consortium, "The International HapMap Project," 792; Altshuler, and the International HapMap Consortium, "A Haplotype Map," 1299. The original number of individuals participating was 270, and phase 2 had 270 individuals sampled. In the end, Japan had one less participant in phase 1. See also Bentley and the International HapMap Consortium, "The International HapMap Project," 791; International HapMap Project, "Which Populations Are Being Sampled?," available at http://hapmap.ncbi.nlm.nih.gov/hapmappopulations.html.en, accessed January 25, 2014.

42. Altshuler and the International HapMap Consortium, "A Haplotype Map," 1303–1304.

43. Ibid., 1315.

44. Philippa Brice, "HapMap Project to Expand," *The Phg Foundation: Making Science Work for Health*, February 11, 2005, available at http://www.phgfoundation.org/news/833, accessed January 20, 2014.

45. Gilean McVean and the International HapMap Consortium, "A Second Generation Human Haplotype Map of Over 3.1 Million SNPs," *Nature* 449, no. 7164 (2007): 851–861, here 851.

46. Troy Duster, "Race and Reification in Science," *Science* 307, no. 5712 (2005): 1050–1051, here 1050.

47. Steven Epstein, "Bodily Differences and Collective Identities: The Politics of Gender and Race in Biomedical Research in the United States," *Body and Society* 10, no. 2–3 (2004): 183–203; Epstein, *Inclusion*, 10.

48. Troy Duster, "Theorizing a Difference: A Conceptual Advance," Books Forum: Differences That Matter, *BioSocieties* 3, pt. 2 (2007): 225–226, here 225.

49. Troy Duster, "Buried Alive: The Concept of Race in Science," in *Genetic Nature/ Culture. Anthropology and Science beyond the Two-Culture Divide*, ed. A. H. Goodman, Deborah Heath, and M. Susan Lindee, 257–278, here 265 (Berkeley: University of California Press, 1998), emphasis in the original.

50. Joan H. Fujimura and Ramya Rajagopalan, "Different Differences: The Uses of 'Genetic Ancestry' versus Race in Biomedical Human Genetic Research," *Social Studies of Science* 41, no. 1 (2011): 5–30, here 10. This point was also applicable to the Human Genome Diversity Project. See Jenny Reardon, *Race to the Finish: Identity and Governance in the Age of Genomics* (Princeton, NJ: Princeton University Press, 2005), 118–122.

51. See, for example, Annette Lareau, "Invisible Inequality: Social Class and Child-rearing in Black Families and White Families," *American Sociological Review* 67, no. 5 (2002): 747–776; G. D. Smith, "Individual Social Class, Area-Based Deprivation, Cardiovascular Disease Risk Factors, and Mortality: The Renfrew and Paisley Study," *Journal of Epidemiology and Community Health* 52, no. 6 (1998): 399–405; Marilyn A. Winkleby, S. P. Fortmann, and D. C. Barrett, "Social Class Disparities in Risk Factors for Disease: Eight-Year Prevalence Patterns by Level of Education," *Preventive Medicine* 19, no. 1 (1990): 1–12; Geoffrey Rose and M. G. Marmot, "Social Class and Coronary Heart Disease," *British Heart Journal* 45 (1981): 13–19; C. J. Crespo, B. E. Ainsworth, S. J. Keteyian, et al., "Prevalence of Physical Inactivity and Its Relation to Social Class in U.S. Adults: Results from the Third National Health and Nutrition Survey, 1988–1994," *Medicine and Science in Sports and Exercise* 31, no. 12 (1999): 1821–1827; R. G. Wilkinson and K. E. Pickett, "Income Equality and Population Health: A Review and Explanation of the Evidence," *Social Science and Medicine* 62, no. 7 (2006): 1768–1784.

52. International HapMap Project, "Guidelines for Referring to the HapMap Populations in Publications and Presentations," June 20, 2005, available at http://hapmap .ncbi.nlm.nih.gov/citinghapmap.html, accessed January 25, 2014. See also Foster, "Integrating Ethics and Science," 469.

53. International HapMap Project, "Guidelines for Referring to the HapMap Populations," June 20, 2005, available at http://hapmap.ncbi.nlm.nih.gov/citinghapmap .html.en, accessed January 25, 2014.

54. I would like to thank Troy Duster, who was at the first meeting, for kindly supplying me with this information.

55. Bentley and the International HapMap Consortium, "The International HapMap Project," 793.

56. Altshuler and the International HapMap Consortium, "A Haplotype Map," 1315.

57. Foster, "Integrating Ethics and Science," 468. The fact that the samples should remain anonymous was never questioned.

58. Ibid.

59. Ibid.

60. See, for example, Kimberly Tallbear, "Native-American-DNA.com: In Search of Native American Race and Tribe," in *Revisiting Race in a Genomic Age*, ed. Barbara A. Koenig, Sandra Soo-Jin Lee, and Sarah S. Richardson, 235–252 (New Brunswick, NJ: Rutgers University Press, 2008).

61. Foster, "Integrating Ethics and Science," 470.

62. Ibid., 471.

63. L. Luca Cavalli-Sforza, "Genes, Peoples, and Languages," *Scientific American* 265, no. 5 (1991): 104–110. See also Reardon, *Race to the Finish*, 1.

64. Reardon, *Race to the Finish*, 74–97.

65. Ibid., 102.

66. Ibid., 105–106.

67. Ibid., 107–109.

68. Wellcome Trust: Sanger Institute, "HapMap 3," November 29, 2012, available at http://www.sanger.ac.uk/resources/downloads/human/hapmap3.html, accessed January 25, 2014. See also Nicole Rusk, "Expanding HapMap," *Nature Methods* 7 no. 10 (2010): 780–781.

69. Ann Morning, *The Nature of Race: How Scientists Think and Teach about Human Difference* (Berkeley: University of California Press, 2011), 36–48, 103–141.

70. Lundy Braun, "Race, Ethnicity, and Health: Can Genetics Explain Disparities?," *Perspectives in Biology and Medicine* 45, no. 2 (2002): 159–174, here 165, as quoted in Morning, *The Nature of Race*, 37.

71. Morning, *The Nature of Race*, 104, 113–117.

72. Catherine Lee, "'Race' and 'Ethnicity' in Biomedical Research: How Do Scientists Construct and Explain Differences in Health?," *Social Science and Medicine* 68, no. 6 (2009): 1183–1190.

73. Wilson, Weale, Smith, et al., "Population Genetic Structure of Variable Drug Response."

74. Robert S. Schwartz, "Racial Profiling in Medical Research," *New England Journal of Medicine* 344, no. 18 (2001): 1392–1393.

75. Schwartz, "Racial Profiling," 1392.

76. Ibid., 1393.

77. Ibid.

78. Wilson, Weale, Smith, et al., "Population Genetic Structure," 265.

79. Ibid., 266.

80. Neil J. Risch, Esteban Burchard, Elad Ziv, et al., "Categorization of Humans in Biomedical Research: Genes, Race and Disease," *Genome Biology* 3, no. 7 (2002): 1–12, here 1.

81. Ibid., 4.

82. Neil J. Risch, "Searching for Genetic Determinants in the New Millennium," *Nature* 405, no. 6788 (2000): 847–856, here 855.

83. As quoted in Risch, Burchard, Ziv, et al., "Categorization of Humans," 5; "Editorial: Census, Race and Science," *Nature Genetics* 24, no. 2 (2000): 97–98, original: "The Association of Anthropologists Statement of Race of 1997."

84. Risch, Burchard, Ziv, et al., "Categorization of Humans," 5. See also J. Claiborne Stephens, Julie A. Schneider, Debra A. Tanguay, et al., "Haplotype Variation and Linkage Disequilibrium in 313 Human Genes," *Science* 293, no. 5529 (2001): 489–493; J. L. Mountain and L. L. Cavalli-Sforza. "Multilocus Genotypes, a Tree of Individuals, and Human Evolutionary History," *American Journal of Human Genetics* 61, no. 3 (1997): 705–718.

85. Risch, Burchard, Ziv, et al., "Categorization of Humans," 5. See also Michael J. Bamshad, "Genetic Influences on Health: Does Race Matter?," *Journal of the American Medical Association* 294, no. 8 (2005): 937–946, here 938.

86. Risch, Burchard, Ziv, et al., "Categorization of Humans," 6.

87. Ibid., 11.

88. Michael J. Bamshad, Stephen Wooding, W. Scott Watkins, et al., "Human Population Genetic Structure and Inference of Group Membership," *American Journal of Human Genetics* 72, no. 3 (2003): 578–589.

89. The Tuskegee syphilis experiment was conducted between 1932 and 1972 by the U.S. Public Health Service. Physicians wished to study the effects of untreated syphilis on humans, so six hundred African American males from rural Tuskegee, Alabama, were never given proper treatment for the disease, even though by the late 1940s penicillin had become the standard treatment for syphilis. See, for example, Susan M. Reverby, ed., *Tuskegee Truths: Rethinking the Tuskegee Syphilis Study* (Chapel Hill: University of North Carolina Press, 2000), and Susan M. Reverby, *Examining Tuskegee: The Infamous Syphilis Study and Its Legacy* (Chapel Hill: University of North Carolina Press, 2009).

90. Esteban González Burchard, Elad Ziv, Natasha Coyle, et al., "The Importance of Race and Ethnic Background in Biomedical Research and Clinical Practice," *New England Journal of Medicine* 348, no. 12 (2003): 1170–1175, here 1171. Similarly, Rosenberg argues that human genome mapping has confirmed the five major groupings—Africans, Caucasians, Pacific Islanders, East Asians, and Native Americans. Noah A. Rosenberg, Jonathan K. Pritchard, James L. Weber, et al., "Genetic Structure of Human Populations," *Science* 298, no. 5602 (2002): 2381–2385. These population groupings were based on the U.S. Census of 2000.

91. Burchard, Ziv, Coyle, et al., "The Importance of Race," 1172.

92. Ibid., 1174.

93. Ibid., 1174–1175.

94. "We were in the Hispanic ghetto ... and we were right on the edge of the black ghetto. So that's where I grew up.... I've always been keenly aware of race, ever since I was a child." Duana Fullwiley's interview with Burchard in Fullwiley, "The Biologistical Construction," 707.

95. Rose, *The Politics of Life*, 157.

96. As cited in "Forum on Race and Genomics," *BioSocieties* 2 (2007): 219.

97. Francis Collins, "What We Do and Don't Know about 'Race,' 'Ethnicity,' Genetics and Health at the Dawn of the Genome," *Nature Genetics Supplement* 36, no. 11 (2004): S13–S15, here S13. See also Fullwiley, "The Biologistical Construction," 728.

98. Kate Berg and The Race, Ethnicity, and Genetics Working Group of the National Human Genome Research Institute, "Review Article: The Use of Racial, Ethnic, and Ancestral Categories in Human Genetics Research," *American Journal of Human Genetics* 77, no. 4 (2005): 519–532; Risch, Burchard, Ziv, et al., "Categorization of Humans," 7.

99. "Therefore, there is no reason to assume that major genetic discontinues exist between different continents." David Serre and Svante Pääло, "Evidence for Gradients of Human Genetic Diversity within and among Continents," *Genome Research* 14, no. 9: 1679–1685, here 1679.

100. Berg and The Race, Ethnicity, and Genetics Working Group of the National Human Genome Research Institute, "Review Article," 520.

101. M. Nei and G. Livshits, "Genetic Relationships of Europeans, Asians, and Africans and the Origin of Modern *Homo Sapiens*," *Human Heredity* 39, no. 5 (1989): 276–281; L. Luca Cavalli-Sforza and W. F. Bodmer, *The Genetics of Human Populations* (San Francisco: Freeman, 1971). See also Lynn B. Jorde and Stephen P. Wooding, "Genetic Variation, Classification and 'Race,'" *Nature Genetics* 36, no. 11S (2004): S28–S33, here S28.

102. Lynn B. Jorde, W. S. Watkins, M. J. Bamshad, "The Distribution of Human Genetic Diversity: A Comparison of Mitochondrial, Autosomal, and Y Chromosome Data," *American Journal of Human Genetics* 66, no. 3 (2003): 979–988; Guido Barbujani, Ariana Magagni, Eric Minch, et al., "An Apportionment of Human DNA Diversity," *Proceedings of the National Academy of Sciences (PNAS) USA* 94, no. 9 (1997): 4516–4519; Jorde and Wooding, "Genetic Variation," S28. See also Berg and The Race, Ethnicity, and Genetics Working Group, "Review," 521 ("The study of genetic variations in *Homo sapiens* shows that there is more genetic variation within populations than between populations. This means that two random individuals from any one group are almost as different as any two random individuals from the entire world"), available at http://www.genome.gov/25019961#al-2, last updated March 29, 2012, accessed January 25, 2014. See also Foster, "Integrating Ethics and Science," 469.

103. Rosenberg, Pritchard, Weber, et al., "Genetic Structure," here 2381–2382.

104. Bamshad, Wooding, Watkins, et al., "Human Population Genetic Structure," 578–589, here 582. See also Bamshad, Wooding, Salisbury, et al., "Deconstructing the Relationship between Genetics and Race," 601.

105. Bamshad, Wooding, Watkins, et al., "Human Population," 587.

106. Bamshad, Wooding, Salisbury, et al., "Deconstructing the Relationship," 605.

107. Berg and the International HapMap Consortium, "Review Article," 521.

108. Rosenberg, Prichard, Weber, et al., "Genetic Structure," 2384.

109. Berg and the International HapMap Consortium, "Review Article," 521; Risch, Burchard, Ziv, et al., "Categorization of Humans." See also M.-C. King and A. G. Motulsky, "Mapping Human History," *Science* 298, no. 5602 (2002): 2342–2343; F. Calafell, "Classifying Humans," *Human Genetics* 33, no. 4 (2003): 435–436; S. A. Tischkoff and K. K. Kidd, "Implications of Biogeography of Human Populations for 'Race' and Medicine," *Nature Genetics* 36, no. 11 supp. (2004): S21–S27.

110. Race, Ethnicity, and Genetics Working Group, "The Use of Racial, Ethnic, and Ancestral Categories in Human Genetics Research," *American Journal of Human Genetics* 77, no. 4 (2005): 519–532. On the politics of the U.S. Census Bureau and Race, see Morning, *The Nature of Race*, 193–201.

111. Pamela Sankar and Mildred K. Cho, "Toward a New Vocabulary of Human Genetic Variation," *Science* 298, no. 5597 (2002): 1337–1338. See also "Editorial: Census, Race and Science," *Nature Genetics* 24, no. 2 (2000): 97–98. here 98.

112. Pamela Sankar, Mildred Cho, and Joanna Mountain. "Race and Ethnicity in Genetic Research," *American Journal of Medical Genetics Part A* 143A, no. 9 (2007): 961–970.

113. Lee, "'Race' and 'Ethnicity' in Biomedical Research," 1183, emphasis in the original. See also 1188.

114. Ibid., 1187.

115. Ibid.

116. Ibid.

117. Ibid., 1189.

118. Ibid.

119. Epstein, *Inclusion*, 79. For a detailed history of the Revitalization Act, see ibid., 79–83, 95–96, 111–114, 130–131, and 183–184.

120. Ibid., 79–82.

121. "NIH Policy and Guidelines on the Inclusion of Women and Minorities as Subjects in Clinical Research," updated October 1, 2001, available at http://grants .nih.gov/grants/funding/women_min/guidelines_amended_10_2001.htm, accessed January 25, 2014.

122. Duana Fullwiley, "The Molecularization of Race: Institutionalizing Human Difference in Pharmacogenetics Practice," *Science in Culture* 16, no. 1 (2007): 1–30, here 3.

123. Duana Fullwiley, "The Molecularization of Race: U.S. Health Institutions, Pharmacogenetics Practice, and Public Science after the Genome," in *Revisiting Race in a Genomic Age: Studies in Medical Anthropology*, ed. Barbara A. Koenig, Sandra Soo-Jin Lee, and Sarah S. Richardson, 149–171, here 151 (New Brunswick, NJ: Rutgers University Press, 2008), emphasis in the original. This view is similar to Nikolas Rose's "framing of explanations at the molecular level." See Rose, "The Politics," 1–30, here 13.

124. Fullwiley, "The Biologistical Construction," 698, italics in the original.

125. Nadia Abu El-Haj, "The Genetic Reinscription of Race," *Annual Review of Anthropology* 36 (2007): 283–300, here 288.

126. Fullwiley, "The Biologistical Construction," 702.

127. Ibid.

128. This argument is similar to Londa Schiebinger's explanation of Linnaeus's classification of plants based on sexual characteristics. There were other classificatory possibilities, yet he viewed organisms through the lens of the sexes as a result of the cultural climate of eighteenth-century Sweden. See Londa Schiebinger, "Gender and Natural History," *Cultures of Natural History*, ed. Nicholas Jardine, James Secord, and Emma Spary, 163–177 (New York: Cambridge University Press, 1996).

129. Fullwiley, "The Biologistical Construction," 702.

130. Fullwiley, "The Molecularization of Race: U.S. Health," 152. Epstein points out that the history of the white male as the standard health model is complicated and convoluted. See Epstein, *Inclusion*, 53–73.

131. As quoted in Epstein, *Inclusion*, 129, original: Center for Drug Evaluation and Research, FDA, "Guideline for the Format and Content of the Clinical and Statistical Sections of New Drug Applications," July 1988, 17.

132. Steven Epstein, "The Rise of 'Recruitmentology': Clinical Research, Racial Knowledge, and the Politics of Inclusion and Difference," *Social Studies of Science* 38, no. 5 (2008): 801–832, here 804; Abu El-Haj, "The Genetic Reinscription," 292–293.

133. Epstein, *Inclusion*, 45.

134. As quoted in Jonathan Kahn, *Race in a Bottle. The Story of BiDil and Racialized Medicine in a Post-Genomic Age* (New York: Columbia University Press, 2013), 25.

135. Epstein, *Inclusion*, 123.

136. Pharmacokinetics studies the history of a drug from the moment that it is delivered into the organism until it has been completely eliminated. Population pharmacokinetics looks at this aspect of pharmacology at members of various subgroups, including race, gender, and age.

137. Kahn, *Race in a Bottle*, 26.

138. Ibid.

139. Epstein, *Inclusion*, 106, 152.

140. As quoted in Montoya, *Making the Mexican Diabetic*, 172.

141. Ibid., 173.

142. As quoted in Epstein, *Inclusion*, 178, original: Fourth Annual Multicultural Pharmaceutical Marketing and Public Relations Conference, sponsored by Strategic Research Institute, held on March 18, 2003, in Princeton, New Jersey, http://www .srinstitute.com.

143. Dorothy Roberts, *Fatal Invention: How Science, Politics, and Big Business and Recreate Race in the Twenty-first Century* (New York: New Press, 2011), 161.

144. As quoted in ibid., 164–165. See also Jonathan Kahn, "From Disparity to Difference: How Race-Specific Medicines May Undermine Policies to Address Inequalities in Health Care," *Southern California Interdisciplinary Law Journal* 15 (2005): 105–129, here 118–119, original: Strategic Research Institute, Sixth Annual Multicultural Pharmaceutical Market Development and Outreach Conference, sponsored by Strategic Research Institute, held on March 18, 2003, in Princeton, New Jersey. See http://www.srinstitute.com/CustomerFiles/upload/brochure/CM453_brochure.pdf.

145. As quoted in Roberts, *Fatal Invention*, 165. See also Timothy Caulfield, "Genesis of Neo-Racism? Biogenetics Discoveries about Race-Specific Idiosyncrasies Have a Dark Side," *Edmonton Journal*, December 22, 2007.

146. Roberts, *Fatal Invention*, 164.

147. Ibid., 151, 163, 166.

148. Epstein, *Inclusion*, 179, 223.

149. Pamela Sankar and Jonathan Kahn, "BiDil: Race Medicine or Race Marketing?," *Health Affairs* 24 (October 2005): W5-455–W5-463. See also Roberts, *Fatal Invention*, 168–201; Kahn, *Race in a Bottle*.

150. Sankar and Kahn, "BiDil." This section on BiDil is derived from Sankar and Kahn's article.

151. Ibid., W5-457.

152. Anne L. Taylor, Susan Ziesche, Clyde Yancy, et al., "Combination of Isosorbide Dinitrate and Hydralazine in Blacks with Heart Failure," *New England Journal of Medicine* 351, no. 20 (2004): 2049–2057, here 2049.

153. Jonathan Kahn, "Exploiting Race in Drug Development: BiDil's Interim Model of Pharmacogenomics," *Social Studies of Science* 38, no. 5 (2008): 737–758, here 739–740.

154. Sankar and Kahn, "BiDil," W5-458.

155. Ibid., W5-461–462.

156. As quoted in Kahn, "Exploiting Race," 742.

157. Epstein, *Inclusion*, 224.

158. Rose, *The Politics of Life*, 180–181.

159. M. Tapper, *In the Blood: Sickle Cell Anemia and the Politics of Race* (Philadelphia: University of Pennsylvania Press, 1999).

160. As cited in Rose, *The Politics of Life*, 175.

161. See, for example, http://www.africanancestry.com/home/, which was cofounded by the African American biologist Rick Kittles, who is currently its scientific director.

162. Steven Epstein, *Impure Science: AIDS, Activism, and the Politics of Knowledge* (Los Angeles: University of California Press, 1996); Shobita Parthasarathy, *Building Genetic Medicine: Breast Cancer, Technology, and the Comparative Politics of Health Care* (Cambridge, MA: MIT Press, 2007).

163. Fätkenheuer, Nelson, Lazzarin, et al., "Subgroup Analyses: 1442–1455, particularly 1444 and 1446. See also Roy M. Gulick, Jacob Lalezari, James Goodrich, et al.,

"Maraviroc for Previously Treated Patients with R5 HIV-1 Infection," *New England Journal of Medicine* 359, no. 14 (2008): 1429–1441, particularly 1434; Michael Saag, James Goodrich, Gerd Fätkenheuer, et al., "A Double-Blind, Placebo Controlled Trial of Maraviroc in Treatment-Experienced Patients Infected with Non R5 HIV-1," *Journal of Infectious Diseases* 199 no. 11 (2009): 1638–1647, particularly 1642; "Highlights of Prescribing Information- Selzentry," https://www.gsksource.com/gskprm/htdocs/documents/SELZENTRY-PI-MG.PDF, p. 16, accessed on 1 March 2014.

164. That changed in December 2013, when the Food and Drug Administration forced 23andMe to discontinue giving out information on alleles that predispose clients to particular diseases or predict their clients' responses to medications based on their genomes until the company received FDA approval. See the epilogue. The company still offers ancestry testing.

165. https://www.23andme.com/health/Resistance-to-HIV-AIDS/, accessed October 11, 2013. After the FDA prohibited the company from offering medical information based on genetic testing, it changed its Web site. See https://www.23andme.com/health/, accessed January 25, 2014. See also https://customercare.23andme.com/entries/23102321-Does-the-23andMe-service-include-analysis-of-the-CCR5-gene-, accessed January 25, 2014.

166. http://www.xygene.com/hiv.php, site last updated in 2007, accessed February 11, 2014.

167. Ibid.

168. Roberts, *Fatal Invention*, 160–161.

169. http://www.familytreedna.com/advanced-test-results.aspx, accessed January 25, 2014.

170. http://www.familytreedna.com/news-letter.aspx?v=8&i=1, accessed January 25, 2014.

171. Ibid.

172. Their World Wide Web address is clever: http://www.delta-32.com, accessed December 18, 2013.

173. Burchard, Ziv, Coyle, et al., "The Importance of Race," 1173.

174. Michael J. Bamshad and Steve E. Olson, "Does Race Exist?," *Scientific American* 289 no. 6 (December 2003): 78–85.

175. Ibid., 80.

176. Ibid., 83–84.

177. Enrique Gonzalez, Michael Bamshad, Naoko Sato, et al., "Race-Specific HIV-1 Disease-Modifying Effects Associated with *CCR5* Haplotypes," *Proceedings of the National Academy of Sciences (PNAS) USA* 96, no. 21 (1999): 12,004–12,009.

178. Bamshad, "Genetic Influences on Health," 937–947.

179. Ibid., 937.

180. Ibid.

181. Ibid., 938.

182. Ibid., 940; Mark D. Shriver, Esteban Parra, Sonia Dios, et al., "Skin Pigmentation, Biographical Ancestry, and Admixture Mapping," *Human Genetics* 112, no. 4 (2003): 387–399.

183. Bamshad, "Genetic Influences on Health," 940; Shriver et al., "Skin Pigmentation," 387–399.

184. Bamshad, "Genetic Influences on Health," 941. See also Enrique Gonzalez, Hemant Kulkarni, Hector Bolivar, et al., "The Influence of *CCL3L1* Gene-Containing Segmental Duplications on HIV-1/AIDS Susceptibility," *Science* 307, no. 5715 (2005): 1434–1440.

185. Bamshad, "Genetic Influences on Health," 941.

186. Nadia Abu El-Haj, "The Genetic Reinscription of Race," *Annual Review of Anthropology* 36 (2007): 283–300, here 287; Snait B. Gissis, "When Is 'Race' a Race? 1946–2003," *Studies in History and Philosophy of Science Part C* 39, no. 4 (2008): 437–450.

187. Jorde and Wooding, "Genetic Variation," S28, S32.

188. Fujimura and Rajagopalan, "Different Differences," 6.

189. Deborah A. Bolnick, "Individual Ancestry Inference and Reification of Race as a Biological Phenomenon," in *Revisiting Race in a Genomic Age: Studies in Medical Anthropology*, ed. Barbara A. Koenig, Sandra Soo-Jin Lee, and Sarah S. Richardson, 70–85, particularly 80–81 (New Brunswick, NJ: Rutgers University Press, 2008).

190. Ibid., 81.

191. Alkes L. Price, Nick J. Patterson, Robert M. Plenge, et al., "Principal Components Analysis Corrects for Stratification in Genome-Wide Association Studies," *Nature Genetics* 38, no. 8 (2006): 904–909.

192. Fujimura and Rajagopalan, "Different Differences," 12. See also 19.

193. See the interviews with medical geneticists in ibid., 12–13.

194. Ibid., 20.

195. Jacques Fellay, Dongliang Ge, Kevin V. Shianna, et al., "Common Genetic Variation and the Control of HIV-1 in Humans," *PLoS Genetics* 5, no. 12 (2007): 1–12, here 1.

196. Ibid.

197. See, for example, Jacques Fellay, Kevin V. Shianna, Dongliang Ge, et al., "A Whole-Genome Association Study of Major Determinants for Host Control of HIV-1," *Science* 317, no. 5840 (2007): 944–947, here 946. In this study, they created "an independent replication cohort of 140 Caucasian patients, drawn from the same participating cohorts."

198. Kimberly Pelak, David B. Goldstein, Nicole M. Walley, et al., "Host Determinants of HIV-1 Control in African Americans," *Journal of Infectious Diseases* 201, no. 8 (2010): 1141–1149.

199. Ibid., 1141.

200. M. Gregg Bloche, "Race-Based Therapeutics," *New England Journal of Medicine* 351, no. 20 (2004): 2035–2037, as cited in Epstein, *Inclusion*, 224.

Epilogue

1. No. 12-398. The case is now referred to as *Association for Molecular Pathology v. Myriad Genetics* because the U.S. Patent and Trademark Office was no longer a defendant after Judge Sweet's ruling.

2. Arguably, *Amgen v. Chugai* indirectly addressed the topic of gene patenting, but the case was about patent infringement, not patentability. 927 F.2d 1200 (1991).

3. Robert E. Kohler, *Lords of the Fly: Drosophila Genetics and the Experimental Life* (Chicago: University of Chicago Press, 1994).

4. Doll, "Biotechnology," 689–690.

5. Ibid., 689.

6. Ibid., 690.

7. Regalado, "The Great Gene Grab," 55.

8. Dutfield, *Intellectual Property Rights*, 76.

9. Ibid., 79.

10. Ibid., 93–94.

11. John P. Walsh, Charlene Cho, and Wesley M. Cohen, "View from the Bench: Patents and Material Transfers," *Science* 309, no. 5743 (2005): 2002–2003; John P. Walsh and Wei Hong, "Secrecy Is Increasing in Step with Competition," *Nature* 422, no. 6934 (2003): 801–802; Timothy Caulfield, Robert M. Cook-Deegan, F. Scott Kief, et al., "Evidence and Anecdotes: An Analysis of Human Gene Patenting Controversies," *Nature Biotechnology* 24, no. 9 (2006): 1091–1094, here 1092; Eric G. Campbell, Brian R. Clarridge, Manjusha Gokhate, et al., "Data Withholding in Academic

Genetics," *Journal of the American Medical Association* 287, no. 4 (2002): 473–480; D. Blumenthal, E. G. Campbell, N. Causino, et al., "Withholding Research Results in Academic Life Science: Evidence from a National Survey of Faculty," *Journal of the American Medical Association* 277, no. 15 (1997): 1224–1228.

12. Cho, Illangasekare, Weaver, et al., "Effects of Patents," 7.

13. Ibid.

14. John F. Merz, Antigone G. Kriss, D. G. B. Lenard, et al., "Diagnostic Testing Fails the Test: The Pitfalls of Patents Are Illustrated by the Case of Haemochromatosis," *Nature* 415, no. 6872 (2002): 577–579.

15. Cho, Illangasekare, Weaver, et al., "Effects of Patents," 3.

16. I. Rabino, "How Human Geneticists in U.S. View Commercialization of the Human Genome Project," *Nature Genetics* 29, no. 1 (2001): 15–16.

17. Julia Carbone, E. Richard, Bhaven Sampat, et al., "DNA Patents and Diagnostics: Not a Pretty Picture," *Nature Biotechnology* 28, no. 8 (2010): 784–791, here 786. As noted in chapter 6, long QT syndrome is a potentially lethal condition in which a delayed repolarization of the heart muscle results in an irregular heartbeat.

18. Ibid.

19. Ibid.

20. Ibid., 785. See also Steven Teutsch and the Secretary's Advisory Committee on Genetics, Health, and Society, "Gene Patents and Licensing Practices and Their Impact on Patient Access to Genetic Tests: Report of the Secretary's Advisory Committee on Genetics, Health, and Society," March 2010, available at http://osp .od.nih.gov/sites/default/files/SACGHS_patents_report_2010.pdf, accessed January 21, 2014, here particularly 3–4, 21, H6, E12–E13.

21. Teutsch and the Secretary's Advisory Committee on Genetics, Health, and Society, "Gene Patents and Licensing Practices."

22. Ibid., v, 8–9.

23. Ibid., 1–2. See also "Science and Engineering Indicators 2008," January 2008, National Science Foundation, available at http://www.nsf.gov/statistics/seind08/c4/ c4h.htm#c4hs, accessed January 25, 2014.

24. Katie Skeehan, Christopher Heaney, and Robert Cook-Deegan, "Impact of Gene Patents on Access to Genetic Testing for Alzheimer Disease," in Steven Teutsch and the Secretary's Advisory Committee on Genetics, Health, and Society, "Gene Patents and Licensing Practices," appendix, B-14, http://osp.od.nih.gov/sites/default/files/ SACGHS_patents_report_2010.pdf, accessed on 30 March 2014.

25. Teutsch and the Secretary's Advisory Committee on Genetics, Health, and Society, "Gene Patents and Licensing Practices," 22.

26. Ibid., 26.

27. Ibid., 27. See also K. G. Huang and F. E. Murray, "Does Patent Strategy Shape the Long-Run Supply of Public Knowledge? Evidence from Human Genetics," *Academy of Management Journal* 52, no. 6 (2009): 1193–1221.

28. Subhashini Chandrasekharan, Christopher Heaney, Tamara James, et al., "Impact of Gene Patents and Licensing Practices on Access to Genetic Testing for Cystic Fibrosis," *Genetic Medicine* 12, no. 4 supp. (2010): S194–S211 and Merrill and Mazza, eds., *Reaping the Benefits*, 67.

29. Teutsch and the Secretary's Advisory Committee on Genetics, Health, and Society, "Gene Patents and Licensing Practices," 2.

30. Ibid., 30.

31. As quoted in ibid., emphasis in the original.

32. Ibid., 30–31.

33. Ibid., 33.

34. Ibid., 3.

35. Ibid.

36. Ibid., 35.

37. Ibid., 42–43.

38. Ibid., 43–44.

39. Ibid., 42.

40. Ibid., 4–6, emphasis in the original.

41. Ségolène Aymé, Gert Matthijs, Sirpa Soini, et al., "Patenting and Licensing in Genetic Testing: Recommendations of the European Society of Human Genetics," *European Journal of Human Genetics* 16, no. 8 (2008): 405–411. See also Sirpa Soini, Ségolène Aymé, and Gert Matthijs, "Patenting and Licensing in Genetic Testing: Ethical, Legal and Social Issues," *European Journal of Human Genetics* 16, no. 1 supp. (2008): S10–S50.

42. Aymé, Matthijs, Soini, et al., "Patenting and Licensing," 407.

43. Ibid., 408.

44. Ibid.

45. Ibid.

46. Ibid., 410.

47. Ibid., 408–411.

48. As quoted in Regalado, "The Great Gene Grab," 53.

49. Hopkins, Mahdi, Patel, et al., "DNA Patenting," 185.

50. Ibid., 186.

51. Ibid.

52. Ibid.

53. Gregory D. Graff, Devon Phillips, Zhen Lei, et al., "Not Quite a Myriad of Gene Patents," *Nature Biotechnology* 31, no. 5 (2013): 404–410, here 408. Other nucleotide sequences include those of other mammals, other animals, plants, microorganisms, and synthetic. See ibid., 406.

54. Hopkins, Mahdi, Patel, et al., "DNA Patenting," 186.

55. Ibid.

56. Ibid., 187.

57. United States District Court, Southern District of New York, *Association for Molecular Pathology et al., Plaintiffs-Appellees v. U.S. Patent and Trademark Office, Defendant, Myriad Genetics et al., Defendant-Appellant*, appeal of case no. 09-CV-4515-RWS, document 255, Senior Judge Robert W. Sweet, March 29, 2010, case 1:09-cv-04515-RWS Document 255, filed on March 29, 2010, p. 107, available at http://www.aclu.org/files/assets/2010-3-29-AMPvUSPTO-Opinion.pdf, accessed January 25, 2014.

58. Alison Frankel, "U.S. Solicitor General to Make Unprecedented Federal Circuit Appearance in Myriad Case," *American Lawyer*, February 24, 2011, available at http://www.americanlawyer.com/id=1202483155902, accessed January 20, 2014.

59. U.S. Court of Appeals for the Federal Circuit: *Association for Molecular Pathology et al., v. U.S. Patent and Trademark Office and Myriad Genetics et al.*, decided July 29, 2011, opinion for the court filed by Circuit Court Judge Lourie, p. 38, available at http://www.genomicslawreport.com/wp-content/uploads/2011/07/Decision-in-USPTO-vs-MYGN.pdf, accessed January 25, 2014.

60. U.S. Supreme Court, *Mayo Collaborative Services v. Prometheus Laboratories*, no. 10-1150, slip op. at 16.

61. U.S. Supreme Court, *Association for Molecular Pathology, Petitioners v. Myriad Genetics et al.*, June 13, 2013, available at http://www.supremecourt.gov/opinions/12pdf/12-398_1b7d.pdf, accessed January 25, 2014.

62. Ibid., syllabus, 2 and no. 12-398, 2.

63. Ibid., no. 12-398, 11.

64. As quoted in ibid., no. 12-398, 12.

65. Ibid., no. 12-398, 13.

66. Ibid., syllabus, 2 and no. 12-398, 16–17.

67. Ibid., no. 12-398, 17.

68. Gero Hütter, Daniel Nowak, Maximilian Mossner, et al., "Long-Term Control of HIV by *CCR5* Delta 32/Delta 32 Stem-Cell Transplantation," *New England Journal of Medicine* 360, no. 7 (2009): 692–698.

69. Maggie Fox, "German Doctors Declare 'Cure' in HIV Patient," Reuters, December 15, 2010, available at http://www.reuters.com/article/2010/12/15/us-aids -transplant-idUSTRE6BE68220101215, accessed January 20, 2014.

70. Rachael Rettner, "Cure for HIV Claimed, but Not Proved: Bone Marrow Transplant Credited with Wiping Out German Man's Infection," *NBC News*, December 15, 2010, available at http://www.nbcnews.com/id/40666443/#.Uq-HAv1wp4M, accessed January 21, 2014.

71. As quoted in Fox, "German Doctors Declare 'Cure.'"

72. See, for example, Fujimura and Rajagopalan, "Different Differences," 6.

73. Scott Hensley, "FDA Tells 23andMe to Stop Selling Popular Genetic Test," *NRP Health News*, November 25, 2013, available at http://www.npr.org/blogs/ health/2013/11/25/247198237/fda-tells-23andme-to-stop-selling-popular-genetic -test, accessed January 20, 2014.

74. Scott Hensley, "23andMe Bows to FDA's Demands, Drops Health Claims," *NPR Health News*, December 6, 2013, available at http://www.npr.org/blogs/health/ 2013/12/06/249231236/23andme-bows-to-fdas-emands-drops-health-claims, accessed January 20, 2014.

Science Glossary

agonist   a molecule that binds to a particular receptor and elicits a physiological response

allele   one of multiple forms of the same gene or group of genes

***Alu* insertion polymorphisms/repeats**   short stretches of DNA that can be cut by the *Alu* restriction endonuclease. They can be used as genetic markers.

amino acid   the building blocks of proteins

ancestry informative markers   single nucleotide polymorphisms that occur in a disproportionate number among various populations

antagonist   a molecule that binds to a particular receptor and does not elicit a physiological response but rather blocks or abates agonist-triggered responses. Antagonists compete with agonists for the binding of a receptor.

antibody   also known as an immunoglobulin, a protein produced by B cells of the immune system that identifies foreign invaders, such as viruses, bacteria, or fungi

antigen   a substance that binds to a particular antibody

antiligand   a molecule that blocks a ligand

antisense oligonucleotide   a synthesized nucleotide (either DNA or RNA) sequence that is complementary to and therefore binds to the mRNA produced by a gene. As a result, the gene's protein product cannot be produced.

CD4 cell   a lymphocyte, or a type of white blood cell, that possesses a CD4 receptor on its cell surface and recognizes specific portions of foreign pathogens. Examples of CD4 cells include T helper cells, monocytes, macrophages, and dendritic cells.

cDNA   complementary DNA, or a stretch of DNA that is made from mRNA by using reserve transcriptase

chemokines   small proteins that attract and activate leukocytes, or white blood cells

CCR5   a chemokine receptor that HIV-1 recognizes as its coreceptor

CCR5   the wild-type (normal) gene for the CCR5 receptor protein

Δ32   an allele or mutation of the *CCR5* gene, in which 32 nucleotides are deleted. Therefore, the receptor is not expressed on the CD4-cell membrane in those who have two copies of (i.e. are homozygous for) the allele. In that case, the individual has a greatly reduced risk of contracting AIDS.

DNA ligase   an enzyme that is involved in DNA replication. It seals the nicks in the phosphodiester backbone of a single strand of DNA.

epitope   the part of an antigen that is recognized by an immune cell, such as a T or B cell

exons   nucleotide sequences of a gene that remain in the mRNA after the introns are removed by RNA splicing

expressed sequence tags (ESTs)   short sequences of cDNA that can be used to identify gene transcripts

genetic marker   a gene or sequence of DNA that has a known location on a chromosome and that is associated with a particular phenotype, such as a disease. Examples include SNPs, *Alu* insertion polymorphisms/repeats, and microsatellites.

genome   all of an organism's genetic information

genomics   the branch of biotechnology that uses techniques from molecular biology and genetics to map DNA sequences and genes, construct genomes, and organize the information in databanks

genotype   the genetic information of an organism's particular trait or allele

glycoprotein   a protein with a sugar (oligosaccharide) attached. The outer-coat protein of HIV-1 is a glycoprotein.

G protein   a family of proteins that is associated with the intracellular membrane and activated by a G protein-coupled receptor. These proteins transmit signals from stimuli outside a cell to inside the cell.

G protein-coupled receptors   receptors that bind to G proteins and are found on the surface of cells. They have seven domains, which are embedded in the cell's membrane. CCR5 and CXCR4 are examples of G protein-coupled receptors.

haplotype   a combination of alleles near each other on a chromosome. As a result of their proximity, they are inherited together.

HeLa cells   an immortal human-cell line used for experimentation in biomedical research

heteroduplex of DNA   a double-stranded DNA molecule that possesses nearly complementary strands. One strand contains one or more mismatched or unpaired nucleotides.

heteroduplex tracking assay   a method to detect and estimate genetic divergence between HIV-1 strains based on DNA heteroduplexes formed between related but not identical nucleic acid sequences

heterozygous   possessing one dominant and one recessive allele for a particular trait

highly active antiretroviral therapy (HAART)   treatment regimes that suppress the replication of HIV and halt the progression of AIDS

high-throughput screening (HTS)   a technique that is used in drug discovery by which a large number of compounds are tested for their ability to bind to and elicit biological activity against target molecules. HTS is used to test molecules that can inhibit enzymatic activity, compete for binding of a ligand to its receptor, or act as agonists or antagonists for receptor-mediated processes.

HIV-1 tropism   refers to the type of chemokine receptor that HIV-1 recognizes and binds to during infection. Two examples are X4-tropic HIV-1, which infects CD4 cells via the chemokine receptor CXCR4, and R5-tropic HIV-1, which infects CD4 cells via CCR5.

homozygous   possessing two copies of the same allele for a particular trait

hydrophilic amino acid   an amino acid with polar side chains. They usually are found on cell surfaces.

hydrophobic amino acid   an amino acid with nonpolar side chains. They normally are embedded in cell membranes.

introns   stretches of DNA within a gene that are removed by RNA splicing. They do not code for a protein.

leucokytes (leucocytes)   white blood cells, which are responsible for an organism's immune system. They include neutrophils, eosinophils, basophils, lymphocytes, and monocytes.

ligand   a molecule that binds to a specific site of a targeted protein triggering some sort of signal

linkage disequilibrium   the nonrandom association of alleles at two or more locations (called loci) in a population

messenger RNA (mRNA)   a type of RNA that codes for a protein. It is the product of DNA transcription by an RNA polymerase after the introns are excised by RNA splicing.

MIP-1α and β macrophage inflammatory proteins, or chemokines, which (in addition to RANTES) are the natural ligands of CCR5. They are now called CCL3 and CCL4.

monoclonal antibody (mAB) a highly specific protein that is produced by immune cells. Monoclonal antibodies are identical because they are produced by the same immune cells, which are the clone of a parent cell. They have a specific affinity for a target cell's epitope.

M-tropic HIV-1 the strains of HIV-1 that use CCR5 as a coreceptor for CD4 cell entry; also called R5-tropic HIV-1

nonnucleoside reverse-transcriptase inhibitors a class of antiretroviral drugs that interfere with the ability of HIV's reserve transcriptase to make a DNA copy of its RNA genome

nucleotide and nucleoside analogue reverse-transcriptase inhibitors a class of antiretroviral drugs that contain an incorrect version of the nucleotides that are used by reverse transcriptase to convert RNA to DNA. With these analogues, HIV's genetic material cannot be incorporated into the healthy genetic material of the cell thereby halting the spread of the virus.

nucleotides the building blocks of DNA and RNA. They include adenine, thymine, cytosine, thymine, and uracil.

open reading frame (ORF) a stretch of DNA that does not have a stop codon and therefore has the potential to code for a protein

peptide a short chain of amino acids

pharmacogenomics the technology of determining how a person's genome affects her or his response to drugs

phenotype the physical manifestation of an organism

polymerase chain reaction (PCR) an in vitro technique to amplify dramatically the copies of a piece of DNA

polymorphism (genetic) two or more different alleles that are present at a particular chromosomal locus within a population

protease an enzyme that cleaves the peptide bonds of a protein. In HIV, the protease cleaves the polyprotein, creating the mature portions of an HIV virion.

protease inhibitors (PIs) a class of antiretroviral drugs used to inhibit HIV's protease, thereby thwarting the formation of new viruses

R5-tropic HIV-1 *See* M-tropic HIV-1

RANTES (regulated on activation, normal T cell expressed and secreted) a chemokine that serves as a natural ligand to CCR5. It is also referred to as CCL5. *See also* MIP-1α and β.

receptors proteins on cell surfaces that bind to specific biomolecules resulting in cellular responses

restriction endonuclease a bacterial enzyme that cuts DNA. They are used as molecular scissors to insert foreign DNA into a cloning vector.

reverse transcriptase an enzyme found in retroviruses that is used by molecular biologists to make a cDNA copy of mRNA

short tandem repeat polymorphism (STR) a microsatellite of DNA comprising two to six nucleotides. They are often used as genetic markers.

single nucleotide polymorphism (SNP) a variation of a DNA sequence involving one nucleotide. For example, one individual might have a guanine nucleotide in a position in the sequence where someone else has an adenine. There are millions of SNPs in the human genome, some of which can be used as genetic markers.

structure-activity relationship (SAR) the relationship between the three-dimensional structure of a chemical or biological molecule and its biological function. Biomedical chemists can alter chemical groups on a particular molecule to determine their biological effects.

T lymphocyte a type of white blood cell that regulates cell-mediated immunity. It possesses a receptor on its cell surface.

T-tropic HIV-1 HIV-1 strains that use CXCR4 as a coreceptor for CD4 cell entry. It is also known as X4-tropic HIV-1.

yeast artificial chromosome a genetically engineered chromosome that is derived from yeast DNA and then inserted into a bacteria plasmid

Yersinia pestis the bacterium that gave rise to the bubonic plague (the Black Death)

X4-tropic HIV-1 *See* T-tropic HIV-1

Bibliography

Abate, Tom. "Call It the Gene Rush: Patent Stakes Run High." *San Francisco Chronicle*, April 20, 2000, A8.

Abbott, Alison. "Europe to Pay Royalties for Cancer Gene: *BRCA1* Patent Decision May Be Ignored in Clinics." *Nature* 456 (2008): 556.

Abu El-Haj, Nadia. "The Genetic Reinscription of Race." *Annual Review of Anthropology* 36 (2007): 283–300.

Achilladelis, Basil. "The Dynamics of Technological Innovation: The Sector of Antibacterial Medicines." *Research Policy* 22 (4) (1993): 279–308.

Adams, M. D., Jenny M. Kelley, Jeannine D. Gocayne, et al. "Complementary DNA Sequencing: Expressed Sequence Tags and Human Genome Project." *Science* 252 (5013) (1991): 1651–1656.

Adler, Reid G. "Biotechnology as an Intellectual Property." *Science* 224 (4647) (1984): 357–363.

Adler, Reid G. "Genome Research: Fulfilling the Public's Expectation for Knowledge and Commercialization." *Science* 257 (5072) (1992): 908–914.

"The Age of AIDS." Frontline/PBS, New York, 2006. Available at http://www.pbs.org/wgbh/pages/frontline/aids, accessed January 20, 2014.

Ahmed, Rumman. "Update: Natco Pharma Seeks 'Compulsory License' for Copy of Pfizer Drug." January 5, 2011. Available at http://in.advfn.com/news_UPDATE-Natco-Pharma-Seeks-Compulsory-License-For-Copy-Of-Pfizer-Drug_45882508.html http://online.wsj.com/article/BT-CO-20110105-703261.htmlUPDATE, accessed January 20, 2014.

Alberts, Bruce. *Report of the Committee on Mapping and Sequencing the Human Genome of the Board on Basic Biology, Commission on Life Sciences, National Research Council.* Washington, DC: National Academy Press, 1988.

Alberts, Bruce, and Aaron Klug. "The Human Genome Itself Must Be Freely Available to All Humankind." *Nature* 404 (325) (2000): 325.

Alkhatib, Ghalib, Christophe Combadiere, Yu Feng, et al. "CC CKR5: A RANTES, MIP-1α, MIP-1β Receptor as a Fusion Cofactor for Macrophage-tropic HIV-1." *Science* 272 (5270) (1996): 1955–1958.

Alonzo, Francis III, Lina Kozhaya, Stephen A. Rawlings, et al. "CCR5 Is a Receptor for *Staphylococcus aureus* Leukotoxin ED." *Nature* 493 (7430) (2013): 51–55.

Altschul, S. F., W. Gish, W. Miller, et al. "Basic Local Alignment Search Tool." *Journal of Molecular Biology* 215 (3) (1990): 403–410.

Altshuler, David A., and The International HapMap Consortium. "A Haplotype Map of the Human Genome." *Nature* 437 (7063) (2005): 1299–1320.

Amernick, Burton A. *Patent Law for the Nonlawyer: A Guide for the Engineer, Technologist, and Manager.* 2nd ed. New York: Van Nostrand Reinhold, 1991.

Andrews, Lori B. "Genes and Patent Policy: Rethinking Intellectual Property Rights." *Nature Reviews: Genetics* 3 (10) (2002): 803–807.

Angell, Marcia. *The Truth about Drug Companies: How They Deceive Us and What to Do about It.* New York: Random House, 2005.

Ansari-Lari, M. A., X. M. Liu, M. L. Metzker, et al. "The Extent of Genetic Variation in the *CCR5* Gene." *Nature Genetics* 16 (3) (1997): 221–222.

Apriatin, S. A., E. R. Rakhmanaliev, I. A. Nikolaeva, et al. "Comparison [of] *CCR5del32* Mutation[s] in the *CCR5* Gene Frequencies in Russians, Tuvinians, and in Different Groups of HIV-Infected Individuals." *Genetika* 41 (2005): 1559–1562.

Arabatzis, Theodore. "Towards a Historical Ontology?" *Studies in History and Philosophy of Science* 34 (2) (2003): 431–442.

Arabatzis, Theodore. *Representing Electrons: A Biographical Approach to Theoretical Entities.* Chicago: University of Chicago Press, 2006.

Arenzana-Seisdedos, Fernando, and Marc Parmentier. "Genetics of Resistance to HIV Infection: Role of Co-receptors and Co-receptor Ligands." *Seminars in Immunology* 18 (6) (2006): 387–403.

Armour, Duncan. "The Discovery of CCR5 Receptor Antagonists for the Treatment of HIV Infection: Hit-to-Lead Studies." *ChemMedChem* 1 (7) (2006): 706–709.

Ashburn, Ted T., and Karl B. Thor. "Drug Repositioning: Identifying and Developing New Uses for Existing Drugs." *Nature Reviews. Drug Discovery* 3 (2004): 673–683.

Aymé, Ségolène, Gert Matthijs, and Sirpa Soini. "Patenting and Licensing in Genetic Testing: Recommendations of the European Society of Human Genetics." *European Journal of Human Genetics* 16 (8) (2008): 405–411.

Baba, Masanori, Osamu Nishimura, Naoyuki Kanzaki, et al. "A Small-Molecule Nonpeptide CCR5 Antagonist with Highly Potent and Selective Anti-HIV-1 Activity."

Proceedings of the National Academy of Sciences (PNAS) USA 96, no. 10 (1999): 5698–5703.

Baba, Masanori, Katsunori Takashima, Hiroshi Miyake, et al. "TAK-652 Inhibits CCR5-Mediated Human Immunodeficiency Virus Type 1 Infection in Vitro and Has Favorable Pharmacokinetics in Humans." *Antimicrobial Agents and Chemotherapy* 49 (11) (2005): 107–116.

Baggiolini, Marco. "Introduction." In *Chemokine Biology: Basic Research and Clinical Application,* ed. Bernhard Moser, Gordon L. Letts, and Kuldeep Neote, 3–15. Basel: Birkhäuser, 2006.

Bailey, Wendy J., William B. Vanti, Susan R. George, et al. "Patent Status of Therapeutically Important G Protein-Coupled Receptors." *Expert Opinion on Therapeutic Patents* 11 (12) (2001): 1861–1887.

Baker, Ronald. "HIVandHepatitis.com." Originally posted November 12, 2007. Available at http://web.archive.org/web/20071112031341/http://www.hivandhepatitis .com/recent/2007/091807_a.html, accessed January 20, 2014.

Bamshad, Michael J. "Genetic Influences on Health: Does Race Matter?" *Journal of the American Medical Association* 294 (8) (2005): 937–946.

Bamshad, Michael J., and Steve E. Olson. "Does Race Exist?" *Scientific American* 289 (6) (December 2003): 78–85.

Bamshad, Michael J., Stephen Wooding, Benjamin A. Salisbury, et al. "Deconstructing the Relationship between Genetics and Race." *Nature Reviews. Genetics* 5 (8) (2004): 598–609.

Bamshad, Michael J., Stephen Wooding, W. Scott Watkins, et al. "Human Population Genetic Structure and Inference of Group Membership." *American Journal of Human Genetics* 72 (3) (2003): 578–589.

Barbujani, Guido, Ariana Magagni, Eric Minch, et al. "An Apportionment of Human DNA Diversity." *Proceedings of the National Academy of Sciences (PNAS) USA* 94, (9) (1997): 4516–4519.

Barton, John H. "Patents, Genomics, Research and Diagnostics." *American Medicine* 77 (12) (1997): 1339–1347.

Batzer, M. A. "African Origin of Human-Specific Polymorphic *Alu* Insertions." *Proceedings of the National Academy of Sciences (PNAS) USA* 91, no. 25 (1994): 12,288–12,292.

Beauchamp, Christopher. "Patenting Nature: A Problem of History." *Stanford Technology Law Review* 16 (2) (2013): 257–311.

Begley, Sharon. "As Top Court Invalidates Some Gene Patents, Biotech Has Moved On." Reuters, June 13, 2013. Available at http://www.reuters.com/article/2013/06/13/ us-usa-court-genes-industry-idUSBRE95C1GD20130613, accessed January 20, 2014.

Benjamin, Walter. *The Arcades Project*. Translated by Howard Eiland and Kevin McLaughlin. Cambridge, MA: Belknap Press of Harvard University Press, 1999.

Bensaude-Vincent, Bernadette, and William R. Newman, eds. *The Artificial and the Natural: An Evolving Polarity*. Cambridge, MA: MIT Press, 2007.

Bentley, David R., and The International HapMap Consortium. "The International HapMap Project." *Nature* 426 (6968) (2003): 789–796.

Berg, Kate, and The Race, Ethnicity, and Genetics Working Group of the National Human Genome Research Institute. "Review Article: The Use of Racial, Ethnic, and Ancestral Categories in Human Genetics Research." *American Journal of Human Genetics* 77 (4) (2005): 519–532.

Berger, Edward A., Robert W. Doms, E.-M. Fenyö, et al. "A New Classification for HIV-1." *Nature* 391 (6664) (1998): 240.

Berger, Edward A., Philip M. Murphy, and Joshua M. Farber. "Chemokine Receptors as HIV-1 Coreceptors: Roles in Viral Entry, Tropism, and Disease." *Annual Review of Immunology* 17 (1999): 657–700.

Biehuoy, Shieh, Yao-Pei Yan, Nai-Ling Ko, et al. "Detection of Elevated Serum ß-Chemokine Levels in Seronegative Chinese Individuals Exposed to Human Immunodeficiency Virus Type 1." *Clinical Infectious Diseases* 33 (3) (2001): 273–279.

Biti, Robyn, Rosemary Ffrench, Judy Young, et al. "HIV-1 Infection in an Individual Homozygous for the *CCR5* Deletion Allele." *Nature Medicine* 3 (3) (1997): 252–253.

Blaak, Hetty, Angélique B. van't Wout, Margreet Brouwer, et al. "*In vivo* HIV-1 Infection of CD45RA+ CD4+ T Cells Is Established Primarily by Syncytium-Inducing Variants and Correlates with the Rate of CD4+ T Cell Decline." *Proceedings of the National Academy of Sciences (PNAS) USA* 97, no. 3 (2000): 1269–1274.

Blaug, Sasha, Michael Shuster, and Henry Su. "*Enzo Biochem v. Gen-Probe*: Complying with the Written Description Requirement under U.S. Patent Law." *Nature Biotechnology* 21, no. 1 (2003): 97–99.

Bloche, M. Gregg. "Race-Based Therapeutics." *New England Journal of Medicine* 351 (20) (2004): 2035–2037.

Blumenthal, D., E. G. Campbell, N. Causino, et al. "Withholding Research Results in Academic Life Science: Evidence from a National Survey of Faculty." *Journal of the American Medical Association* 277 (15) (1997): 1224–1228.

Bolnick, Deborah A. "Individual Ancestry Inference and Reification of Race as a Biological Phenomenon." In *Revisiting Race in a Genomic Age: Studies in Medical Anthropology*, ed. Barbara A. Koenig, Sandra Soo-Jin Lee, and Sarah S. Richardson, 70–85. New Brunswick, NJ: Rutgers University Press, 2008.

Botstein, D., R. L. White, M. Skolnick, et al. "Construction of a Genetic Linkage Map in Man Using Restriction Fragment Length Polymorphisms." *American Journal of Human Genetics* 32 (1980): 314–331.

Boyce, Nell, and Andy Coghlan. "Your Genes in Their Hands." *New Scientist* 2239 (May 15, 2000): 15.

Braun, Lundy. "Race, Ethnicity, and Health: Can Genetics Explain Disparities?" *Perspectives in Biology and Medicine* 45 (2) (2002): 159–174.

Brice, Philippa. "HapMap Project to Expand." *Phg Foundation: Making Science Work for Health*. February 11, 2005. Available at http://www.phgfoundation.org/news/833, accessed January 20, 2014.

Brinckerhoff, Courtenay C. "Protecting Invention in the U.S. and Europe: Inventors Need to Be Cognizant of Patent Laws on Both Sides of the Atlantic." *Genetic Engineering Biotechnology News* 28 (2008). Available at http://www.genengnews.com/gen-articles/protecting-inventions-in-the-u-s-and-europe/2385/, accessed January 20, 2014.

Broder, Samuel. "The Development of Antiretroviral Therapy and Its Impact on the HIV-1/AIDS Pandemic." *Antiretroviral Research* 85 (1) (2010): 1–38.

Brown, Bill. "Thing Theory." *Critical Inquiry* 28 (1) (2001): 1–22.

Bruttig, Stephen P., Garnette D. Draper, and Murray P. Hamlet. "Platelet-Endothelial Function in Relation to Environmental Temperature." *Medical Research and Development to Environmental Temperature* 84 (1983): 1–27.

Bugos, Glenn E., and Daniel J. Kevles. "Plants as Intellectual Property: American Practice, Law, and Policy in World Context." *Osiris*, 2nd ser., 7 (1992): 75–104.

Burchard, Esteban González, E. K. Silverman, L. R. Rosenwasser, et al. "Association between a Sequence Variant in the *IL-4* Gene Promoter and FEV_1 in Asthma." *American Journal of Respiratory and Critical Care Medicine* 160 (3) (1999): 919–922.

Burchard, Esteban González, Elad Ziv, Natasha Coyle, et al. "The Importance of Race and Ethnic Background in Biomedical Research and Clinical Practice." *New England Journal of Medicine* 348 (12) (2003): 1170–1175.

Burchfiel, Kenneth J. *Biotechnology and the Federal Circuit*. Washington, DC: Bureau of National Affairs, 1995/2001.

Burchfiel, Kenneth J. *Biotechnology and the Federal Circuit: 2005 Cumulative Supplement*. Washington, DC: Bureau of National Affairs, 2005.

Burger, Harold, and Donald Hoover. "HIV-1 Tropism, Disease Progression, and Clinical Management." *Journal of Infectious Diseases* 198 (8) (2008): 1095–1097.

Calafell, F. "Classifying Humans." *Human Genetics* 33 (4) (2003): 435–436.

Caledron, Tina M., and Joan W. Berman. "Overview and History of Chemokines and Their Receptors." In *Chemokines, Chemokine Receptors, and Disease*, ed. Lisa M. Schwiebert, 1–17. London: Elsevier, 2005.

Calvert, Jane, and Pierre-Benoît Joly. "How Did the Gene Become a Chemical Compound? The Ontology of the Gene and the Patenting of DNA." *Social Sciences Information. Information Sur les Sciences Sociales* 50 (2) (2011): 1–21.

Campbell, Eric G., Brian R. Clarridge, Manjusha Gokhate, et al. "Data Withholding in Academic Genetics." *Journal of the American Medical Association* 287 (4) (2002): 473–480.

Cao, Yunzhen, Limo Qin, Linqi Zhang, et al. "Virologic and Immunologic Characterization of Long-Term Survivors of Human Immunodeficiency Virus Type 1 Infection." *New England Journal of Medicine* 332 (4) (1995): 201–208.

Carbó-Droca, Ramon, Xavier Gironés, and Paul G. Mezey, eds. *Fundamentals of Molecular Similarity*. New York: Kluwer Academic / Plenum, 2001.

Carbone, Julia, E. Richard, Bhaven Sampat, et al. "DNA Patents and Diagnostics: Not a Pretty Picture." *Nature Biotechnology* 28 (8) (2010): 784–791.

Carfí, Andrea, Craig A. Smith, Pamela J. Smolak, et al. "Structure of a Soluble Secreted Chemokine Inhibitor vCCI (p35) from Cowpox Virus." *Proceedings of the National Academy of Sciences (PNAS) USA* 96, (22) (1999): 12,379–12,383.

Carrington, Mary, Michael Dean, Maureen P. Martin, et al. "Genetics of HIV-1 Infection: Chemokine Receptor *CCR5* Polymorphism and Its Consequences." *Human Molecular Genetics* 8 (10) (1999): 1939–1945.

Carrington, Mary, Terri Kissner, Bernard Gerrard, et al. "Novel Alleles of the Chemokine-Receptor Gene *CCR5*." *American Journal of Human Genetics* 61 (6) (1997): 1261–1267.

Carvalhaes, Fernanda Andreza de Pinho Lott, Greice Lemos Cardoso, Igor Guerreiro Hamoy, et al. "Distribution of *CCR5-Δ32, CCR2-64I, and SDF1-3'A* Mutations in Populations from the Brazilian Amazon Region." *Human Biology* 76, (4) (2004): 643–646.

Caulfield, Timothy. "Genesis of Neo-Racism? Biogenetics Discoveries about Race-Specific Idiosyncrasies Have a Dark Side." *Edmonton Journal*, December 22, 2007.

Caulfield, Timothy, Robert M. Cook-Deegan, F. Scott Kief, et al. "Evidence and Anecdotes: An Analysis of Human Gene Patenting Controversies." *Nature Biotechnology* 24 (9) (2006): 1091–1094.

Cavalli-Sforza, L. Luca. "Genes, Peoples, and Languages." *Scientific American* 265 (5) (1991): 104–110.

Cavalli-Sforza, L. Luca, and W. F. Bodmer. *The Genetics of Human Populations*. San Francisco: Freeman, 1971.

Chandrasekharan, Subhashini, Christopher Heaney, Tamara James, et al. "Impact of Gene Patents and Licensing Practices on Access to Genetic Testing for Cystic Fibrosis." *Genetics in Medicine* 12 (4 supp.) (2010): S194–S211.

Charo, Israel F., Scott J. Myers, Ann Herman, et al. "Molecular Cloning and Functional Expression of Two Monocyte Chemoattractant Protein 1 Receptors Reveals Alternative Splicing of the Carboxyl-Terminal Tails." *Proceedings of the National Academy of Sciences (PNAS) USA* 91, (7) (1994): 2752–2756.

Chartrand, Sabra. "A Human Gene Is Patented as a Potential Tool against AIDS, but Ethical Questions Remain." *New York Times*, March 6, 2000. Available at http://www.nytimes.com/2000/03/06/business/patents-human-gene-patented-potential-tool-against-aids-but-ethical-questions.html?pagewanted=all&src=pm, accessed January 20, 2014.

Cho, Mildred K., Samantha Illangasekare, Meredith A. Weaver, et al. "Effects of Patents and Licenses on the Provision of Clinical Genetic Testing Services." *Journal of Molecular Diagnostics* 5 (1) (2003): 3–8.

Choe, Hyeryun, Michael Farzan, Ying Sun, et al. "The β-Chemokine Receptors CCR3 and CCR5 Facilitate Infection by Primary HIV-1 Isolates." *Cell* 85 (7) (1996): 1135–1148.

Christodoulou, Christina, Marios Poullikas, Avidan U. Neumann, et al. "Low Frequency of *CCR5Δ32* Allele among Greeks in Cyprus." *AIDS Research and Human Retroviruses* 13 (16) (1997): 1373–1374.

Clerici, Mario, J. V. Giorgi, C. C. Chou, et al. "Cell-Mediated Immune Response to Human Immunodeficiency Virus (HIV) Type 1 in Seronegative Homosexual Men with Recent Sexual Exposure to HIV-1." *Journal of Infectious Diseases* 165 (6) (1992): 1012–1019.

Cocchi, Fiorenza, Anthony L. DeVico, Alfredo Garzino-Demo, et al. "Identification of RANTES, MIP-1α, and MIP-1β as the Major HIV-Suppressive Factors Produced by CD8+ T Cells." *Science* 270 (5243) (1995): 1811–1815.

Cohen, Jordan J. Public Comments on the United States Patent and Trademark Office, "Revised Interim Guidelines for Examination of Patent Applications under the 35 U.S.C. § 112, ¶1 'Written Description' Requirement." 64 *Federal Register* 71,427, December 21, 1999, comment 53. Available at http://www.uspto.gov/web/offices/com/sol/comments/utilitywd/aamc.pdf, accessed January 23, 2014.

Cohn, S. K., Jr., and L. T. Weaver. "The Black Death and AIDS: *CCR5-Δ32* in Genetics and History." *Quarterly Journal of Medicine* 99 (8) (2006): 497–503.

Collins, Francis. "What We Do and Don't Know about 'Race,' 'Ethnicity,' Genetics and Health at the Dawn of the Genome." *Nature Genetics Supplement* 36 (11) (2004): S13–S15.

Combadiere, Christophe, Sunil K. Ahuja, and Philip M. Murphy. "Cloning and Functional Expression of a Human Eosinophil CC Chemokine Receptor." *Journal of Biological Chemistry* 270 (27) (1995): 16,491–16,494.

Combadiere, Christophe, Sunil K. Ahuja, H. L. Tiffany, et al. "Cloning and Functional Expression of CC-CKR5, a Human Monocyte CC-Chemokine Receptor-Selective for MIP-1-α, MIP-1-β, and RANTES." *Journal of Leukocyte Biology* 60 (1) (1996): 147–152.

Comerford, Iain, and Shaun R. McColl. "Mini Review Series: Focus on Chemokines." *Immunology and Cell Biology* 89 (2011): 183–184.

Conley, John M., and Roberte Makowski. "Back to the Future: Rethinking the Product of Nature Doctrine as a Barrier to Biotechnology Patents." *Journal of the Patent and Trademark Office Society* 85 (2003): 301–370 (pt. 1) and 371–398 (pt. 2).

Connor, Ruth I., Kristine E. Sheridan, Daniel Ceradini, et al. "Change in Coreceptor Use Correlates with Disease Progression in HIV-1–Infected Individuals." *Journal of Experimental Medicine* 185 (4) (1997): 621–628.

Cook-Deegan, Robert. *The Gene Wars: Science, Politics, and the Human Genome.* New York: Norton, 1994.

Cook-Deegan, Robert, and Christopher Heaney. "Patents in Genomics and Human Genetics." *Annual Review of Genomics and Human Genetics* 11 (2010): 383–425.

Corey, George. Letter to the U.S. Patent and Trademark Office, March 22, 2000, in Public Comments on the United States Patent and Trademark Office, "Revised Interim Guidelines for Examination of Patent Applications under the 35 U.S.C. § 112, ¶1 'Written Description' Requirement," 64 *Federal Register* 71,427, December 21, 1999, comment 12, http://www.uspto.gov/web/offices/com/sol/comments/utilitywd/gcorey.pd, accessed January 23, 2014.

Creager, Angela N. H. *The Life of a Virus: Tobacco Mosaic Virus as an Experimental Model.* Chicago: University of Chicago Press, 2002.

Crespi, R. Stephen. "Patenting and Ethics: A Dubious Connection." *Journal of the Patent and Trademark Office Society* 85 (2003): 31–43.

Crespo, C. J., B. E. Ainsworth, S. J. Keteyian, et al. "Prevalence of Physical Inactivity and Its Relation to Social Class in U.S. Adults: Results from the Third National Health and Nutrition Survey, 1988–1994." *Medicine and Science in Sports and Exercise* 31 (12) (1999): 1821–1827.

Crouch, Dennis. "Patent Reform Act of 2011: An Overview." 2011. Available at http://www.patentlyo.com/patent/2011/02/patent-reform-act-of-2011-an-overview.html, accessed January 23, 2014.

Cui, Can. "Patentability of Molecules: Product of Nature Doctrine after Myriad." *Journal of Intellectual Property and Entertainment Law.* 2013. Available at http://jipel

.law.nyu.edu/2011/04/patent-eligibility-of-molecules-%E2%80%9Cproduct-of -nature%E2%80%9D-doctrine-after-myriad/#FN21, accessed January 20, 2014.

Cumming, J. G., A. E. Cooper, K. Grime, et al. "Modulators of the Human CCR5 Receptor. Part 2, SAR of Substituted 1-(3,3-Diphenylpropyl)-Piperidinyl Phenylacetamides." *Bioorganic and Medicinal Chemistry Letters* 15 (22) (2005): 5012–5015.

Daston, Lorraine, ed. *Biographies of Scientific Objects*. Chicago: University of Chicago Press, 2000.

Daston, Lorraine. "The Coming into Being of Scientific Objects." In *Biographies of Scientific Objects*, ed. Lorraine Daston, 1–14. Chicago: University of Chicago Press, 2000.

Davies, Kevin. *Cracking the Genome: Inside the Race to Crack the Human Genome*. Baltimore, MD: Johns Hopkins University Press, 2001.

Dean, Michael, Mary Carrington, Cheryl Winkler, et al. "Genetic Restriction of HIV-1 Infection and Progression to AIDS by a Deletion Allele of the *CKR5* [*CCR5*] Structural Gene." *Science* 273 (5283) (1996): 1856–1862.

De Clercq, Erik. "The History of Antiretrovirals: Key Discoveries over the Past Twenty-five Years." *Reviews in Medical Virology* 19 (5) (2009): 287–299.

Degerli, N., E. Yilmaz, F. Bardakci, et al. "The *Δ32* Allele Distribution of the *CCR5* Gene and Its Relationship with Certain Cancers in a Turkish Population." *Clinical Biochemistry* 28 (2005): 248–252.

DeGiulio, James. "The Genomic Research and Accessibility Act: More Science Fiction Than Fact." *Northwestern Journal of Technology and Intellectual Property* 8 (2010): 292–306.

Delwart, Eric L., Haynes W. Sheppard, Bruce D. Walker, et al. "Human Immunodeficiency Virus Type 1 in Vivo Tracked by DNA Heteroduplex Mobility Assays." *Journal of Virology* 68 (10) (1994): 6672–6683.

Delwart, Eric L., Eugene G. Shpaer, Joost Louwagie, et al. "Genetic Relationships Determined by a DNA Heteroduplex Mobility Assay Analysis of HIV-1 *env* Genes." *Science* 262 (5137) (1993): 1257–1261.

Demaine, L. J., and A. X. Fellmeth. "Reinventing the Double Helix: A Novel and Nonobvious Reconceptualization of the Biotechnology Patent." *Stanford Law Review* 55 (2) (2002): 303–462.

Deng, Hongkui, Rong Liu, Willfried Ellmeier, et al. "Identification of a Major Co-receptor for Primary Isolates of HIV-1." *Nature* 381 (6584) (1996): 661–666.

Desgranges, Claude, Patricia Carvajal, Alejandro Afani, et al. "Frequency of *CCR5* Gene 32-Basepair Deletion in Chilean HIV-1 Infected and Non-infected Individuals." *Immunology Letters* 76 (2) (2001): 115–117.

de Silva, Eric, and Michael P. H. Stumpf. "HIV and the *CCR5-Δ32* Resistance Allele." *FEMS Microbiology Letters* 241 (1) (2004): 1–12.

De Waal, Edmund. *The Hare with Amber Eyes: A Family's Century of Art and Loss*. New York: Farrar, Straus, and Giroux, 2010.

Dickinson, Q. Todd. "Guidelines for Examination of Patent Applications under the 35 U.S.C. 112, paragraph 1, 'Written Description' Requirement, USPTO." 66 *Federal Register* 1099–1111, January 5, 2001, notices.

Dickson, David. "NIH Opposes Plans for Patenting 'Similar' Gene Sequences." *Nature* 405 (6782) (2000): 3.

Diner, Byran C., and David S. Forman. "Emerging New Biotechnologies and the Patent Attorneys' Struggle to Best Protect Them." *Trends in Biotechnology*, January 2001. Available at http://www.finnegan.com/resources/articles/articlesdetail.aspx?news=7a7fdfb3-ce6a-4656-813d-9754f3a5d3af, accessed January 20, 2014.

Doll, John J. "Biotechnology: The Patenting of DNA." *Science* 280 (5364) (1998): 689–690.

Dood, Kendall J. "Patent Models and the Patent Law: 1790–1880 (Part I)" and "Patent Models and the Patent Law: 1790–1880 (Part II–Conclusion)." *Journal of the Patent Office Society* 65 (1983): 187–216, 234–274.

Doranz, Benjamin J., J. Rucker, F. R. Jirik, et al. "A Dual-Tropic Primary HIV-1 Isolate That Uses Fusin and the Beta-Chemokine Receptors CKR-5, CKR-3, and CKR-2b as Fusion Cofactors." *Cell* 85 (7) (1996): 1149–1158.

Dorn, Conrad P., Paul E. Finke, Bryan Oates, et al. "Antagonists of the Human CCR5 Receptor as Anti-HIV-1 Agents. Part 1, Discovery and Initial Structure-Activity Relationships for 1-Amino-2-Phenyl-4-(Piperidin-1-yl)Butanes." *Bioorganic and Medicinal Chemistry Letters* 11 (2) (2001): 259–264.

Dorr, Patrick, Mike Westby, S. Dobbs, et al. "Maraviroc (UK-427,857): A Potent, Orally Bioavailable, and Selective Small-Molecule Inhibitor of Chemokine Receptor CCR5 with Broad-Spectrum Anti-Human Immunodeficiency Virus Type 1 Activity." *Antimicrobial Agents and Chemotherapy* 49 (11) (2005): 4721–4732.

Downer, M. V., T. Dodge, D. K. Smith, et al. "Regional Variation in the *CCR5-Δ32* Distribution among Women from the U.S. HIV Epidemiology Research (HERS)." *Genes and Immunity* 3 (5) (2002): 295–298.

Dragic, Tatjana, Virginia Litwin, Graham P. Allaway, et al. "HIV-1 Entry into CD4+ Cells Is Mediated by the Chemokine Receptor CC-CKR-5." *Nature* 381 (6584) (1996): 667–673.

Drahos, Peter. *The Global Governance of Knowledge: Patent Offices and Their Clients*. New York: Cambridge University Press, 2010.

Drahos, Peter, with John Braithwaite. *Information Feudalism: Who Owns the Knowledge Economy?* New York: New Press, 2002.

Duncan, Scott R., Susan Scott, and C. J. Duncan. "Reappraisal of the Historical Selective Pressures for the *CCR5-Δ32* Mutation." *Journal of Medical Genetics* 42 (3) (2005): 205–208.

Durack, Katherine T. "Tacit Knowledge in Patent Applications: Observations on the Value of Models to Early U.S. Patent Office Practice and Potential Implications for the Twenty-first Century." *World Patent Information* 26 (2) (2004): 131–136.

Duster, Troy. "Buried Alive: The Concept of Race in Science." In *Genetic Nature/ Culture. Anthropology and Science beyond the Two-Culture Divide*, ed. A. H. Goodman, Deborah Heath, and M. Susan Lindee, 257–278. Berkeley: University of California Press, 1998.

Duster, Troy. "Race and Reification in Science." *Science* 307 (5712) (2005): 1050–1051.

Duster, Troy. "Theorizing a Difference: A Conceptual Advance. Books Forum: Differences That Matter." *Biosocieties* 3 (pt. 2) (2007): 225–226.

Dutfield, Graham. *Intellectual Property Rights and the Life Science Industries: Past, Present and Future.* 2nd ed. Hackensack, NJ: World Scientific, 2009.

Editorial Board of the New York Times. "India's Novartis Decision." *New York Times*, April 4, 2013. Available at http://www.nytimes.com/2013/04/05/opinion/the-supreme-court-in-india-clarifies-law-in-novartis-decision.html?_r=0, accessed January 24, 2014.

"Editorial: Census, Race and Science." *Nature Genetics* 24 (2) (2000): 97–98.

Eisenberg, Rebecca S. "Genes, Patents, and Product Developments." *Science* 257 (5072) (1992): 903–908.

Eisenberg, Rebecca S. "Patenting the Human Genome." *Emory Law Journal* 39 (3) (1990): 721–745.

Eisenberg, Rebecca S. "Re-Examining the Role of Patents in Appropriating the Value of DNA Sequences." *Emory Law Journal* 49 (3) (2000): 783–800.

Eisenberg, Rebecca S., and Robert P. Merges. "Opinion Letter as to the Patentability of Certain Inventions Associated with the Identification of Partial cDNA Sequences." *AIPLA Quarterly Journal* 23 (1) (1995): 1–52.

Elharti, Elmir, R. Elaouad, M. J. Simons, et al. "Letter to the Editor: Frequency of the *CCR5Δ32* Allele in the Moroccan Population." *AIDS Research and Human Retroviruses* 16 (1) (2000): 87–89.

Elvin, S. J., E. D. Williamson, J. C. Scott, et al. "Evolutionary Genetics: Ambiguous Role of CCR5 in *Y. pestis* Infection." *Nature* 430 (6998) (2004): 417.

Engelfriet, Arnoud. "Differences between U.S. and European Patents." *Ius Mentis: Law and Technology Explained*, October 1, 2005 Available at http://www.iusmentis .com/patents/uspto-epodiff/, accessed January 20, 2014.

Enserink, Martin. "Patent Office May Raise Bar on Gene Claims." *Science* 287 (5456) (2000): 1196–1197.

Epstein, Steven. "Bodily Differences and Collective Identities: The Politics of Gender and Race in Biomedical Research in the United States." *Body and Society* 10 (2–3) (2004): 183–203.

Epstein, Steven. *Impure Science: AIDS, Activism, and the Politics of Knowledge.* Berkeley: University of California Press, 1996.

Epstein, Steven. *Inclusion: The Politics of Difference in Medical Research.* Chicago: University of Chicago Press, 2007.

Epstein, Steven. "The Rise of 'Recruitmentology': Clinical Research, Racial Knowledge, and the Politics of Inclusion and Difference." *Social Studies of Science* 38 (5) (2008): 801–832.

Equils, Ozlem, Eileen Garratty, Lian S. Wei, et al. "Recovery of Replication-Competent Virus from CD4 T Cell Reservoirs and Change in Coreceptor Use in Human Immunodeficiency Virus Type 1–Infected Children Responding to Highly Active Antiretroviral Therapy." *Journal of Infectious Diseases* 182 (3) (2000): 751–757.

Esté, José A., Cecilia Cabrera, Julià Blanco, et al. "Shift of Clinical Human Immunodeficiency Virus Type 1 Isolates from X4 to R5 and Prevention of Emergence of the Syncytium-Inducing Phenotype by Blockade of CXCR4." *Journal of Virology* 73 (7) (1999): 5577–5585.

"The Fate of Gene Patents under the New Utility Guidelines." *Duke Law and Technology Review* 8, February 28, 2001. Available at http://www.law.duke.edu/journals/dltr/articles/2001dltr0008.html, accessed January 20, 2014.

Fätkenheuer, Gerd, Mark Nelson, Adriano Lazzarin, et al. "Subgroup Analyses of Maraviroc in Previously Treated R5 HIV-1 Infection." *New England Journal of Medicine* 359 (14) (2008): 1442–1455.

Faure, Eric, and Manuela Royer-Carenzi. "Is the European Spatial Distribution of the HIV-1 Resistant *CCR5-Δ32* Allele Formed by a Breakdown of the Pathocenosis Due to the Historical Roman Expansion?" *Infection, Genetics and Evolution* 8 (2008): 864–874.

"FDA Panel OKs Pfizer's Selzentry for Broader Us [sic] in HIV Naïve Patients, but Drug Criticized for Cost." *The Pharma Letter*, December 10, 2009, available at http://www.thepharmaletter.com/article/fda-panel-oks-pfizer-s-selzentry-for-broader-us-in-hiv-naive-patients-but-drug-criticized-for-its-cost, accessed January 20, 2014.

Federico, Pasquale J. "Patents for New Chemical Compounds." *Journal of the Patent Office Society* 21 (1939): 544–549.

Fellay, Jacques, Dongliang Ge, Kevin V. Shianna, et al. "Common Genetic Variation and the Control of HIV-1 in Humans." *PLoS Genetics* 5 (12) (2007): 1–12.

Fellay, Jacques, Kevin V. Shianna, Dongliang Ge, et al. "A Whole-Genome Association Study of Major Determinants for Host Control of HIV-1." *Science* 317 (5840) (2007): 944–947.

Feng, Tao, Anping Ni, Guocui Yang, et al. "Distribution of the *CCR5* Gene 32-Base Pair Deletion and *CCR5* Expression in Chinese Minorities." *Journal of Acquired Immune Deficiency Syndromes* 32 (2) (2003): 131–134.

Feng, Yu, Christopher C. Broder, Paul E. Kennedy, et al. "HIV-1 Entry Cofactor: Functional cDNA Cloning of a Seven-Transmembrane, G Protein-Coupled Receptor." *Science* 272 (5263) (1996): 872–877.

Fleischer, Arndt. *Patentgesetzgebung und chemisch-pharmazeutische Industrie im deutschen Kaiserreich (1871–1918). Mit einem Geleitwort von Rudolf Schmitz.* Stuttgart: Deutscher Apotheker Verlag, 1984.

Flexner, Charles. "HIV-Protease Inhibitors." *New England Journal of Medicine* 338 (18) (1998): 1281–1292.

Fortun, Michael. *Promising Genomics: Iceland and deCODE Genetics in a World of Speculation.* Berkeley: University of California Press, 2009.

"Forum on Race and Genomics." *Biosocieties* 2 (2007): 219.

Foster, Morris W. "Integrating Ethics and Science in the International HapMap Project." *Nature Reviews. Genetics* 5 (6) (2004): 467–475.

Foucault, Michel. *The History of Sexuality.* Vol. 1. New York: Vintage, 1978.

Foucault, Michel. "Nietzsche, la généalogie, l'histoire." In *Hommage à Jean Hyppolite*, 145–172. Paris: Presses Universitaires de France, 1971.

Foucault, Michel. "Nietzsche, Genealogy, History." In *The Foucault Reader*, ed. Paul Rabinow. New York: Pantheon Books, 1984.

Foucault, Michel. In *Work of Foucault: Ethics, Subjectivity, and Truth.* Vol. 1. Ed. Paul Rabinow. London: Penguin, 1997.

Fox, James M., and James E. Pease. "The Molecular and Cellular Biology of CC Chemokines and Their Receptors." In *Chemokines, Chemokine Receptors, and Disease: Current Topics in Membranes*, ed. Lisa M. Schwiebert, 73–102. San Diego: Academic Press, 2005.

Fox, Maggie. "German Doctors Declare 'Cure' in HIV Patient." Reuters, December 15, 2010. Available at http://www.reuters.com/article/2010/12/15/us-aids-transplant-idUSTRE6BE68220101215, accessed January 20, 2014.

Frankel, Alison. "U.S. Solicitor General to Make Unprecedented Federal Circuit Appearance in Myriad Case." *American Lawyer*, February 24, 2011. Available at http://www.americanlawyer.com/id=1202483155902, accessed January 20, 2014.

Freitas, Tamara, António Brehm, and Tedresa Fernandes. "Frequency of the *CCR5-Δ32* Mutation in the Atlantic Island Populations of Madeira, the Azores, Cabo Verde, and Sao Tomé e Príncipe." *Human Biology* 78 (6) (2006): 697–703.

Fujimura, Joan H., Troy Duster, and Ramya Rajagopalan. "Race, Human Genomics, and Biomedicine." *Social Studies of Science* 38 (5) (2008): 643–656.

Fujimura, Joan H., and Ramya Rajagopalan. "Different Differences: The Uses of 'Genetic Ancestry' versus Race in Biomedical Human Genetic Research." *Social Studies of Science* 41 (1) (2011): 5–30.

Fullwiley, Duana. "The Biologistical Construction of Race: 'Admixture Technology' and the New Genetic Medicine." *Social Studies of Science* 38 (5) (2008): 695–735.

Fullwiley, Duana. "The Molecularization of Race: Institutionalizing Human Difference in Pharmacogenetics Practice." *Science in Culture* 16 (1) (2007): 1–30.

Fullwiley, Duana. "The Molecularization of Race: U.S. Health Institutions, Pharmacogenetics Practice, and Public Science after the Genome." In *Revisiting Race in a Genomic Age: Studies in Medical Anthropology*, ed. Barbara A. Koenig, Sandra Soo-Jin Lee, and Sarah S. Richardson, 149–171. New Brunswick, NJ: Rutgers University Press, 2008.

Gallant, Joel E. "VICTOR-E3 and VICTOR-E4: Vicriviroc Plus PI-Based Optimized Background Regimen in Treatment-Experienced Patients." In *The CCO Independent Conference Coverage of the 2010 Conference on Retroviruses and Opportunistic Infections*, San Francisco, CA, 2010, available at http://www.clinicaloptions.com/login.aspx?item=%2fhiv%2fconference+coverage%2fretroviruses+2010%2fpodium%2fpodium%2fpages%2fpage+11&user=extranet%5cAnonymous&site=website&qs=, accessed January 20, 2014.

Galvani, Alison P., and Montgomery Slatkin. "Evaluating Plague and Smallpox as Historical Selective Pressures for the *CCR5-Δ32* HIV-Resistance Allele." *Proceedings of the National Academy of Sciences (PNAS) USA* 100 (25) (2003): 15,276–15,279.

Garnier, J.-B. "Rebuilding the R&D Engine in Big Pharma." *Harvard Business Review* 86 (5) (2008): 68–76.

Gaudillière, Jean-Paul. "Professional or Industrial Order? Patents, Biological Drugs, and Pharmaceutical Capitalism in Early Twentieth Century Germany." *History and Technology* 24 (2) (2008): 107–133.

Gibbons, Gary H., Choong Chin Liew, Mark O. Goodarzi, et al. "Markers of Malign across the Cardiovascular Continuum: Interpretation and Application." *Circulation* 109 (2004): IV-47–IV-58.

Giovannetti, A., F. Ensoli, F. Mazzetti, et al. "CCR5 and CXCR4 Chemokine Receptor Expression and β-Chemokine Production during Early T Cell Repopulation Induced by Highly Active Anti-retroviral Therapy." *Clinical and Experimental Immunology* 118 (1) (1999): 87–94.

Gissis, Snait B. "When Is 'Race' a Race? 1946–2003." *Studies in History and Philosophy of Science Part C* 39 (4) (2008): 437–450.

Gitter, Donna M. "International Conflicts over Patenting Human DNA Sequences in the United States and the European Union: An Argument for Compulsory Licensing and a Fair-Use Exemption." *NYU Law Review* 76 (6) (2001): 1623–1691.

Glushakova, Svetlana, Yanjie Yi, Jean-Charles Grivel, et al. "Preferential Coreceptor Utilization and Cytopathicity by Dual-Tropic HIV-1 in Human Lymphoid Tissue ex Vivo." *Journal of Clinical Investigation* 104 (5) (1999): R7–R11.

Gold, E. Richard, and Alain Gallochat. "The European Biotech Directive: Past as Prologue." *European Law Journal* 7 (3) (2001): 331–366.

Goldman, Bonnie. "A New Way to Fight HIV: CCR5 Inhibitors. An Interview with David Hardy, M.D." In *The Body: The Complete HIV/AIDS Resource*, April 30, 2008, available at http://www.thebody.com/content/art46473.html, accessed January 20, 2014.

Gonzalez, Enrique, Michael Bamshad, Naoko Sato, et al. "Race-Specific HIV-1 Disease-Modifying Effects Associated with *CCR5* Haplotypes." *Proceedings of the National Academy of Sciences (PNAS) USA* 96 (21) (1999): 12,004–12,009.

Gonzalez, Enrique, Rahul Dhanda, Mike Bamshad, et al. "Global Survey of Genetic Variation in *CCR5*, *RANTES*, and *MIP-1α*: Impact on the Epidemiology of the HIV-1 Pandemic." *Proceedings of the National Academy of Sciences (PNAS) USA* 98 (9) (2001): 5199–5204.

Gonzalez, Enrique, Hemant Kulkarni, Hector Bolivar, et al. "The Influence of *CCL3L1* Gene-Containing Segmental Duplications on HIV-1/AIDS Susceptibility." *Science* 307 (5715) (2005): 1434–1440.

Gosden, Chris, and Yvonne Marshall. "The Cultural Biography of Objects." *World Archaeology* 31 (2) (1999): 169–178.

Graff, Gregory D., Devon Phillips, Zhen Lei, et al. "Not Quite a Myriad of Gene Patents." *Nature Biotechnology* 31 (5) (2013): 404–410.

Greely, Henry T. "Genetic Genealogy: Genetics Meets the Marketplace." In *Revisiting Race in a Genomic Age*, ed. Barbara A. Koenig Sandra Soo-Jin Lee, and Sarah S. Richardson, 215–234. New Brunswick, NJ: Rutgers University Press, 2008.

Grisham, Julie. "New Rules for Gene Patents." *Nature Biotechnology* 18 (9) (2000): 921.

Grodzicker, T., J. Williams, P. Sharp, et al. "Physical Mapping of Temperature Sensitive Mutations." *Cold Spring Harbor Symposium Quarterly Biology* 39 (1) (1975): 439–446.

Gulick, Roy M., Jacob Lalezari, James Goodrich, et al. "Maraviroc for Previously Treated Patients with R5 HIV-1 Infection." *New England Journal of Medicine* 359 (14) (2008): 1429–1441.

Gutting, Gary. "Foucault's Genealogical Method." *Midwest Studies in Philosophy* 15 (15) (1990): 327–343.

Hamdan, Fadi F., Martin Audet, Philippe Garneau, et al. "High-Throughput Screening of G Protein-Coupled Receptor Antagonists Using a Bioluminescence Resonance Energy Transfer 1-Based ß-Arrestin2 Recruitment Assay." *Journal of Biomolecular Screening* 10 (5) (2005): 463–475.

Hamilton, Joan O. "How SmithKline and Incyte Became Lab Partners." *Signals Magazine*, December 22, 1997.

Hardy, W. David, Roy M. Gulick, Howard Mayer, et al. "Two-Year Safety and Virologic Efficacy of Maraviroc in Treatment-Experienced Patients with CCR5-Tropic HIV-1 Infection: Ninety-six-Week Combined Analysis of MOTIVATE 1 and 2." *Journal of Acquired Immune Deficiency Syndromes* 55 (5) (2010): 558–564.

Harkness, Jon M. "Dicta on Adrenalin(e): Myriad Problems with Learned Hand's Product-of-Nature Pronouncements in *Parke-Davis v. Mulford*." *Journal of the Patent and Trademark Office Society* 93 (4) (2011): 363–399.

He, Jianglin, Youzhi Chen, Michael Farzan, et al. "CCR3 and CCR5 Are Co-receptors for HIV-1 Infection of Microglia." *Nature* 385 (6617) (1997): 645–649.

Heath, Heidi, S. Qin, P. Rao, et al. "Chemokine Receptor Usage by Human Eosinophils: The Importance of CCR3 Demonstrated Using an Antagonistic Monoclonal Antibody." *Journal of Clinical Investigation* 99 (2) (1997): 178–184.

Hedrick, Philip W., and Brian C. Verrelli. "'Ground Truth' for Selection on *CCR5-Δ32*." *Trends in Genetics* 22 (6) (2006): 293–296.

Heller, M., and R. Eisenberg. "Can Patents Deter Innovation? The Anti-Commons in Biomedical Research." *Science* 280 (5364) (1998): 698–701.

Helmreich, Stefan. "Species of Biocapital." *Science as Culture* 17 (4) (2008): 463–478.

Hensley, Scott. "FDA Tells 23andMe to Stop Selling Popular Genetic Test." *NRP Health News*, November 25, 2013. Available at http://www.npr.org/blogs/health/2013/11/25/247198237/fda-tells-23andme-to-stop-selling-popular-genetic-test, accessed January 20, 2014.

Hensley, Scott. "23andMe Bows to FDA's Demands, Drops Health Claims." *NPR Health News*, December 6, 2013. Available at http://www.npr.org/blogs/health/

2013/12/06/249231236/23andme-bows-to-fdas-emands-drops-health-claims, accessed January 20, 2014.

"HGS Patent on HIV Sequence Found to Contain Sequence Errors: Is It or Is It Not Valid?" *Biotechnology Law Report* 19 (2000): 602–603. Available at http://online .liebertpub.com/doi/pdf/10.1089/073003100750036717, accessed January 20, 2014.

Highleyman, Liz. "MERIT Reanalysis with More Sensitive Trofile Test Shows Miraviroc (Selzentry) Works as well as Efaviren (Sustiva) in Patients New to Therapy." Paper presented at the Fifth-eighth Annual ICAAC and Forty-sixth Annual IDSA Meeting, October 25–28, 2008, in Washington, D.C., October 28, 2008. Available at http://www.hivandhepatitis.com/2008icr/icaac_idsa/docs/102808_c.html, accessed January 20, 2014.

Highleyman, Liz. "Monoclonal Antibody PRO 140 Suppresses HIV Viral Load with Once-Weekly Dosing," May 7, 2010. Available at http://www.hivandhepatitis.com/ recent/2010/0507_2010_b.html, accessed January 20, 2014.

Highleyman, Liz. "Vicriviroc Fails to Beat Stiff Competition, Merck Will Not File for Treatment-Experienced Approval." Paper presented at the Seventeenth Conference on Retroviruses and Opportunistic Infections (CROI 2010), February 16–19, 2010, San Francisco, California, February 19, 2010. Available at http://www .hivandhepatitis.com/2010_conference/croi/docs/0219_2010_f.html, accessed January 20, 2014.

Hilts, Philip J. *Scientific Temperaments: Three Lives in Contemporary Science.* New York: Simon & Schuster, 1982.

Hitti, Miranda. "Selzentry Is First in a New Class of HIV Drugs Made to Slow HIV's Advance, Says FDA." August 7, 2007. Available at http://www.webmd .com/hiv-aids/news/20070807/fda-oks-new-hiv-drug-selzentry, accessed January 20, 2014.

Hoke, Franklin. "Gene Patenting Is on the Rise, But Scientists Are Unimpressed." *The Scientist* 9 (1995): 1, 6–7.

Holman, Chris. "Holman's Biotech IP Blog, Genomics-Based Patents: Are Prophetic Assertions of Utility Enough?" December 1, 2008. Available at http:// holmansbiotechipblog.blogspot.com/2008/12/genomics-based-patents-are-prophetic .html, accessed January 20, 2014.

Holtzman, David. "Gene Patenting Guidelines: 'Magna Carta of Biotechnology.'" *Genetic Engineering News*, February 1, 2001. Available at http://www.mindfully .org/GE/Biotech-Magna-Carta.htm, accessed January 20, 2014.

Hope, Thomas J., and Didier Trono. "Structure, Expression, and Regulation of the HIV Genome." *UCSF HIVInSite*, November 2000. Available at http://hivinsite.ucsf .edu/InSite?page=kb-02-01-02, accessed January 20, 2014.

Hopkins, Michael M., Surya Mahdi, Pari Patel, et al. "DNA Patenting: The End of an Era?" *Nature Biotechnology* 25 (2) (2007): 185–187.

Horn, Tim. "Encouraging Data from Two Maraviroc Studies." *AIDSMEDS*, February 28, 2007. Available at http://www.aidsmeds.com/articles/1961_11404.shtml, accessed January 20, 2014.

Horuk, Richard. "Chemokine Receptors and HIV-1: The Fusion of Two Major Research Fields." *Immunology Today* 20 (2) (1999): 89–94.

Howell, R. Rodney. Public Comments on the United States Patent and Trademark Office, "Revised Interim Guidelines for Examination of Patent Applications under the 35 U.S.C. § 112, ¶1 'Written Description' Requirement," 64 *Federal Register* 71,427, December 21, 1999, comment 50, available at http://www.uspto.gov/web/offices/com/sol/comments/utilitywd/acmg.pdf, accessed January 23, 2014.

Huang, K. G., and F. E. Murray. "Does Patent Strategy Shape the Long-Run Supply of Public Knowledge? Evidence from Human Genetics." *Academy of Management Journal* 52 (6) (2009): 1193–1221.

Huang, Yaoxing, William A. Paxton, Steven M. Wolinsky, et al. "The Role of Mutant *CCR5* Allele in HIV-1 Transmission and Disease Progression." *Nature Medicine* 2 (11) (1996): 1240–1243.

"Human Genome Sciences Receives Patent on AIDS Virus Entry Point," February 16, 2000, available at http://www.prnewswire.com/news-releases/human-genome-sciences-receives-patent-on-aids-virus-entry-point-72613242.html, last accessed on January 24, 2014.

Hummel, S., D. Schmidt, B. Kremeyer, et al. "Detection of the *CCR5-Δ32* HIV Resistance Gene in Bronze Age Skeletons." *Genes and Immunity* 6 (2005): 371–374.

Hütter, Gero, Daniel Nowak, Maximilian Mossner, et al. "Long-Term Control of HIV by *CCR5* Delta 32/Delta 32 Stem-Cell Transplantation." *New England Journal of Medicine* 360 (7) (2009): 692–698.

Hyde, Lewis. *Common as Air: Revolution, Art, and Ownership.* New York: Farrar, Straus and Giroux, 2010.

Idemyor, Vincent. "Human Immunodeficiency Virus (HIV) Entry Inhibitors (CCR5 Specific Blockers) in Development: Are They the Next Novel Therapies?" *HIV Clinical Trials* 6 (5) (2005): 272–277.

Imagawa, David T., and R. Detels. "HIV-1 in Seronegative Homosexual Men." *New England Journal of Medicine* 325 (17) (1991): 1250–1251.

Imagawa, David T., Moon H. Lee, Steven M. Wolinsky, et al. "Human Immunodeficiency Virus Type 1 in Homosexual Men Who Remain Seronegative for Prolonged

Periods." *New England Journal of Medicine* 320 (22) (1989): 1458–1462 and 321 (24) (1989): 1681.

Jackson, Catherine M. "Re-examining the Research School: August Wilhelm Hoffmann and the Re-creation of a Creation of a Liebigian Research School in London." *History of Science* 44 (2006): 281–319.

Jacobs, Paul, and Peter G. Gosselin. "Profiteering and Shoddy Science: Errors Found in Patent of AIDS Gene, Scientists Say; News Comes amid Concerns That Genomics Race Could Lead to Shoddy Science and Profiteering." *Los Angeles Times*, March 21, 2000. Available at http://www.commondreams.org/headlines/032100-02.htm, accessed January 21, 2014.

Jacobs, Paul, and Peter G. Gosselin. "'Robber Barons of the Genetic Age': Experts Fret over the Effect of Gene Patents of Research." *Los Angeles Times*, February 28, 2000. Available at http://articles.latimes.com/2000/feb/28/news/mn-3512, accessed January 21, 2014.

Jacobson, Jeffrey M., Melanie A. Thompson, Jacob P. Lalezari, et al. "Anti-HIV-1 Activity of Weekly or Biweekly Treatment with Subcutaneous PRO 140, a CCR5 Monoclonal Antibody." *Journal of Infectious Diseases* 201 (10) (2010): 1481–1487.

Janeway, Charles A., Jr., Paul Travers, Mark Walport, et al. *Immunobiology*. New York: Garland, 1994.

Jasanoff, Sheila. *Designs on Nature: Science and Democracy in Europe and the United States*. Princeton, NJ: Princeton University Press, 2005.

Jasanoff, Sheila. *The Fifth Branch: Science Advisers as Policymakers*. Cambridge, MA: Harvard University Press, 1990.

Jasanoff, Sheila. "The Idiom of Co-Production." In *States of Knowledge: The Co-Production of Science and the Social Order*, ed. Sheila Jasanoff, 1–12. London: Routledge, 2004.

Jasanoff, Sheila. "Introduction." In *Reframing Rights: Bioconstitutionalism in the Genetic Age*, ed. Sheila Jasanoff, 1–28. Cambridge, MA: MIT Press, 2011.

Jasanoff, Sheila. *Science at the Bar: Law, Science, and Technology in America*. Cambridge, MA: Harvard University Press, 1995.

Jeffrey, A. J. "DNA Sequence Variants in the $^G\gamma$-, $^A\gamma$-, δ- and β-Globin Genes of Man." *Cell* 18 (1) (1979): 1–10.

Jensen, Kyle, and Fiona Murray. "Intellectual Property Enhanced: Intellectual Property Landscape of the Human Genome." *Science* 310 (5746) (2005): 239–240.

Jiang, Jian-Dong, Yue Wang, Z.-Z. Wang, et al. "Low Frequency of the $CCR5\Delta32$ HIV-Resistance Allele in Mainland China: Identification of the First Case of

CCR5Δ32 Mutation in the Chinese Population." *Scandinavian Journal of Infectious Diseases* 31 (4) (1999): 345–348.

Johnson, Jeffrey Alan. *The Kaiser's Chemists: Science and Modernization in Imperial Germany*. Chapel Hill, NC: University of North Carolina Press, 1990.

Johnston, Sean A. Public Comments on the United States Patent and Trademark Office, "Revised Interim Guidelines for Examination of Patent Applications under the 35 U.S.C. § 112, ¶1 'Written Description' Requirement." Letter to Mark Nagumo, Steven Walsh, Linda Therkorn, March 22, 2000, 64 *Federal Register* 71,427, December 21, 1999, comment 59. Available at http://www.uspto.gov/web/offices/com/sol/comments/utilitywd/genentech.pdf, accessed January 24, 2014.

Jorde, Lynn B., W. S. Watkins, and M. J. Bamshad. "The Distribution of Human Genetic Diversity: A Comparison of Mitochondrial, Autosomal, and Y Chromosome Data." *American Journal of Human Genetics* 66 (3) (2003): 979–988.

Jorde, Lynn B., and Stephen P. Wooding. "Genetic Variation, Classification and 'Race.'" *Nature Genetics* 36 (no. 11S) (2004): S28–S33.

Kahn, Jonathan. "Exploiting Race in Drug Development: BiDil's Interim Model of Pharmacogenomics." *Social Studies of Science* 38 (5) (2008): 737–758.

Kahn, Jonathan. "From Disparity to Difference: How Race-Specific Medicines May Undermine Policies to Address Inequalities in Health Care." *Southern California Interdisciplinary Law Journal* 15 (2005): 105–129.

Kahn, Jonathan. *Race in a Bottle: The Story of BiDil and Racialized Medicine in a Post-Genomic Age*. New York: Columbia University Press, 2013.

Kaiser, Joseph. *Das Deutsche Patentgesetz vom 7. April 1891*. Leipzig: A. Deichert'sche Verlagsbuchhandlung Nachf. Georg Böhme, 1907.

Kalev, I., A.-V. Mikelsaar, L. Beckman, et al. "High Frequency of the HIV-1 Protective *CCR5Δ32* Deletion in Native Estonians." *European Journal of Epidemiology* 16 (2000): 1107–1109.

Kantor, R., and J. M. Gershoni. "Distribution of the *CCR5* Gene 32-Base Pair Deletion in Israeli Ethnic Groups." *Journal of Acquired Immune Deficiency Syndromes and Human Retrovirology* 20 (1) (1999): 81–84.

Kaplan, Warren A., and Sheldon Krimsky. "Patentability of Biotechnology Inventions and the PTO Utility Guidelines: Still Uncertain after All These Years?" 2001. Available at http://www.tufts.edu/~skrimsky/PDF/patentability.PDF, accessed January 21, 2014.

Kaslow, Richard A. "The Multicenter AIDS Cohort Study: Rationale, Organization, and Selected Characteristics of the Participants." *American Journal of Epidemiology* 126 (2) (1986): 310–318.

Katznelson, Ron D. "Bad Science in Search of 'Bad' Patents." *Federal Circuit Bar Journal* 17 (1) (2007): 1–30.

Kevles, Daniel J. "Ananda M. Chakrabarty Wins a Patent: Biotechnology, Law, and Society." *Historical Studies in the Physical and Biological Sciences* 25 (1) (1994): 111–135.

Kevles, Daniel J. "Inventions, Yes: Nature, No: The Birth of the Products-of-Nature Doctrine in the American Colonies and Courts." Forthcoming in *Perspectives on Science* 23 (1) (2014).

Kevles, Daniel J. "Of Mice and Money: The Story of the World's First Animal Patent." *Daedalus* 131 (2) (2002): 78–88.

Kevles, Daniel J. "Out of Eugenics: The Historical Politics of the Human Genome." In *The Code of Codes: Scientific and Social Issues in the Human Genome Project*, ed. Daniel J. Kevles and Leroy Hood, 3–36. Cambridge, MA: Harvard University Press, 1992.

Kevles, Daniel J. "Patents, Protections, and Privileges: The Establishment of Intellectual Property in Animals and Plants." *Isis* 98 (2) (2007): 323–331.

Kiley, Thomas D. "Patent on Random Complementary DNA Fragments?" *Science* 257 (5072) (1992): 915–918.

King, M.-C., and A. G. Motulsky. "Mapping Human History." *Science* 298 (5602) (2002): 2342–2343.

Kingston, W. "Removing Some Harm from the World Trade Organization." *Oxford Development Studies* 32 (2) (2004): 309–320.

Klitz, William, Chaim Brautbar, Anna M. Schito, et al. "Evolution of the *CCR5 Δ32* Mutation Based on Haplotype Variation in Jewish and Northern European Population Samples." *Human Immunology* 62 (5) (2001): 530–538.

Knudson, William A. "An Introduction to Patents, Brands, Trade Secrets, Trademarks, and Intellectual Property Rights Issues." August 2006, 2–3. Available at http://productcenter.msu.edu/uploads/files/ippaper%202.pdf, accessed January 21, 2014.

Kock, Michael A. "Purpose-Bound Protection for DNA Sequences: In through the Back Door?" *Journal of Intellectual Property Law and Practice* 5 (7) (2010): 495–513.

Kohl, N. E., E. A. Emini, W. A. Schleif, et al. "Active Human Immunodeficiency Virus Protease Is Required for Viral Infectivity." *Proceedings of the National Academy of Sciences (PNAS) USA* 85, (13) (1988): 4686–4690.

Kohler, Robert E. *Lords of the Fly: Drosophila Genetics and the Experimental Life*. Chicago: University of Chicago Press, 1994.

Kondru, Rama, Jun Zhang, Changhua Ji, et al. "Molecular Interactions of CCR5 with Major Classes of Small-Molecule Anti-HIV CCR5 Antagonists." *Molecular Pharmacology* 73 (3) (2008): 789–800.

Kopytoff, Igor. "The Cultural Biography of Things." In *The Social Life of Things: Commodities in Cultural Perspective*, ed. Arjun Appadurai, 64–91. New York: Cambridge University Press, 1988.

Kreitman, Martin, and Anna Di Rienzo. "Balancing Claims for Balancing Selection." *Trends in Genetics* 20 (7) (2004): 300–304.

Krimsky, Sheldon. *Science in the Private Interest: Has the Lure of Profits Corrupted Biomedical Research?* Lanham, MD: Rowman & Littlefield, 2003.

Kruglyak, Leonid. "The Road to Genome-Wide Association Studies." *Nature Reviews. Genetics* 9 (4) (2008): 314–318.

Kruglyak, Leonid. "The Use of a Genetic Map of Biallelic Markers in Linkage Studies." *Nature Genetics* 17 (1) (1997): 21–24.

Kuritzkes, Daniel, Santwana Kar, and Peter Kirkpatrick, et al. "Maraviroc." *Nature Reviews. Drug Discovery* 7 (1) (2008): 15–16.

Kurlansky, Mark. *Salt: A World History*. New York: Penguin, 2002.

Lahana, Roger. "Who Wants to Be Irrational?" *Drug Discovery Today* 8 (15) (2003): 655–656.

Lalani, Alshad S., Jennefer Masters, Wei Zeng, et al. "Use of Chemokine Receptors by Poxviruses." *Science* 286 (5446) (1999): 1968–1971.

Lalezari, J. P., J. J. Eron, M. Carlson, et al. "A Phase II Clinical Study of the Long-Term Safety and Antiviral Activity of Enfuvirtide-Based Antiretroviral Therapy." *AIDS* 17 (5) (2003): 691–698.

Lalezari, J. P., G. K. Yadavalli, M. Para, et al. "Safety, Pharmacokinetics, and Antiviral Activity of HGS004, a Novel Fully Human IgG4 Monoclonal Antibody against CCR5, in HIV-1-Infected Patients." *Journal of Infectious Diseases* 197 (5) (2008): 721–727.

LaMattina, John L. *Drug Truths: Dispelling the Myths about Pharma R&D*. Hoboken, NJ: Wiley, 2009.

Landecker, Hannah. *Culturing Life: How Cells Became Technologies*. Cambridge, MA: Harvard University Press, 2007.

Landers, Jim. "Trouble Impending in Patent Process." *Dallas Morning News*, May 1, 2007. Available at http://www.inventionstatistics.com/Patent_Office.html and http://www.inventionstatistics.com/Patent_Backlog_Patent_Office_Backlog.html, both accessed January 21, 2014.

Landers, P. "Drug Industry's Big Push into Technology Falls Short: Testing Machines Were Built to Streamline Research—but May Be Stifling It." *Wall Street Journal*, February 24, 2004, A1.

Langlade-Demoyen, P., N. Ngo-Giang-Huong, F. Ferchal, et al. "Human Immunodeficiency Virus (HIV) Nef-Specific Cytotoxic T Lymphocytes in Noninfected Heterosexual Contact of HIV-Infected Patients." *Journal of Clinical Investigation* 93 (3) (1994): 1293–1297.

Langreth, Robert. "Beyond Talk." *Forbes* 172 (2003): 72–75.

Lareau, Annette. "Invisible Inequality: Social Class and Childrearing in Black Families and White Families." *American Sociological Review* 67 (5) (2002): 747–776.

Latinovic, Olga, Marvin Reitz, Nhut M. Le, et al. "CCR5 Antibodies HGS004 and HGS101 Preferentially Inhibit Drug-Bound CCR5 Infection and Restore Drug Sensitivity of Maraviroc-Resistant HIV-1 in Primary Cells." *Virology* 411 (1) (2011): 32–40.

Latour, Bruno. "On the Partial Existence of Existing and Nonexisting Objects." In *Biographies of Scientific Objects*, ed. Lorraine Daston, 247–269. Chicago: University of Chicago Press, 2000.

Latour, Bruno. *Science in Action: How to Follow Scientists and Engineers through Society*. Cambridge, MA: Harvard University Press, 1987.

Leboute, A. P. M., M. W. P. de Carvalho, and A. L. Simoes, et al. "Absence of the *Δccr5* Mutation in Indigenous Populations of the Brazilian Amazon." *Human Genetics* 105 (5) (1999): 442–443.

Lee, Catherine. "'Race' and 'Ethnicity' in Biomedical Research: How Do Scientists Construct and Explain Differences in Health?" *Social Science and Medicine* 68 (6) (2009): 1183–1190.

Lesch, John E. *The First Miracle Drugs: How the Sulpha Drugs Transformed Medicine*. New York: Oxford University Press, 2007.

Levin, Jules. "Efficacy and Safety of Maraviroc Plus Optimized Background Therapy in Treatment-Experienced Patients Infected with CCR5-Tropic HIV-1: Forty-eight-Week Combined Analysis of the MOTIVATE Studies—Pooled Analysis of MOTIVATE 1 and 2." Paper presented at the Fifteenth Annual Meeting of CROI, February 3–6, 2008, Boston, MA. Available at http://www.natap.org/2008/CROI/croi_43.htm, accessed January 21, 2014.

Levy, Jay A., Carl E. Mackewicz, and Edward Barker. "Controlling HIV Pathogenesis: The Role of the Noncytotoxic Anti-HIV Response of CD8(+) T Cells." *Immunology Today* 17 (5) (1996): 217–224.

Levy, Samuel, Granger Sutton, Pauline C. Ng, et al. "The Diploid Genome Sequence of an Individual Human." *PLoS Biology* 5 (10) (2007): 2113–2144.

Li, C., S. C. Lu, P. S. Hsieh, et al. "Distribution of Human Chemokine (C-X3-C) Receptor 1 (*CX3CR1*) Gene Polymorphisms and Haplotypes of the CC Chemokine

Receptor 5 (*CCR5*) Promoter in Chinese People, and the Effects of CCR5 Haplotypes on CCR5 Expression." *International Journal of Immunogenetics* 32 (2) (2005): 99–106.

Li, C., Y. P. Yan, B. Shieh, et al. "Frequency of the *CCR5 Delta 32* Mutant Allele in HIV-1-Positive Patients, Female Sex Workers, and a Normal Population in Taiwan." *Journal of the Formosan Medical Association* 96 (12) (1997): 979–984.

Libert, Frédérick, Pascale Cochaux, Gunhild Beckman, et al. "The *Δccr5* Mutation Conferring Protection against HIV-1 in Caucasian Populations Has a Single and Recent Origin in Northeastern Europe." *Human Molecular Genetics* 7 (3) (1998): 399–406.

Liebenau, Jonathan. "Industrial R&D in Pharmaceutical Firms in the Early Twentieth Century." *Business History* 26 (3) (1984): 329–346.

Liebenau, Jonathan. "Patents and the Chemical Industry: Tools of Business Strategy." In *The Challenge of New Technology: Innovation in British Business since 1850*, ed. Jonathan Liebenau, 135–150. Brookfield, VT: Gower, 1988.

Lin, Nina H., and Daniel R. Kuritzkes. "Tropism Testing in the Clinical Management of HIV-1 Infection." *Current Opinions in HIV and AIDS* 4 (6) (2009): 481–487.

Liu, H., E. E. Nakayama, I. Theodorou, et al. "Polymorphisms in *CCR5* Chemokine Receptor Gene in Japan." *International Journal of Immunogenetics* 34 (5) (2007): 325–335.

Liu, Rong, William A. Paxton, Sunny Choe, et al. "Homozygous Defect in HIV-1 Coreceptor Accounts for Resistance of Some Multiply-Exposed Individuals to HIV-Infection." *Cell* 86 (3) (1996): 367–377.

Lucotte, Gérard. "Frequencies of the CC Chemokine Receptor 5 *Δ32* Allele in Various Populations of Defined Racial Background." *Biomedicine and Pharmacotherapy* 51 (10) (1997): 469–473.

Lucotte, Gérard. "Frequencies of 32 Base Pair Deletion of the (*Δ32*) Allele of the *CCR5* HIV-1 Co-receptor Gene in Caucasians: A Comparative Analysis." *Infection, Genetics and Evolution* 1 (3) (2002): 201–205.

Lucotte, Gérard, and Florent Dieterlen. "More about the Viking Hypothesis of Origin of the *Δ32* Mutation in the *CCR5* Gene Conferring Resistance to HIV-1 Infection." *Infection, Genetics and Evolution* 3 (4) (2003): 293–295.

Lucotte, Gérard, and Géraldine Mercier. "*Δ32* Mutation Frequencies of the CCR5 Coreceptor in Different French Regions." Comptes rendus de l'Academie des Sciences, Series III. *Sciences de la Vie* 321 (5) (1998): 409–413.

Lucotte, Gérard, and Géraldine Mercier. "Distribution of the *CCR5* Gene 32-bp Deletion in Europe." *Journal of Acquired Immune Deficiency Syndromes and Human Retrovirology* 19 (2) (1998): 174–177.

Lucotte, Gérard, and P. Smets. "*CCR5-Δ32* Allele Frequencies in Ashkenazi Jews." *Genetic Testing* 7 (4) (2003): 333–337.

Ludlam, Charles E. Public Comments on the United States Patent and Trademark Office, "Revised Interim Guidelines for Examination of Patent Applications under the 35 U.S.C. § 112, ¶1 'Written Description' Requirement." 64 *Federal Register* 71,427, December 21, 1999, comment 55, http://www.uspto.gov/web/offices/com/ sol/comments/utilitywd/bio.pdf, accessed January 23, 2014.

Ma, Liying, Michael Marmor, Ping Zhong, et al. "Distribution of *CCR2-64I* and *SDF1-3'A* Alleles and HIV Status in Seven Ethnic Populations of Cameroon." *Journal of Acquired Immune Deficiency Syndromes and Human Retrovirology* 40 (1) (2005): 89–95.

Maayan, S., L. Zhang, E. Shinar, et al. "Evidence for Recent Selection of the *CCR5-delta 32* Deletion from Differences in Its Frequency between Ashkenazi and Sephardic Jews." *Genes and Immunity* 1 (6) (2000): 358–361.

Macarron, Ricardo, Martyn N. Banks, Dejan Bojanic, et al. "Impact of High-Throughput Screening in Biomedical Research." *Nature Reviews: Drug Discovery* 10 (3) (2011): 188–195.

MacGregor, Neil. *A History of the World in One Hundred Objects*. New York: Viking Penguin, 2011.

MacKenzie, Donald. *Inventing Accuracy: A Historical Sociology of Nuclear Missile Guidance*. Cambridge, MA: MIT Press, 1990.

Magierowska, Magda, Virginia Lepage, Ludmila Boubnova, et al. "Distribution of the *CCR5* Gene 32 Base Pair Deletion and *SDF1-3'A* Variant in Healthy Individuals from Different Populations." *Immunogenetics* 48 (6) (1998): 417–419.

Mangano, A., G. Theiler, L. Sala, et al. "Distribution of *CCR5-Δ32* and *CCR2-64I* Alleles in an Argentine Amerindian Population." *Tissue Antigens* 58 (2) (2001): 99–102.

Marshall, Eliot. "HIV Experts vs. Sequencers in Patent Race." *Science* 275 (5304) (1997): 1263.

Marshall, Eliot. "Patent on HIV Receptor Provokes Outcry." *Science* 287 (5457) (2000): 1375–1377.

Martin, Brian, and Evelleen Richards. "Scientific Knowledge, Controversy, and Public Decision Making." In *Handbook of Science and Technology Studies*, ed. Sheila Jasanoff, Gerald E. Markle, James C. Petersen, et al., 506–522. Newbury Park, CA: Sage, 1995.

Martin, Maureen P., Michael Dean, Michael W. Smith, et al. "Genetic Acceleration of AIDS Progression by a Promoter Variant of *CCR5*." *Science* 282 (5395) (1998): 1907–1911.

Martinson, Jeremy J., Nicola H. Chapman, David C. Rees, et al. "Global Distribution of the *CCR5* Gene 32-Basepair Deletion." *Nature Genetics* 16 (1) (1997): 100–103.

Martinson, Jeremy J., Lily Hong, Rose Karanicolas, et al. "Global Distribution of the *CCR2-64I/CCR5-59653T* HIV-1 Disease-Protective Haplotype." *AIDS* 14 (5) (2000): 483–489.

Mason, Matt. *The Pirate's Dilemma: How Youth Is Reinventing Capitalism.* New York: Free Press, 2009.

Masquelier, Cecile, Jean-Yves Servais, Emmanuel Rusanganwa, et al. "A Novel 24-Base Pair Deletion in the Coding Region of *CCR5* in African Population." *AIDS* 21 (1) (2007): 111–113.

McCabe, Linda L., and Edward R. B. McCabe. *DNA: Promise and Peril.* Berkeley: University of California Press, 2008.

McGarrigle, Philip, and Vern Norviel. "Laws of Nature and the Business of Biotechnology." *Santa Clara Computer and High-Technology Law Journal* 24 (2) (2008): 275–334.

McGowan, Joseph P., and Sanjiv Shah. "Understanding HIV Tropism." *Physicians Research Network (PRN) Notebook* 15 (January 2010). Available at http://www.prn .org/index.php/management/article/hiv_tropism_1002, accessed January 21, 2014.

McVean, Gilean, and The International HapMap Consortium. "A Second Generation Human Haplotype Map of Over 3.1 Million SNPs." *Nature* 449 (7164) (2007): 851–861.

Mecsas, Joan, Greg Franklin, William A. Kuziel, et al. "Evolutionary Genetics: CCR5 Mutation and Plague Protection." *Nature* 427 (6975) (2004): 606.

Merges, Robert P. "As Many as Six Impossible Patents before Breakfast: Property Rights for Business Concepts and Patent System Reform." *Berkeley Technology Law Journal* 14 (1999): 577–615.

Merges, Robert P., Peter S. Menell, and Mark A. Lemley. et al. *Intellectual Property in the New Technological Age.* 4th ed. New York: Aspen, 2004.

Merrill, Stephen A., and Anne-Marie Mazza, eds. *Reaping the Benefits of Genomic and Proteomic Research.* Washington, DC: National Academies Press, 2006.

Merz, John F., Antigone G. Kriss, D. G. B. Lenard, et al. "Diagnostic Testing Fails the Test: The Pitfalls of Patents Are Illustrated by the Case of Haemochromatosis." *Nature* 415 (6872) (2002): 577–579.

Miller, Arthur R., and Michael H. Davis. *Intellectual Property: Patents, Trademarks, and Copyrights in a Nutshell.* 2nd ed. St. Paul, MN: West, 1990.

Montoya, Michael. *Making the Mexican Diabetic: Race, Science, and the Genetics of Inequality.* Berkeley: University of California Press, 2011.

Morning, Ann. *The Nature of Race: How Scientists Think and Teach about Human Difference*. Berkeley: University of California Press, 2011.

Moses, Hamilton III, E. R. Dorsey, D. H. Matheson, et al. "Financial Anatomy of Biomedical Research." *Journal of the American Medical Association* 294 (3) (2005): 1333–1342.

Mountain, J. L., and L. L. Cavalli-Sforza. "Multilocus Genotypes, a Tree of Individuals, and Human Evolutionary History." *American Journal of Human Genetics* 61 (3) (1997): 705–718.

Mowery, D. C., and N. Rosenberg. *Paths of Innovation: Technological Change in Twentieth-Century America*. New York: Cambridge University Press, 1988.

Mull, William C. "Note: Using the Written Description Requirement to Limit Broad Patent Scope, Allow Competition, and Encourage Innovation in Biotechnology." *Health Matrix* 14 (2004): 393–435.

Mullin, Rick. "As High-Throughput Screening Draws Fire, Researchers Leverage Science to Put Automation into Perspective." *Chemical and Engineering News* 82 (30) (2004): 23–32.

Mummidi, Srinivas, Seema S. Ahuja, Enrique Gonzalez, et al. "Genealogy of the *CCR5* Locus and Chemokine System Gene Variants Associated with Altered Rates of HIV-1 Disease Progression." *Nature Medicine* 4 (7) (1998): 786–793.

Mummidi, Srinivas, Mike Bamshad, Seema S. Ahuja, et al. "Evolution of Human and Non-human Primate CC Chemokine Receptor 5 Gene and mRNA: Potential Roles for Haplotype and mRNA Diversity, Differential Haplotype-Specific Transcriptional Activity, and Altered Transcription Factor Binding to Polymorphic Nucleotides in the Pathogenesis of HIV-1 and Simian Immunodeficiency Virus." *Journal of Biological Chemistry* 275 (25) (2000): 18,946–18,961.

Murray, Fiona. "Patenting Life: The Oncomouse." In *Making and Unmaking Intellectual Property: Creative Production in Legal and Cultural Perspective*, ed. Mario Biagioli, Peter Jaszi, and Martha Woodmansee et al., 399–411. Chicago: University of Chicago Press, 2011.

Muxel, S. M., S. D. Borelli, M. K. Amarante, et al. "Association Study of *CCR5 delta 32* Polymorphism among the HLA-DRB1 Caucasian Population in Northern Paraná, Brazil." *Journal of Clinical Laboratory Analysis* 22 (4) (2008): 229–233.

Nagashima, Kirsten A. "Human Immunodeficiency Virus Type 1 Entry Inhibitors PRO 542 and T-20 Are Potently Synergistic in Blocking Virus-Cell and Cell-Cell Fusion." *Journal of Infectious Diseases* 183 (7) (2001): 1121–1125.

Nakano, Toru, Ken-ichi Higashino, Norihisa Kikuchi, et al. "Vascular Smooth Muscle Cell-Derived, Gla-Containing Growth-Potentiating Factor for Ca (2+)-Mobilizing Growth Factors." *Journal of Biological Chemistry* 270 (11) (1995): 5702–5705.

Nasioulas, G., M. Dean, E. Koumbarelis, et al. "Allele Frequency of the CCR5 Mutant Chemokine Receptor in Greek Caucasians." *Journal of Acquired Immune Deficiency Syndromes and Human Retrovirology* 17 (2) (1998): 181–182.

Neel, James V. "Diabetes Mellitus: A 'Thrifty' Genotype Rendered Detrimental by 'Progress'?" *American Journal of Human Genetics* 14 (4) (1962): 353–362.

Nei, M., and G. Livshits. "Genetic Relationships of Europeans, Asians, and Africans and the Origin of Modern *Homo Sapiens*." *Human Heredity* 39 (5) (1989): 276–281.

Newman, William R. *Promethean Ambitions: Alchemy and the Quest to Perfect Nature*. Chicago: University of Chicago Press, 2004.

Nietzsche, Friedrich. *Zur Genealogie der Moral*. Leipzig: Naumann, 1887.

Noble, David F. *America by Design: Science, Technology and the Rise of Corporate Capitalism*. New York: Oxford University Press, 1977.

Novembre, John, Alison P. Galvani, and Montgomery Slatkin. "The Geographic Spread of the *CCR5 Δ32* HIV-Resistance Allele." *PLoS Biology* 3 (11) (2005): 1554–1562.

O'Brien, Stephen J., and Michael Dean. "In Search of AIDS-Resistance Genes." *Scientific American* (September 1997). Available at http://www.ncoic.com/0997obrien .html, accessed January 21, 2014.

O'Brien, Thomas R., Cheryl Winkler, Michael Dean, et al. "HIV-1 Infection in a Man Homozygous for *CCR5Δ32*." *Lancet* 349 (9060) (1997): 1219.

O'Dowd, Niall. "Harvard Professor Gates Is Half-Irish, Related to Cop Who Arrested Him." *ABC News*, July 28, 2009. Available at http://abcnews.go.com/Politics/ story?id=8195564#.T0AXL1F9m-8, accessed January 21, 2014.

Office of Technology Assessment. U.S. Congress. *Mapping Our Genes: The Genome Projects—How Big, How Fast?* OTA-BA-373. Washington, DC: U.S. Government Printing Office, 1988.

O'Hara, Bryan M., and William C. Olson. "HIV Entry Inhibitors in Clinical Development." *Current Opinion in Pharmacology* 2 (5) (2002): 523–528.

Olson, William C., Gwénaël E. E. Rabut, Kirsten A. Nagashimi, et al. "Differential Inhibition of Human Immunodeficiency Virus Type 1 Fusion, gp120 Binding, and CC-Chemokine Activity by Monoclonal Antibodies to CCR5." *Journal of Virology* 73 (5) (1999): 4145–4155.

Oppermann, Martin. "Chemokine Receptor CCR5: Insights into Structure, Function, and Replication." *Cellular Signaling* 16 (11) (2004): 1201–1210.

Oreskes, Naomi, and Erik M. Conway. *Merchants of Doubt: How a Handful of Scientists Obscured the Truth on Issues from Tobacco Smoke to Global Warming*. New York: Bloomsbury Press, 2010.

Organisation for Economic Co-operation and Development. *Genetic Inventions, Intellectual Property Rights and Licensing Practices: Evidence and Policies.* Paris: Organisation for Economic Co-operation and Development, 2002.

Pai, Jennifer C., Jamie N. Sutherland, and Jennifer Maynard. "Progress towards Recombinant Anti-Infective Antibodies." *Recent Patents on Anti-infective Drug Discovery* 4 (1) (2007): 1–17.

Palani, Anandan, Sherry Shapiro, John W. Clader, et al. "Discovery of 4-[(Z)-(4-Bromophenyl)- (Ethoxyimino)Methyl]-1'-[(2,4-Dimethyl-3- Pyridinyl)Carbonyl]-4'-Methyl-1,4'- Bipiperidine N-Oxide (SCH 351125): An Orally Bioavailable Human CCR5 Antagonist for the Treatment of HIV Infection." *Journal of Medicinal Chemistry* 44 (21) (2001): 3339–3342.

Palmer, Eric. "Natco May Attack Pfizer, Roche Drugs with Compulsory License." *Fierce Pharma,* July 20, 2012. Available at http://www.fiercepharma.com/story/natco-may-next-attack-pfizer-roche-drugs-compulsory-license/2012-07-20, accessed January 21, 2014.

Palombi, Luigi. "The Patenting of Biological Materials in the Context of the Agreement on Trade-Related Aspects of Intellectual Property Rights." Ph.D. dissertation, Law School of the University of New South Wales, Australia, 2004.

Pan, Ying. "A Post-*KSR* Consideration of Gene Patenting: The 'Obvious To Try' Standard Limits the Patentability of Genes." *Marquette Law Review* 93 (1) (2009): 285–308.

Pantaleo, Giuseppe, Stefano Menzo, Mauro Vaccarezza, et al. "Studies in Subjects with Long-Term Nonprogressive Human Immunodeficiency Virus Infection." *New England Journal of Medicine* 332 (4) (1995): 209–216.

Parthasarathy, Shobita. *Building Genetic Medicine: Breast Cancer, Technology, and the Comparative Politics of Health Care.* Cambridge, MA: MIT Press, 2007.

Patani, G. A., and E. J. LaVoie. "Bioisosterism: A Rational Approach in Drug Design." *Chemical Reviews* 96 (8) (1996): 3147–3176.

Paxton, William A., Scott R. Martin, Doris Tse, et al. "Relative Resistance to HIV-1 Infection of CD4 Lymphocytes from Persons Who Remain Uninfected Despite Multiple High-Risk Sexual Exposures." *Nature Medicine* 2 (4) (1996): 412–417.

Pelak, Kimberly, David B. Goldstein, Nicole M. Walley, et al. "Host Determinants of HIV-1 Control in African Americans." *Journal of Infectious Diseases* 201 (8) (2010): 1141–1149.

Pereira, Dennis A., and John A. Williams. "Origin and Evolution of High Throughput Screening." *British Journal of Pharmacology* 152 (1) (2007): 53–61.

Perna, N. T., M. A. Batzer, P. L. Deininger, et al. "*Alu* Insertion Polymorphism: A New Type of Marker for Human Population Studies." *Human Biology* 64 (5) (1992): 641–648.

Perros, Manos. "CCR5 Antagonists for the Treatment of HIV Infection and AIDS." In *Advances in Antiviral Drug Design*, vol. 5, ed. Erik De Clercq, 185–213. Oxford, UK: Elsevier, 2007.

Petersen, Desiree C., Maritha J. Kotze, Michele D. Zeier, et al. "Novel Mutations Identified Using a Comprehensive *CCR5*-Denaturing Gradient Gel Electrophoresis Assay." *AIDS* 15 (2) (2001): 171–177.

"Phase 2 Clinical Trials Started on PRO 140." *AIDS Patient Care and STDs* 22 (2) (2008): 159–160.

Philpott, Sean, Barbara Weiser, Kathryn Anastos, et al. "Preferential Suppression of CXCR4-Specific Strains of HIV-1 by Antiviral Therapy." *Journal of Clinical Investigation* 107 (4) (2001): 431–437.

Philpott, Sean, Barbara Weiser, and Harold Burger. "Heteroduplex Tracking Assay." U.S. Patent 7,344,830 awarded March 18, 2008. Available at http://www.google.com/patents/us7344830, accessed January 21, 2014.

Philpott, Sean, Barbara Weiser, Harold Burger, et al. "Analysis of HIV-1 Coreceptor Use in the Clinical Care of HIV-1-Infected Patients." U.S. Patent 7,943,297 awarded May 17, 2011. Available at http://patents.com/us-7943297.html, accessed January 21, 2014.

Philpott, Sean, Barbara Weiser, Harold Burger, et al. 2010. "Heteroduplex Tracking Assay Description/Claims." U.S. Patent and Trademark Office Patent Application 20100323341. Available at http://www.freshpatents.com/-dt20101223ptan20100323341.php, accessed January 21, 2014.

Picton, Anabela C. P., Maria Paximadis, and Caroline T. Tiemessen, et al. "Genetic Variation within the Gene Encoding the HIV-1 CCR5 Coreceptor in Two South African Populations." *Infection, Genetics and Evolution* 10 (4) (2010): 487–494.

Ping, An, George Nelson, Mary Carrington, et al. "Influence of *CCR5* Promoter Haplotypes on AIDS Progression in African-Americans." *AIDS* 14 (14) (2000): 2117–2122.

Porter, Theodore M. "Life Insurance, Medical Testing, and the Management of Morality." In *Biographies of Scientific Objects*, ed. Lorraine Daston, 226–246. Chicago: University of Chicago Press, 2000.

Pottage, Alain. "Law Machines: Scale Models, Forensic Materiality and the Making of Modern Patent Law." *Social Studies of Science* 41 (5) (2011): 621–643.

Power, Christine A., Alexandra Meyer, Karin Nemeth, et al. "Molecular Cloning and Functional Expression of a Novel CC Chemokine Receptor cDNA from a Human Basophilic Cell Line." *Journal of Biological Chemistry* 270 (33) (1995): 19,495–19,500.

Price, Alkes L., Nick J. Patterson, Robert M. Plenge, et al. "Principal Components Analysis Corrects for Stratification in Genome-Wide Association Studies." *Nature Genetics* 38 (8) (2006): 904–909.

Price, David. "Maraviroc (Selzentry): The First-in-Class CCR5 Antagonist for the Treatment of HIV." In *Modern Drug Synthesis*, ed. Jie Jack Li and Douglas S. Johnson, 17–27. New York: Wiley, 2010.

Proctor, Robert N. *Cancer Wars: How Politics Shapes What We Know and Don't Know about Cancer.* New York: Basic Books, 1996.

Pulley, Shon R. "CCR5 Antagonists: From Discovery to Clinical Efficacy." In *Chemokine Biology: Basic Research and Clinical Application*, ed. Kuldeep Neote, L. Gordon Letts, and Bernhard Moser. 2 vols. (2006–2007), vol. 2 (2007), 145–163.

Rabino, I. "How Human Geneticists in U.S. View Commercialization of the Human Genome Project." *Nature Genetics* 29 (1) (2001): 15–16.

Race, Ethnicity, and the Genetics Working Group. "The Use of Racial, Ethnic, and Ancestral Categories in Human Genetics Research." *American Journal of Human Genetics* 77 (4) (2005): 519–532.

Radetsky, Peter. "Immune to a Plague." *Discover*, June 1997. Available at http://discovermagazine.com/1997/jun/immunetoaplague1147, accessed January 21, 2014.

Rajan, Kaushik Sunder. *Biocapital: The Constitution of Postgenomic Life.* Rayleigh, NC: Duke University Press, 2006.

Raport, Carol J., Jennifa Gosling, Vicki L. Schweickart, et al. "Molecular Cloning and Functional Characterization of a Novel Human CC Chemokine Receptor (CCR5) for RANTES, MIP-1β, and MIP-1α." *Journal of Biological Chemistry* 271 (29) (1996): 17,161–17,166.

Reardon, Jenny. *Race to the Finish: Identity and Governance in the Age of Genomics.* Princeton, NJ: Princeton University Press, 2005.

Regalado, Antonio. "The Great Gene Grab." *MIT Technology Review* 103 (5) (September–October 2000). Available at http://www.technologyreview.com/featuredstory/400800/the-great-gene-grab/, accessed January 21, 2014.

"Report from the Commission to the Council and the European Parliament: Development and Implications of Patent Law in the Field of Biotechnology and Genetic Engineering (SEC (2005) 943)." July 14, 2005. Available at http://eur-lex.europa.eu/LexUriServ/LexUriServ.do?uri=COM:2005:0312:FIN:EN:PDF, access January 21, 2014.

Restaino, Leslie Gladstone, and Theresa Tackeuchi. "Gene Patents and Global Competition Issues: Protection of Biotechnology under Patent Law." *Legal Affairs* 26 (1). Available at http://www.genengnews.com/articles/chitem.aspx?aid=1163&chid=0, accessed January 21, 2014.

Rettner, Rachael. "Cure for HIV Claimed, but Not Proved: Bone Marrow Transplant Credited with Wiping Out German Man's Infection." *NBCNews*, December

15, 2010, available at http://www.nbcnews.com/id/40666443/#.Uq-HAv1wp4M, accessed January 21, 2014.

Reverby, Susan M. *Examining Tuskegee: The Infamous Syphilis Study and Its Legacy.* Chapel Hill: University of North Carolina Press, 2009.

Reverby, Susan M., ed. *Tuskegee Truths: Rethinking the Tuskegee Syphilis Study.* Chapel Hill: University of North Carolina Press, 2000.

Reynolds, Tom. "Gene Patent Race Speeds Ahead amid Controversy." *Journal of the National Cancer Institute* 92 (8) (2000): 184–186.

Rheinberger, Hans-Jörg. "Cytoplasmic Particles." In *Biographies of Scientific Objects,* ed. Lorraine Daston, 270–294. Chicago: University of Chicago Press, 2000.

Rheinberger, Hans-Jörg. *Toward a History of Epistemic Things: Synthesizing Proteins in the Test Tube.* Stanford, CA: Stanford University Press, 1994.

Risch, Neil J. "Searching for Genetic Determinants in the New Millennium." *Nature* 405 (6788) (2000): 847–856.

Risch, Neil J., Esteban Burchard, Elad Ziv, et al. "Categorization of Humans in Bio-medical Research: Genes, Race and Disease." *Genome Biology* 3 (7) (2002): 1–12.

Rivoli, Pietra. *The Travels of a T-Shirt in the Global Economy.* 2nd ed. Hoboken, NJ: Wiley, 2009.

Roberts, Dorothy. *Fatal Invention: How Science, Politics, and Big Business and Re-create Race in the Twenty-first Century.* New York: New Press, 2011.

Rocke, Alan. *The Quiet Revolution: Hermann Kolbe and the Science of Organic Chemistry.* Berkeley: University of California Press, 1993.

Rose, Geoffrey, and M. G. Marmot. "Social Class and Coronary Heart Disease." *British Heart Journal* 45 (1981): 13–19.

Rose, Nikolas. "The Politics of Life Itself." *Theory, Culture and Society* 18 (6) (2001): 1–30.

Rose, Nikolas. *The Politics of Life Itself: Biomedicine, Power, and Subjectivity in the Twenty-first Century.* Princeton, NJ: Princeton University Press, 2007.

Rosenberg, Noah A., Jonathan K. Pritchard, James L. Weber, et al. "Genetic Structure of Human Populations." *Science* 298 (5602) (2002): 2381–2385.

Rosenfeld, Jeffrey, and Christopher E. Mason. "Pervasive Sequence Patents Cover the Entire Human Genome." *Genome Medicine* 5 (3) (2013): 27–33.

Rowland-Jones, S., J. Sutton, K. Ariyoshi, et al. "HIV-Specific Cytotoxic T-Cells in HIV-Exposed but Infected Gambian Women." *Nature Medicine* 9 (1) (1995): 59–64.

Rucker, Joseph, Michel Samson, Benjamin J. Doranz, et al. "Regions in β-Chemokine Receptors CCR5 and CCR2b That Determine HIV-1 Cofactor Specificity." *Cell* 87 (3) (1996): 437–446.

Rusk, Nicole. "Expanding HapMap." *Nature Methods* 7 (10) (2010): 780–781

Saag, Michael, James Goodrich, Gerd Fätkenheuer, et al. "A Double-Blind, Placebo Controlled Trial of Maraviroc in Treatment-Experienced Patients Infected with Non R5 HIV-1." *Journal of Infectious Diseases* 199 (11) (2009): 1638–1647.

Saag, Michael, J. Heera, J. Goodrich, et al. "Reanalysis of the MERIT Study with the Enhanced Trofile™ Assay (MERIT ES)." Paper presented at the 2008 ICAAC/IDSA Annual Meeting, Washington, DC, October 28, 2008. Available at http://www .natap.org/2008/ICAAC/ICAAC_19.htm, accessed January 24, 2014.

Sabeti, Pardis C., Emily Walsh, Steve F. Schaffner, et al. "The Case for Selection at CCR5-Δ32." *PLoS Biology* 3 (11) (2005): 1963–1969.

Salem, Abdel-Halim, and Mark A. Batzer. "Distribution of the HIV Resistance CCR5-Δ32 Allele among Egyptians and Syrians." *Mutation Research/Fundamental and Molecular Mechanisms of Mutagenesis* 616 (1–2) (2007): 175–180.

Samson, Michel, Olivier Labbe, Catherine Mollereau, et al. "Molecular Cloning and Functional Expression of a New Human CC-Chemokine Receptor Gene." *Biochemistry* 35 (11) (1996): 3362–3367.

Samson, Michel, Frédérick Libert, Benjamin J. Doranz, et al. "Resistance to HIV-1 Infection in Caucasian Individuals Bearing Mutant Alleles of the CCR-5 Chemokine Receptor Gene." *Nature* 382 (6593) (1996): 722–725.

Sankar, Pamela, and Mildred K. Cho. "Toward a New Vocabulary of Human Genetic Variation." *Science* 298 (5597) (2002): 1337–1338.

Sankar, Pamela, Mildred K. Cho, and Joanna Mountain. "Race and Ethnicity in Genetic Research." *American Journal of Medical Genetics Pt. A* 143A (9) (2007): 961–970.

Sankar, Pamela, and Jonathan Kahn. "BiDil: Race Medicine or Race Marketing?" *Health Affairs* 24 (October 2005): W5-455–W5-463.

Sayre, L. E. "Patent Laws in Regard to the Protection of Chemical Industry." *Transactions of the Kansas Academy of Science* 30 (1919): 39–44.

Scarlatti, Gabriella, Eleonora Tresoldi, Asa Björndal, et al. "In Vivo Evolution of HIV-1 Co-receptor Usage and Sensitivity to Chemokine-Mediated Suppression." *Nature Medicine* 3 (11) (1997): 1259–1265.

Scheinfeld, Robert C. "Enzo Biochem: What Direction Is Written Description Taking?" *Baker Botts Publications*, September 25, 2002. Available at http://www

.bakerbotts.com/infocenter/publications/detail.aspx?id=345304c2-ff97-4fde-a023 -909338bd2d57, accessed January 21, 2014.

Schiebinger, Londa. "Gender and Natural History." In *Cultures of Natural History*, ed. Nicholas Jardine, James Secord, and Emma Spary, 163–177. New York: Cambridge University Press, 1996.

Schulman, Robert M., Parker H. Bagley, and Tara Agnew. "The Written Description Requirement: Federal Circuit May Be Recognizing That Biotechnology Is Not Amenable to the Same Rules as Chemistry." *National Law Journal*, May 31, 2004. Available at http://www.bakerbotts.com/infocenter/publications/detail .aspx?id=345304c2-ff97-4fde-a023-909338bd2d57, accessed January 21, 2014.

Schwartz, Robert S. "Racial Profiling in Medical Research." *New England Journal of Medicine* 344 (18) (2001): 1392–1393.

Scott, Susan, and Christopher J. Duncan. *Biology of Plagues: Evidence from Historical Populations*. Cambridge, UK: Cambridge University Press, 2005.

Secko, David. "Phase I of HapMap Complete." *News from The Scientist* 6 (October 26, 2005): 1026.

"Secrets of the Dead: Mystery of the Black Death." Produced and written by Emma Faure Whitlock. A Tigress Production. New York: WNET New York, Educational Broadcasting Corporation, 2002.

Serre, David, and Svante Päälo. "Evidence for Gradients of Human Genetic Diversity within and among Continents." *Genome Research* 14 (9) (2004): 1679–1685.

Shankarappa, Raj, Joseph B. Margolick, Stephen J. Gange, et al. "Consistent Viral Evolutionary Changes Associated with the Progression of Human Immunodeficiency Virus Type 1 Infection." *Journal of Virology* 73 (12) (1999): 10,489–10,502.

Shapin, Steven. *The Scientific Life: A Moral History of a Late Modern Vocation*. Chicago: University of Chicago Press, 2008.

Shapin, Steven, and Simon Schaffer. *Leviathan and the Air-Pump: Hobbes, Boyle, and the Experimental Life*. Princeton, NJ: Princeton University Press, 1987.

Shen, Dong-Ming, Min Shu, Sander G. Mills, et al. "Antagonists of Human CCR5 Receptor Containing 4-(Pyrazolyl)Piperdine Side Chains. Part 1, Discovery and SAR Study of 4-Pyrazolylpiperdine Side Chains." *Bioorganic and Medicinal Chemistry Letters* 14 (4) (2004): 935–939.

Shen, Dong-Ming, Min Shu, Christopher A. Willoughby, et al. "Antagonists of Human CCR5 Receptor Containing 4-(Pyrazolyl)Piperdine Side Chains. Part 2, Discovery of Potent, Selective, and Orally Bioavailable Compounds." *Bioorganic and Medicinal Chemistry Letters* 14 (4) (2004): 941–945.

Sheridan, C. "Curie's Victory over *BRCA1*." *Nature Biotechnology* 22 (7) (2004): 797.

Shimmings, Alex. "2008 Scrip Awards Celebrate Industry's Achievement." December 11, 2008. Available at http://www.scripintelligence.com/home/2008-Scrip-Awards -celebrate-industrys-achievements-22020, accessed January 21, 2014.

Shin, Niu, Kim Solomon, Naiming Zhou, et al. "Identification and Characterization of INCB9471, an Allosteric Noncompetitive Small-Molecule Antagonist of C-C Chemokine Receptor 5 with Potent Inhibitory Activity against Monocyte Migration and HIV-1 Infection." *Journal of Pharmacology and Experimental Therapeutics* 338 (1) (2011): 228–239.

Shioda, Tatsuo, Emi E. Nakayama, Yuetsu Takana, et al. "Naturally Occurring Deletional Mutation in the C-Terminal Cytoplasmic Tail of CCR5 Affects Surface Trafficking of CCR5." *Journal of Virology* 75 (7) (2001): 3462–3468.

Shiraishi, M., Y. Aramaki, M. Seto, et al. "Discovery of Novel, Potent, and Selective Small-Molecule CCR5 Antagonists as Anti-HIV-1 Agents: Synthesis and Biological Evaluation of Anilide Derivatives with a Quaternary Ammonium Moiety." *Journal of Medicinal Chemistry* 43 (10) (2000): 2049–2063.

Shreeve, James. *The Genome War: How Craig Venter Tried to Capture the Code of Life and Save the World*. New York: Knopf, 2004.

Shriver, Mark D., and Rick A. Kittles. "Genetic Ancestry and the Search for Personalized Genetic Histories." In *Revisiting Race in a Genomic Age*, ed. Barbara Koenig, Sandra Soo-Jin Lee, and Sarah S. Richardson, 201–214. New Brunswick, NJ: Rutgers University Press, 2008.

Shriver, Mark D., Esteban Parra, Sonia Dios, et al. "Skin Pigmentation, Biographical Ancestry, and Admixture Mapping." *Human Genetics* 112 (4) (2003): 387–399.

Shu, M., J. L. Loebach, K. A. Parker, et al. "Antagonists of Human CCR5 Receptor Containing 4-(Pyrazolyl)Piperdine Side Chains. Part 3, SAR Studies on the Benzylpyrazole Segment." *Bioorganic and Medicinal Chemistry Letters* 14 (4) (2004): 947–952.

Sidoti, A., R. D'Angelo, C. Rinaldi, et al. "Distribution of the Mutated Delta 32 Allele of the *CCR5* Gene in a Sicilian Population." *International Journal of Immunogenetics* 32 (3) (2005): 193–198.

Singh, Khoma. "Natco Seeks Pfizer Nod for Drug Clone." *Economic Times*, January 5, 2011. Available at http://articles.economictimes.indiatimes.com/2011-01-05/news/ 28426847_1_natco-pharma-pfizer-hiv-patients, accessed January 21, 2014.

Skeehan, Katie, Christopher Heaney, and Robert Cook-Deegan. "Impact of Gene Patents on Access to Genetic Testing for Alzheimer Disease." In Steven Teutsch and the Secretary's Advisory Committee on Genetics, Health, and Society, "Gene Patents and Licensing Practices," appendix, B-14, 2010. Available at http://osp.od.nih.gov/ sites/default/files/SACGHS_patents_report_2010.pdf, accessed on March 30, 2014.

Skloot, Rebecca. *The Immortal Life of Henrietta Lacks*. New York: Broadway Paperbacks, 2010.

Skrabal, Katharina, Virginie Trouplin, Béatrice Labrosse, et al. "Impact of Antiretroviral Treatment on the Tropism of HIV-1 Plasma Virus Populations." *AIDS* 17 (6) (2003): 809–814.

Smaglik, Paul. "Could AIDS Treatments Slip through Patents Loophole?" *Nature* 404 (6776) (2000): 322.

Smith, G. D. "Individual Social Class, Area-Based Deprivation, Cardiovascular Disease Risk Factors, and Mortality: The Renfrew and Paisley Study." *Journal of Epidemiology and Community Health* 52 (6) (1998): 399–405.

Smith, Michael W., Michael Dean, Mary Carrington, et al. "Contrasting Genetic Influence of *CCR2* and *CCR5* Variants on HIV-1 Infection and Disease Progression." *Science* 277 (5328) (1997): 959–965.

Soini, Sirpa, Ségolène Aymé, and Gert Matthijs. "Patenting and Licensing in Genetic Testing: Ethical, Legal and Social Issues." *Nature* 16 (no. 1S) (2008): S10–S50.

Spencer, John. "Case Study on Maraviroc." In *An Introduction to Medicinal Chemistry*, ed. Graham L. Patrick. New York: Oxford University Press, 2009. Online update. Available at http://fdslive.oup.com/www.oup.com/orc/resources/chemistry/patrick4e/01student/updates/sep09maraviroc.pdf, accessed January 21, 2014.

Spiegel, Jack. Public Comments on the United States Patent and Trademark Office, "Revised Interim Guidelines for Examination of Patent Applications under the 35 U.S.C. § 112, ¶1 'Written Description' Requirement." 64 *Federal Register* 71, 427, December 21, 1999, comment 64 on the Interim Utility Guidelines 10–11, March 22, 2000. Available at http://www.uspto.gov/web/offices/com/sol/comments/utilitywd/nihjs.pdf

Stallybrass, Peter. "Marx's Coat." In *Border Fetishisms: Material Objects in Unstable Spaces*, ed. Patricia Spyer, 183–207. New York: Routledge, 1998.

Stephens, J. Claiborne, David E. Reich, David B. Goldstein, et al. "Dating the Origin of the *CCR5-Δ32* AIDS-Resistance Allele in the Coalescence of Haplotypes." *American Journal of Human Genetics* 62 (6) (1998): 1507–1515.

Stephens, J. Claiborne, Julie A. Schneider, Debra A. Tanguay, et al. "Haplotype Variation and Linkage Disequilibrium in 313 Human Genes." *Science* 293 (5529) (2001): 489–493.

"The Story of Selzentry." 2010. Available at http://www.innovation.org/index.cfm/Storiesofinnovation/InnovatorStories/The_Story_of_Selzentry, accessed January 21, 2014.

Strizki, Julie M., Cecile Tremblay, Serena Xu, et al. "Discovery and Characterization of Vicriviroc (SCH 417690), a CCR5 Antagonist with Potent Activity against Human

Immunodeficiency Virus Type 1." *Antimicrobial Agents and Chemotherapy* 49 (12) (2005): 4911–4919.

Struyf, Frank, et al. "Prevalence of *CCR5* and *CCR2* HIV-Coreceptor Gene Polymorphisms in Belgium." *Human Heredity* 50 (5) (2000): 304–307.

Stryer, Lubert. *Biochemistry.* 3rd ed. New York: Freeman, 1988.

Stumpf, Michael P. H., and Hilde M. Wilkinson-Herbots. "Allelic Histories: Positive Selection on a HIV-Resistance Allele." *Trends in Ecology and Evolution* 19 (4) (2004): 166–168.

Sulston, John. "Heritage of Humanity." *Le Monde diplomatique*, December 2002. Available at http://mondediplo.com/2002/12/15genome, accessed January 21, 2014.

Szalai, C., A. Czinner, A. Császár, et al. "Frequency of the HIV-1 Resistance *CCR5* Deletion Allele in Hungarian Newborns." *European Journal of Pediatrics* 157 (9) (1999): 782.

Tagat, Jayaram R., Stuart W. McCombie, Dennis Nazareno, et al. "Piperazine-Based CCR5 Antagonists as HIV-1 Inhibitors. IV, Discovery of 1-[(4,6-Dimethyl-5-Pyrimidinyl)Carbonyl]- 4-[4-[2-Methoxy-1(R)-4-(Trifluoromethyl)Phenyl]ethyl-3(S) -Methyl-1-Piperazinyl]- 4-Methylpiperidine (Sch-417690/Sch-D), a Potent, Highly Selective, and Orally Bioavailable CCR5 Antagonist." *Journal of Medicinal Chemistry* 47 (10) (2004): 2405–2408.

Tallbear, Kimberly. "Native-American-DNA.com: In Search of Native American Race and Tribe." In *Revisiting Race in a Genomic Age*, ed. Barbara A. Koenig, Sandra Soo-Jin Lee, and Sarah S. Richardson, 235–252. New Brunswick, NJ: Rutgers University Press, 2008.

Tang, Jianming, Brent Sheldon, Nina J. Makhatadze, et al. "Distribution of Chemokine Receptor *CCR2* and *CCR5* Genotypes and Their Relative Contribution to Human Immunodeficiency Virus Type 1 (HIV-1) Seroconversion, Early HIV-1 RNA Concentration in Plasma, and Later Disease Progression." *Journal of Virology* 76 (2) (2002): 662–672.

Tapper, M. *In the Blood: Sickle Cell Anemia and the Politics of Race.* Philadelphia: University of Pennsylvania Press, 1999.

Taylor, Anne L., Susan Ziesche, Clyde Yancy, et al. "Combination of Isosorbide Dinitrate and Hydralazine in Blacks with Heart Failure." *New England Journal of Medicine* 351 (20) (2004): 2049–2057.

Teutsch, Steven, and the Secretary's Advisory Committee on Genetics, Health, and Society. "Gene Patents and Licensing Practices and Their Impact on Patient Access to Genetic Tests: Report of the Secretary's Advisory Committee on Genetics, Health, and Society," March 2010, available at http://osp.od.nih.gov/sites/default/files/SACGHS_patents_report_2010.pdf, accessed January 21, 2014.

Theodorou, Ioannis, Laurence Meyer, Magdalena Magierowskia, et al. "HIV-1 Infection in an Individual Homozygous for *CCR5 Δ32*: Seroco Study Group." *Lancet* 349 (9060) (1997): 1219–1220.

Thoma, Gebhard, François Nuninger, Marc Schaefer, et al. "Orally Bioavailable Competitive CCR5 Antagonists." *Journal of Medicinal Chemistry* 47 (8) (2004): 1939–1955.

Thumm, N. "Patents for Genetic Inventions: A Tool to Promote Technological Advance or a Limitation for Upstream Inventions?" *Technovation* 25 (12) (2005): 1410–1417.

Tilton, John C., and Robert W. Doms. "Entry Inhibitors in the Treatment of HIV-1 Infection." *Antiviral Research* 85 (1) (2010): 91–100.

Tischkoff, S. A., and K. K. Kidd. "Implications of Biogeography of Human Populations for 'Race' and Medicine." *Nature Genetics* 36 (11 Suppl) (2004): S21–S27.

Tolbert, Margaret E. M., Johnston A. Ramalu, and Garnette D. Draper. "Effects of Cadmium, Zinc, Copper, and Manganese on Hepatic Parenchymal Cell Gluconeogenesis." *Journal of Environmental Science and Health* 16, 5 pt. B (1981): 575–585.

"Trilateral Co-operation of the U.S., European and Japanese Patent Offices." *Biotechnology Law Review* 7 (1988): 159–193.

United States Statutes at Large, vol. 1, 1st Cong., sess. 2, chap. 7 (April 10, 1790), available at http://en.wikisource.org/wiki/United_States_Statutes_at_Large/Volume_1/1st_Congress/2nd_Session/Chapter_7, accessed on January 20, 2014.

Vaddi, Krishna, Margaret Keller, and Robert C. Newton. *The Chemokine Facts Book.* San Diego, CA: Academic Press, 1997.

Vandekerckhove, Linos, Chris Verhofstede, and Dirk Vogelaers. "Maraviroc: Perspectives for Use in Antiretroviral-Naïve HIV-1-Infected Patients." *Journal of Antimicrobial Chemotherapy* 63 (3) (2009): 1087–1096.

Vargas, A. E., A. R. Marrero, F. M. Salzano, et al. "Frequency of *CCR5Δ32* in Brazilian Populations." *Brazilian Journal of Medical and Biological Research* 39 (3) (2006): 321–325.

Vaughan, Floyd L. "Suppression and Non-Working of Patents, with Special Reference to the Dye and Chemical Industries." *American Economic Review* 9 (4) (1919): 693–700.

Veloso, Sergi, Montserrat Olona, Felipe García, et al. "Effect of *TNF-α* Genetic Variants and *CCR5Δ32* on the Vulnerability to HIV-1 Infection and Disease Progression in Caucasian Spaniards." *BMC Medical Genetics* 11 (2010): 63–73.

Venter, J. Craig. *A Life Decoded. My Genome: My Life.* New York: Viking, 2007.

Vernon, Jules. "MOTIVATE 1 Study: Efficacy and Safety of Maraviroc Plus Optimized Background Therapy in Viremic, ART-Experienced Patients Infected with CCR5-Tropic HIV-1: Twenty-four-Week Results of Phase 2b/3 Studies." Paper presented at the Fourteenth Conference on Retroviruses and Opportunistic Infections (CROI), Los Angeles, California, February 25–28, 2007. Available at http://www.natap .org/2007/CROI/croi_39.htm, accessed January 21, 2014.

Voight, Benjamin, Sridhar Kudaravalli, Xiaoquan Wen, et al. "A Map of Recent Positive Selection in the Human Genome." *PLoS Biology* 4 (3) (2006): 446–458.

Wade, Nicolas. "Assembling of the Genome Is at Hand." *New York Times*, April 7, 2000, A20.

Wagner, Johannes Rudolf. *A Handbook of Chemical Technology*. Trans. William Crookes. New York: Appleton, 1872.

Waldholz, Michael. "Right to Life: Genes Are Patentable; Less Clear Is If Finder Must Know Their Role." *Wall Street Journal*, March 16, 2000, A1.

Walsh, John P., Charlene Cho, and Wesley M. Cohen. "View from the Bench: Patents and Material Transfers." *Science* 309 (5743) (2005): 2002–2003.

Walsh, John P., and Wei Hong. "Secrecy Is Increasing in Step with Competition." *Nature* 422 (6934) (2003): 801–802.

Wang, D. G., J. B. Fan, C. J. Siao, et al. "Large-Scale Identification, Mapping and Genotyping of Single-Nucleotide Polymorphisms in the Human Genome." *Science* 280 (5366) (1998): 1077–1082.

Wang, F., L. Jin, Z. Lei, et al. "Genotypes and Polymorphisms of Mutant *CCR5-Delta 32*, *CCR2-64I*, and *SDF1-3'A* HIV-1 Resistance Alleles in Indigenous Han Chinese." *Chinese Medical Journal* 114 (11) (2001): 1162–1166.

Wang, F., and D. Liu. "Polymorphism of Human Alleles Associated with Genetic Resistance against HIV-1 Infection and Its Implications." *Zhonghua Yi Xue Yi Chuan Xue Za Zhi* 17 (4) (2000): 285–287.

Watkins, Jeff C., P. Krogsgaard-Larsen, and T. Honoré. "Structure-Activity Relationships in the Development of Excitatory Amino Acid Receptor Agonists and Competitive Antagonists." *Trends in Pharmacological Sciences* 11 (1) (1990): 25–33.

Weber, J. L., and P. E. May. "Abundant Class of Human DNA Polymorphisms Which Can Be Typed Using the Polymerase Chain Reaction." *American Journal of Human Genetics* 44 (3) (1989): 388–396.

Wegner, Harold C. "The Disclosure Requirements of the 1952 Patent Act: Looking Back and a New Statute for the Next Fifty Years." *Akron Law Review* 37 (2004): 243–261.

Wei, Robert G., Damian O. Arnaiz, You-Ling Chou, et al. "CCR5 Receptor Antagonists: Discovery and SAR Study of Guanylhydrazone Derivatives." *Bioorganic and Medicinal Chemistry Letters* 17 (1) (2007): 231–234.

Weiser, Barbara. "HIV-1 Receptor Usage and CXCR4-Specific Viral Load Predict Clinical Disease Progression during Combination Antiretroviral Therapy." *AIDS* 22 (4) (2008): 469–479.

Weissenbach, J., G. Gyapay, A. Vignil, et al. "A Second-Generation Linkage Map of the Human Genome Project." *Nature* 359 (6398) (1992): 794–801.

Wensing, Annemarie M. J., Noortje M. van Maarseveen, and Monique Nijhuis. "Fifteen Years of HIV Protease Inhibitors: Raising the Barrier to Resistance." *Antiviral Research* 85 (1) (2010): 59–74.

West, Tony, Beth S. Brinkmann, Scott R. McIntosh, et al. 2010. "In the United States Court of Appeals for the Federal Circuit, the Association for Molecular Pathology, et al. Plaintiffs-Appellees v. United States Patent and Trademark Office, Defendant, Myriad Genetics, Inc., et al., Defendant-Appellant. Appeal of Case No. 09-CV-4515, Senior Judge Robert W. Sweet, Brief for the United States as Amicus Curiae in Support of Neither Party. No. 2010-1406." Available at http://graphics8 .nytimes.com/packages/pdf/business/genepatents-USamicusbrief.pdf, accessed January 21, 2014.

Weston, Ainsley, James Ensey, Kathleen Kreiss, et al. "Racial Differences in Prevalence of a Supratypic HLA-Genetic Marker Immaterial to Pre-Employment Testing for Susceptibility to Chronic Beryllium Disease." *American Journal of Industrial Medicine* 41 (6) (2002): 457–465.

Whitcomb, Jeannette M., Wei Huang, Signe Fransen, et al. "Development and Characterization of a Novel Single-Cycle Recombinant-Virus Assay to Determine Human Immunodeficiency Virus Receptor Tropism." *Antimicrobial Agents and Chemotherapy* 51 (2) (2007): 566–575.

Wilkin, T. J., Zhaohui Su, Daniel R. Kuritzkes, et al. "HIV Type 1 Chemokine Coreceptor Use among Antiretroviral-Experienced Patients Screened for a Clinical Trial of a CCR5 Inhibitor: AIDS Clinical Trial Group A5211." *Clinical Infectious Diseases* 44 (4) (2007): 591–595.

Wilkinson, R. G., and K. E. Pickett. "Income Equality and Population Health: A Review and Explanation of the Evidence." *Social Science and Medicine* 62 (7) (2006): 1768–1784.

Williams-Jones, Bryn. "History of a Gene Patent: Tracing the Development and Application of Commercial BRCA Testing." *Health Law Journal* 10 (2002): 123–146. Available at http://www.academia.edu/634302/History_of_a_Gene_Patent_Tracing _the_Development_and_Application_of_Commercial_BRCA_Testing, accessed January 24, 2014.

Williamson, Carolyn, S. A. Loubser, B. Brice, et al. "Allelic Frequencies of Host Genetic Variants Influencing Susceptibility to HIV-1 Infection and Disease in South African Populations." *AIDS* 14 (4) (2000): 449–451.

Wilson, James F., Michael E. Weale, Alice C. Smith, et al. "Population Genetic Structure of Variable Drug Response." *Nature Genetics* 29 (3) (2001): 265–269.

Winickoff, D., Sheila Jasanoff, Lawrence Busch, et al. "Adjudicating the GM Food Wars: Science, Risk and Democracy in World Trade Law." *Yale Journal of International Law* 30 (1) (2005): 81–123.

Winkleby, Marilyn A., S. P. Fortmann, and D. C. Barrett, et al. "Social Class Disparities in Risk Factors for Disease: Eight-Year Prevalence Patterns by Level of Education." *Preventive Medicine* 19 (1) (1990): 1–12.

Winkler, Cheryl, Ping An, and Stephen J. O'Brien. "Patterns of Ethnic Diversity among the Genes That Influence AIDS." *Human Molecular Genetics* 13 (supp. 1) (2004): R9–R19.

Wood, Anthony, and Duncan Armour. "The Discovery of the CCR5 Receptor Antagonist, UK-427,857: A New Agent for the Treatment of HIV Infection and AIDS." *Progress in Medicinal Chemistry* 43 (2005): 239–271.

Wooley, John C., and Herbert S. Lin, eds. *Catalyzing Inquiry at the Interface of Computing and Biology*. Washington, DC: National Academies Press, 2005.

Worton, Ronald. Public Comments on the United States Patent and Trademark Office, "Revised Interim Guidelines for Examination of Patent Applications under the 35 U.S.C. § 112, ¶1 'Written Description' Requirement," 64 *Federal Register* 71,427, December 21, 1999, comment 52, http://www.uspto.gov/web/offices/com/sol/comments/utilitywd/ashg.pdf, accessed January 23, 2014.

Wynn, Gary H., Michael J. Zapor, Benjamin H. Smith, et al. "Antiretrovirals, Part I: Overview, History, and Focus on Protease Inhibitors." *Psychosomatics* 45 (3) (2004): 262–270.

Wynne, Brian. "Public Engagement as a Means of Restoring Public Trust in Science: Hitting the Notes, but Missing the Music?" *Community Genetics* 9 (3) (2006): 211–220.

Wynne, Brian. "Risky Delusions: Misunderstanding Science and Misperforming Publics in the GE Crops Issue." In *Genetically Engineered Crops: Interim Policies, Uncertain Legislation*, ed. I. E. P. Taylor, 258–281. Vancouver, BC: UBC Haworth Press, 2007.

Xu, Lidan, Yuandong Qiao, Xuelong Zhang, et al. "A Haplotype in the *CCR5* Gene Promoter Was Associated with the Susceptibility to HIV-1 Infection in a Northern Chinese Population." *Molecular Biology Reports* 38 (1) (2011): 327–332.

Xue, Chu-Biao, Lihua Chen, Ganfeng Cao, et al. "Discovery of INCB9471, a Potent, Selective, and Orally Bioavailable CCR5 Antagonist with Potent Anti-HIV-1 Activity." *ACS Medicinal Chemistry Letters* 1 (9) (2010): 483–487.

Yamagami, S., Y. Tokuda, K. Ishii, et al. "cDNA Cloning and Functional Expression of a Human Monocyte Chemoattractant Protein 1 Receptor." *Biochemical and Biophysical Research Communications* 202 (2) (1994): 1156–1162.

Yoxen, Edward. "Life as a Productive Force: Capitalizing upon Research in Molecular Biology." In *Science, Technology and the Labour Process*, ed. L. Levidow and R. Young, 66–122. London: Blackrose Press, 1981.

Zamarchi, Rita, Stefano Indraccolo, Sonia Minuzzo, et al. "Frequency of a Mutated CCR-5 Allele (*Δ32*) among Italian Healthy Donors and Individuals at Risk of Parenteral HIV Infection." *AIDS Research and Human Retroviruses* 15 (4) (1999): 337–344.

Zawicki, Przemysław, and Henryk W. Witas. "HIV-1 Protecting *CCR5-Δ32* Allele in Medieval Poland." *Infection, Genetics and Evolution* 8 (2) (2008): 146–151.

Zhao, Xiu-Ying, Shui-Shan Lee, Ka-Hing Wong, et al. "Functional Analysis of Naturally Occurring Mutations in the Open Reading Frame of *CCR5* in HIV-Infected Chinese Patients and Healthy Controls." *Journal of Acquired Immune Deficiency Syndromes* 38 (5) (2005): 509–517.

Zimmerman, Peter A., Alicia Buckler-White, Ghalib Alkhatib, et al. "Inherited Resistance to HIV-1 Conferred by an Inactivating Mutation in CC Chemokine Receptor 5: Studies in Populations with Contrasting Clinical Phenotypes, Defined Racial Background, and Quantified Risk." *Molecular Medicine* 3 (1) (1997): 23–36.

Index